Critical Thinking

Understanding and Evaluating Dental Research

Second Edition

Critical Thinking

Understanding and Evaluating Dental Research

Second Edition

Donald Maxwell Brunette, PhD
Professor
Department of Oral Biological and Medical Sciences
Faculty of Dentistry
University of British Columbia
Vancouver, BC Canada

Contributors

Kathryn Hornby, MLS, DMD
Medical Liaison Librarian
Woodward Biomedical Library
University of British Columbia
Vancouver, BC, Canada

Carol Oakley, DDS, MSc, PhD
Clinical Assistant Professor
Faculty of Dentistry
University of British Columbia
Vancouver, BC, Canada

NORTHAMPTON
LIBRARY
Bethlehem, PA 18020
COMMUNITY COLLEGE

quintessence
books

Quintessence Publishing Co, Inc

Chicago, Berlin, Tokyo, London, Paris, Milan, Barcelona,
Istanbul, São Paulo, Mumbai, Moscow, Prague, and Warsaw

Library of Congress Cataloging-in-Publication Data

Brunette, Donald Maxwell.
  Critical thinking : understanding and evaluating dental research / Donald
Maxwell Brunette. -- 2nd ed.
     p. ; cm.
  Includes bibliographical references and index.
  ISBN 978-0-86715-426-9 (pbk.)
 1. Dentistry--Research--Evaluation. I. Title.
  [DNLM: 1. Dental Research. WU 20.5 B895c 2007]
  RK80.B78 2007
  617.6'027--dc22
                                    2007021716

© 2007 Quintessence Publishing Co, Inc

Quintessence Publishing Co, Inc
4350 Chandler Drive
Hanover Park, IL 60133
www.quintpub.com

All rights reserved. This book or any part thereof may not be reproduced, stored in a retrieval system, or transmitted
in any form or by any means, electronic, mechanical, photocopying, or otherwise, without prior written permission
of the publisher.

Editors: Bryn Goates and Lisa C. Bywaters
Design: Dawn Hartman
Production: Patrick Penney

Printed in the USA

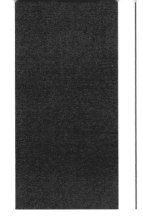

Table of Contents

Preface to the Second Edition

The need for a second edition of *Critical Thinking* was driven by three considerations: the changes taking place in dentistry and dental research, comments from readers, and finally my own determination that the rhetoric of science had to be given more emphasis in the book.

At the time the first edition was published, students and investigators typically searched the literature and index databases only indirectly via a professional librarian, who served as the mediator and search strategist. Today, researchers make searches from their own desktops. While the Internet has made research more convenient, the loss of professional advice has doubtless led to many inefficient and fruitless searches. This edition incorporates a chapter on searching the dental literature (see chapter 4), which is cowritten by Dr Kathryn Hornby, a dentist with qualifications in library science and medical informatics.

Evidence-based dentistry has become a more important topic in the last 10 years, but one obstacle to its implementation is a lack of understanding by dental and other health professionals of the use of diagnostic measures in clinical decision making. The first edition included a chapter on this topic that some readers found to be somewhat abstract. Dr Carol Oakley, who has specialty qualifications in both periodontics and oral medicine, has rewritten this chapter (chapter 14) with an emphasis on practical examples.

I have found that some readers wanted more information on statistics in the book. To that end, I have expanded the sections on statistics to include more information on basic statistical principles (chapters 9–10 and throughout). Readers should know that this book is in no way comprehensive on this topic, but does cover the most common concepts and tests used in dental research. References to more detailed statistical texts and material are also provided.

If you had asked me my profession 15 years ago, I would undoubtedly have answered "scientist" without qualification. Since then, I have come to realize that looking through a microscope, running a polyacrylamide gel, or analyzing data does not actually occupy a large portion of my working day. Instead, I write papers and referee the papers of others. I write grants and evaluate other people's grants. As a department head I evaluated my faculty's pleas for everything from merit increases in salary to early retirement. In turn I pleaded for all manner of things from my dean. As a professor I evaluate students' essays and theses and coach my own students on how to write persuasive papers and theses. In sum, I spend a large part of my day either persuading or being persuaded. To put it another way, scientists today must play the role of rhetorician to be successful. In the same way, consumers of dental research must understand the principles of persuasion as applied to science in order to detect and separate the scientific signal from the rhetorical noise. Chapter 3 of this edition on rhetoric is informed not only by the classical approach to rhetoric, but also by more modern psychological studies as well as my own experiences as a reviewer of grants and publications and as a participant in panels that make decisions about funding.

Other chapters in the book have been updated and expanded with more recent information or more detailed consideration of certain topics, including argument maps (see chapter 21), abductive logic (see chapter 6), real-world research (see chapter 16), and

Simpson's paradox (see chapter 13). In all, the book has expanded some 32%, to make it both broader and more in depth than the previous edition.

Finally, readers are invited to visit the Quintessence website (www.quintpub.com/CriticalThinking), where they can access software programs for performing simple statistical calculations as well as additional information on this subject. The site will be periodically updated, so readers should check back from time to time for more information.

I would like to express my appreciation to the many people involved in the realization of the second edition of this book.

I thank my wife Liz for her continuous support over the many years of my academic career that entailed considerable time away from home and more than a little shirking of domestic responsibilities. My son Max provided advice on aspects of law and logic, and my son Regan contributed some of the illustrations. That I place my family first on this list is no accident given their importance in my life, as well as the unfortunate fact that I egregiously forgot to thank them in the first edition—an omission, I might add, that was noticed, and one that I would not recommend to other authors.

As acknowledged in the preface to the first edition, my colleagues at the University of British Columbia have always been helpful in answering my questions concerning their disciplines. In this edition, I particularly would like to thank Dr Doug Waterfield for his comments on all of the chapters and Dr Babak Chehroudi for his contributions to my thinking on many topics. It was a pleasure to work with Dr Kathryn Hornby and Dr Carol Oakley, who co-authored chapters 4 and 14, respectively; their contributions have made the book much stronger in their respective areas of expertise. Dr Ryan Woods of the HIV Network of Excellence commented on the presentation of statistical concepts and checked them for statistical orthodoxy and accuracy. A number of the members of my lab have been dragooned into various tasks and performed them graciously; in particular, I thank Leon Cheng and Mabel Cho for their help on the new illustrations for this edition and Dr Mandana Nematollahi for the drudgery euphemistically called "library work."

Critical Thinking is an unusual topic for a publisher such as Quintessence, which concentrates on books on clinical dentistry, and I am grateful to Tomoko Tsuchiya, who took the gamble of producing the first edition of this book; its success was a vindication of her judgment. The existence of this second edition is due in no small part to Senior Editor Lisa Bywaters, whose friendly advice and encouragement, as well as her occasional stern admonitions, were instrumental in keeping this book high on my list of priorities. Her skilful editing as well as that of Editor Bryn Goates and the work of Production Editor Patrick Penney have greatly improved the clarity and appearance of this edition.

Preface to the First Edition

The intent of this book is to enable dentists, dental students, and graduate students, as well as allied oral health care professionals, to become sophisticated consumers of dental research. The book directly addresses the information management and critical thinking requirements of the American Dental Association Commission on Accreditation and the National Dental Examining Board of Canada, which require that students be able to locate, understand, and critically evaluate dental literature.

Research is a complex enterprise, but traditional courses ignore this complexity and heavily emphasize statistics. Although statistics is an important aspect of research, one has only to attend research sessions of the International Association of Dental Research, for example, and listen to the questions and comments to realize that statistics often play only a bit role in many discussions. Questions on method and interpretation are more common, and indeed the presentation of scientific data can be considered as a rhetorical exercise designed to convince readers of the truth of the author's interpretation.

Understanding this rhetoric requires an understanding of the elements of logic, including the logic of statistical inference, measurement, elements of statistics, types of errors, research strategies and designs, presentation of results, and lower forms of rhetorical life. The wide range of topics covered in this book more nearly represents, in my view, the intellectual skills and information needed to evaluate biological research.

This book evolved over a 16-year period from notes for a course on the evaluation of dental research given to undergraduate dental students and graduate students. The book has benefited from their comments and reactions. The general approach to evaluating research given here is to encourage a healthy skepticism. Although such an attitude might appear to be unduly negative, it should be recalled that organized skepticism is generally considered to be the appropriate interaction between scientists. I noticed, however, that some students exposed to this material became hypercritical, and to counteract this tendency I added a section on forming balanced judgments. I also noticed that some of the students, while being skeptical about academic research, somehow accepted uncritically claims made by so-called alternative healthcare practitioners. At first this may seem surprising, but as noted by Peter Skrabenek (*Lancet* 1986;1:960) medical (and for that matter dental) education does not provide criteria for the demarcation of the absurd. To rectify this situation, I introduced a chapter on quacks, cranks, and abuses of logic into the book and course.

I am grateful to my clinical colleagues at the University of British Columbia, most particularly Drs Tim Gould, Michael MacEntee, Helen Scott, Babak Chehroudi, and Bob Priddy who commented on various topics, and Dr Ping Ma, formerly of the Department of Statistics at the University of British Columbia, now with Success Consulting, Surrey, BC, for checking the statistical calculations.

Developing and executing a novel course on evaluating dental research into the curriculum required the encouragement and assistance of my academic superiors, most particularly Tony Melcher, director of the MRC Group in Periodontal Physiology at the University of Toronto, and Leon Kraintz and Barry McBride, formerly heads of the Department of Oral Biology, and Dean George Beagrie at the University of British Columbia. Many secretaries and technical personnel were involved in the production of various versions of the manuscript over the years, but I would particularly like to thank Clare Louie, Diane Price, Lesley Weston, and Kathy Wyder for their aid in editing the text and producing illustrations. While acknowledging all this assistance, I must also add that any errors that appear in the book are, of course, my responsibility. Finally I should note that one part of the way students are evaluated in my course is that they must critique a paper found in the dental literature. The problem section is largely based on their submissions, and it is intended to provide concrete examples of how issues of logic, statistics, measurement, design, and argument are actually expressed in research publications. I would appreciate hearing from readers with additional examples.

1 | Reasons for Studying Critical Thinking

It has happened more than once that I found it necessary to say of one or another eminent colleague, "He is a very busy man and half of what he publishes is true but I don't know which half."
—Erwin Chargaff[1]

Critical Thinking

Critical thinking has been defined many ways, from the simple—"Critical thinking is deciding rationally what to or what not to believe"[2]—to the more complex but still not comprehensive—"Critical thinking is concerned with reason, intellectual honesty, and open-mindedness, as opposed to emotionalism, intellectual laziness, and closed-mindedness"[3]—to the comprehensive:

> Critical thinking involves following evidence where it leads; considering all possibilities; relying on reason rather than emotion; being precise; considering a variety of possible viewpoints and explanations; weighing the effects of motives and biases; being concerned more with finding the truth than with being right; not rejecting unpopular views out of hand; being aware of one's own prejudices and biases; and not allowing them to sway one's judgment.[3]

Self-described practitioners of critical thinking range from doctrinaire postmodernists who view the logic of science with its "grand narratives" as inherently subordinating[4] to market-driven dentists contemplating the purchase of laser tooth-whitening systems. In this book, critical thinking, and in particular the evaluation of scientific information, is conceived as "organized common sense" following Bronowski's view of science in general.[5] Of course, common sense

can be quite uncommon. A secondary use of the term *critical thinking* implies that common sense involves a set of unexamined and erroneous assumptions. For example, prior to Galileo, everyone "knew" that heavy objects fell faster than lighter ones. Critical thinking as organized co11mmon sense takes the systematic approach of examining assumptions. The professional use of critical thinking is particularly complex for dental professionals because they live in two different worlds. On the one hand, they are health professionals treating patients who suffer from oral diseases. On the other hand, dentists typically also inhabit the business world, where decisions may be based on the principle of maximizing income from their investment. Dental practice is based only very loosely on responding to disease,[6] less than one third of patient visits result in identifying a need for restorative care.[7] Twenty percent of work is elective, such as most of orthodontics, tooth whitening, and veneers, and typically that work comprises the most lucrative aspects of practice. Thus, the information that must be evaluated in performing these disparate roles covers the spectrum from advertisements to financial reports to systematic meta-analysis of health research.

Dentists are health professionals, people with specialized training in the delivery of scientifically sound health services. The undergraduate dental curriculum is designed to give dental students the basic knowledge to practice dentistry scientifically, at least to the extent allowed by the current state of knowledge. But if any guarantee can be made to dental students, it is that dentistry will change, because the knowledge base of biomedical and biomaterial sciences grows exponentially. Most dentists today have had to learn techniques and principles that were not yet known when they were in dental school. In the future, as the pace of technological innovation continues to increase and the pattern of dental diseases shifts, the need to keep up-to-date will be even more pressing. Means of staying current include interacting with colleagues, reading the dental literature, and attending continuing education courses—activities that require dentists to evaluate information. Yet, there is abundant historical evidence that dentists have not properly evaluated information. Perhaps the best documented example in dentistry of a widely accepted yet erroneous hypothesis is the focal infection theory. Proposed in 1904 and accepted by some clinicians until the Second World War, this untested theory resulted in the extraction of millions of sound teeth.[8] But errors are not restricted to the past; controversial topics exist in dentistry today, because new products or techniques are continually introduced and their usefulness debated. Ideally, dentists should become sophisticated consumers of research who can distinguish between good and bad research and know when to suspend judgment. This is different from proposing that dentists become research workers. One objective of this book is to provide a systematic method for the evaluation of scientific papers and presentations.

A systematic approach to analyzing scientific papers has to be studied, because this activity requires more rigor than the reasoning used in everyday life. Faced with an overabundance of information and limited time, most of us adopt what is called a *make-sense epistemology*. The truth test of this epistemology or theory of knowledge is whether propositions make superficial sense.[9] This approach minimizes the cognitive load and often works well for day-to-day short-term decision making. In 1949, Zipf[10] of Harvard University published *Human Behaviour and the Principle of Least Effort,* in which he stated:

> The Principle of Least Effort means, for example that in solving his immediate problems he will view these against a background of his probable future problems, *as estimated by himself*. Moreover, he will strive to solve his problems in such a way as to minimize the *total work* that he must expend in solving *both* his immediate problems *and* his probable future problems.[10]

Zipf used data from diverse sources ranging from word frequencies to sensory sampling to support his thesis. Although the methods and style of psychological research have changed, some more recent discoveries, such as the concept of *cognitive miser* in studies of persuasion,[11] coincide with Zipf's concept. Many of us minimize our mental effort when evaluating persuasive arguments.

But in science, the objective is not to make easy short-term decisions but rather to explain the phenomena of the physical world. The goal is accuracy, not necessarily speed, and a different, more sophisticated, more rigorous approach is required. Perkins et al[9] have characterized the ideal skilled reasoner as a critical epistemologist who can challenge and elaborate hypothetical models. Where the makes-sense epistemologist or naive reasoner asks only that a given explanation or model makes intuitive sense, the critical epistemologist moves beyond that stage and asks why a model may be inadequate. That is, when evaluating and explaining, the critical epistemologist asks both *why* and *why not* a postulated model may work. The critical epistemologist arrives at models of reality, using practical tactics and skills and drawing upon a large repertoire of logical and heuristic methods.[9]

A second objective of the book is to inculcate the habits of thought of the critical epistemologist in readers concerned with dental science and clinical dentistry.

The scope of the problem

In brief, the problems facing anyone wishing to keep up with developments in dentistry or other health professions are that (1) there is a huge amount of literature, (2) it is growing fast, and (3) much of it is useless. If measured by their influence on subsequent research, many papers are failures. Less than 25% of all papers will be cited 10 times in all eternity,[12] and a large number are never cited at all.

The actual rate of growth of the scientific literature has been estimated to be 7% per year of the extant literature, which in 1976 comprised close to 7.5 million items.[11] This rate of growth means that the biomedical literature doubles every 10 years. In dentistry, there are about 500 journals available today.[13] Many dental articles are found in low-impact journals, but, ignoring these, there were still 2,401 articles published in 1980 in the 30 core journals.[14] More recently, it has been estimated that about 43,000 dental-related articles are published per year.

However, the problem is not intractable. Relman,[15] a former editor of the *New England Journal of Medicine,* believes that most of the important business of scientific communication in medicine is conducted in a very small sector of top-quality journals. The average practitioner needs to read only a few well-chosen periodicals.[15] The key to dealing with the problem of the information explosion is in choosing what to read and learning to evaluate the information.

Dentists are exposed to diverse information sources, and the important issues vary depending on the source. For example, a dentist may wish to determine whether potassium nitrate toothpastes reduce dentin hypersensitivity. One approach would be to look up a systematic review on this topic in the Cochrane Library,[16] which many regard as the highest level in the hierarchy of evidence. The skills required to understand the review would include a basic knowledge of statistics and research design. The same dentist, facing the competitive pressures of his local market, might also want to determine whether a particular laser-bleaching instrument should be purchased for the practice. In that instance, there likely would not be a relevant Cochrane review, and there may not even be a relevant paper in a refereed journal to support a decision. Available evidence might consist of advertising brochures and anecdotes of colleagues. The dentist may have to employ a different set of skills, ranging from evaluating the lie factor in graphics (see chapter 13) to disentangling rhetoric (see chapter 3) from fact. Advertisements and salesmanship are persuasive exercises; the chapter on rhetoric (chapter 3) deals with means of persuasion.

Typically, dentists acquire information on innovative procedures through participation in networks in which their colleagues supply informal data on the effectiveness of the innovations. Nevertheless, dentists cite reading peer-reviewed dental literature and experimental studies as the gold standard for determining the quality of innovations.[17] New technology is often introduced into their practices through trial and error; dentists take the pragmatic approach of directly determining what works in their hands in their practice.[17] Doubtless, some of the personal and financial expenses typical of the trial-and-error approach could be reduced with more effective evaluation of information prior to selecting a material or technique for testing.

This book focuses on evaluating refereed scientific papers, but many of the issues of informational quality and questions that should be asked apply equally to other less formal channels of communication.

What is a scientific paper?

The Council of Biology Editors defines a *scientific paper* as follows:

> An acceptable primary scientific publication must be the first disclosure containing sufficient information to enable peers (1) to assess observations; (2) to repeat experiments; and (3) to evaluate intellectual processes; moreover, it must be sensible to sensory perception, essentially permanent, available to the scientific community without restriction, and available for regular screening by one or more of the major recognized secondary services.[18]

Similar ideas were stated more succinctly by De-Bakey,[19] who noted that the contents of an article shall be new, true, important, and comprehensible. A good deal of the literature circulated to dentists does not meet these requirements. But even excluding the throwaway or controlled-circulation magazines that are little more than vehicles for advertisements, the amount of information published annually appears formidable.

One approach to dealing with a large number of papers is to disregard original papers and receive information secondhand. Dental and medical journals present reviews of current research in specific clinical or scientific fields; some journals, such as *Dental Clinics of North America,* are exclusively devoted to this approach. Although this tactic reduces the volume of literature to be covered, it does not solve the problem of evaluating the information contained in the reviews. To perform this task effectively, a researcher must be able to assess the soundness of the reviewer's conclusions. In deciding to accept information secondhand, the researcher is also deciding whether the author of the review is a reliable, objective authority. Thus, the problem of evaluation has been changed, but not eliminated.

This book focuses on the primary literature, where it is hoped that new, true, important, and comprehensible information is published. The systematic review, a relatively new review form, attempts to deal with some of the more glaring problems of traditional reviews and is covered briefly in chapter 4. Although useful for some purposes, the systematic review has its own shortcomings, and the researcher must judge how these affect the conclusions. Journals vary in quality; chapter 4 discusses bibliometric approaches of ranking journals. Below, I present a brief review of how articles get published that may help to explain some of this variation.

The Road to Publication: Refereed vs Nonrefereed Journals

The first hurdle faced by an article submitted for publication is an editor's decision on the article's suitability for the journal. Different journals have different audiences, and the editors are the arbiters of topic selection for their journal. Editors can reject papers immediately if they think the material is unsuited to their particular journal.

In some journals, acceptance or rejection hinges solely on the opinion of the editor. However, this method is problematic, because informed decisions on some papers can only be made by experts in a particular field. Therefore, as a general rule, the most highly regarded journals ask the opinion of such specialists, called *referees* or *editorial consultants*. Referees attempt to ensure that a submitted paper does not demonstrably deviate from scientific method and the standards of the journal. Whether a journal is refereed can be determined by consulting *Ulrich's Index of Periodicals*. Editors usually provide referees with an outline of the type of information that they desire from the referee. The criteria for acceptance will necessarily include both objective (eg, obvious errors of fact or logic) and subjective (eg, priority ratings) components. Unfortunately, the task of refereeing is difficult and typically unpaid. Refereeing is often squeezed in among other academic activities, so it should not be surprising that it sometimes is not done well and that referees often disagree.

Studies of the reliability of peer-review ratings are disappointing for readers wanting to keep faith in the peer-review system. Reliability quotients, which can range from 0 (no reliability) to 1 (perfect reliability), for various attributes of submission to a psychology journal[20] follow:

Probable interest in the problem	0.07
Importance of present contribution	0.28
Attention to relevant literature	0.37
Design and analysis	0.19
Style and organization	0.25
Succinctness	0.31
Recommendation to accept or reject	0.26

Despite problems, there is evidence that the review process frequently raises important issues that, when resolved, improve the manuscript substantially.[21]

After consulting with referees, the editor decides whether the paper should be *a)* published as is—a comparatively rare event; *b)* published after suitable revision; or *c)* rejected. Journals reject papers in proportions varying from 0% to 90%. The literature available to dental health professionals ranges the spectrum of refereed to nonrefereed, from low (or no) rejection rates to high rejection rates. *The Journal of Dental Research,* for example, has a 50% rejection rate (Dawes, personal communication, 1990). Even among the refereed journals, there is no guarantee that the referees did a good job. In fact, these considerations only serve to reinforce the view "caveat lector"—let the reader beware.

Editorial independence

Ideally, the contents of the journal should be independent of economic issues, but this is seldom the case. Publication of color illustrations can be prohibitively expensive, and many respected journals are publications of learned societies that operate on lean budgets. The *Journal of Dental Research,* for example, is published and subsidized by the International Association for Dental Research. Such a journal would be expected not to be influenced by advertisers. Other journals have a need to generate income, and, in some instances, entire issues appear to be sponsored by a commercial interest. It is not unreasonable to wonder whether the advertiser influenced the editorial content, for "he who pays the piper calls the tune."

The components of a scientific paper

Scientific papers are traditionally divided into components, each of which has a different function. Journals vary in the order in which components are arranged, but most journals have a materials and methods section placed before the results. *Science,* however, prints the experimental details as footnotes at the end of the article. The functions of the components are outlined below.

Title

A well-written title is informative, concise, and graceful.[22] It attracts the interest of readers while giving them the topic of the study. The current trend is to present the conclusion in the title as, for example, "Dilantin causes gingival overgrowth," rather than "Studies on the effects of drugs on human gingival tissues Part XII. Dilantin."

On reading the title, the reader should ask why the study was done in the first place, bearing in mind that often what gets studied depends on what gets funded. Agencies fund what interests them. Commercial interests fund research to provide credibility for their products. In such instances, the research may be providing facts for only one side of the argument.

Author

Scientists, like horses, come in various classes and establish track records. The problem is distinguishing the thoroughbreds from the plough horses from the rogues. A technique called *citation analysis,* using the science citation index—which may be likened to the Daily Racing Form in this analogy—is one approach to this problem. Previously unpublished authors present a different challenge, as noted by Sackett,[23] who recommends that the work of unknown scientists, like the work of unknown sculptors, deserves at least a passing glance.

The author's address enables readers to write for reprints, clarification, or discussion of the paper. It will sometimes give clues to the assumptions or traditions behind the research. For example, consider a paper on dental implants published by a group in Gothenburg, Sweden, the site where the Brånemark system was developed. The reader can be confident in a firmly embedded assumption that the most desired form of integration of the implant is through a bony interface. A paper coming from Loma Linda, where blade vents have been used extensively, may not share that assumption.

With the growth of multiauthored papers, the question of what authorship signifies has arisen. At one extreme is the view that an author can justify intellectually the entire contents of an article.[24] But that is a difficult standard to uphold in the world of multidisciplinary research, where a clinician might have trouble justifying complex statistical procedures or where a statistician is held responsible for the molecular biological procedures. Some medical journals require contributors to state explicitly what part they played in the research. A study in which an editor contacted coauthors directly for their views and then compared them with their stated views in the published article reported that published papers rarely

represented the full range of opinions of the coauthors.[25]

Date of submission and acceptance

Ostensibly, these dates are given to establish priority of discovery to the authors. A long delay between submission and acceptance may indicate that referees found serious problems in the initial version and that extensive rewriting was required, or it may indicate inefficiency in the editors, referees, or authors. Many journals have moved from paper-based to electronically based submission and review of articles, and, as a general rule, this change reduces the time between submission and publication. Some variables are associated with the date of the study. For example, the incidence of dental caries in North America will probably be less in the 21st century than it was in the mid 20th century, and this might have an effect on the results of some types of study.

Abstract or summary

The abstract should tell the reader why the study was done, what was done, what was found, and what was concluded, whereas a summary usually focuses on the principal findings and conclusion of the study.[26] Although often overlooked, the abstract should be studied closely by anyone interested either in seriously evaluating a paper or saving time. For example, the abstract should contain the information that enables the reader to answer the Fisher Assertability Question,[27] which asks, "What information would I require to accept the conclusions?" If the methods used in the paper do not provide the appropriate information, the reader may wish to skip reading the paper in closer detail, thus saving time. In answering the assertability question, one has to make a judgment about appropriate standards—that is, how much evidence is required to prove the point. Too severe a standard will suggest that nothing could be known with certainty and nothing is worth reading, but, conversely, lax standards will lead to error and gullibility.[28] Having read the abstract and determined that the paper merits attention, the reader can consider the contents with the author's conclusion in mind, and is thus in a better position to identify weaknesses. In a paper reporting negative results, such as a treatment that did not produce a beneficial effect, a critical question is the size of the sample and the power of the statistical test. On encountering a negative result in the abstract, the reader is forewarned to pay particular attention to the size of the sample. The assertability question, as well as analysis of the relationship between evidence and conclusion, falls into the domain of logic, which is covered in chapters 5 to 8. The logic of statistical inference is of sufficient importance that it is featured in three chapters, 9, 10, and 20.

For medical journals, there has been a movement to structured abstracts, which are required in the CONSORT guidelines adopted by medical editors for reports of randomized controlled trials (RCTs). A structured abstract provides the objective, design, setting, subject, interventions, outcomes, results, and conclusions of a study. In general, structured abstracts provide more—and more easily accessible—information than unstructured abstracts and aid investigators preparing systematic reviews.

Introduction

The introduction states the problem and the current state of knowledge related to it, as well as the reasons for the investigation. Accessing the current state of knowledge through the scientific literature is covered in chapter 4. The introduction also often contains the most significant conclusion of the paper so that the reader can judge the evidence that will be presented in context.

Materials and methods

The materials and methods section should be presented in such sufficient detail that the reader could repeat the investigation. The components to be evaluated here are the measurements and their errors (see chapters 11, 12, and 14) and the investigational strat-

egy, tactics, and design (see chapters 15 to 19). Aspects of measurement include operational definition, precision, accuracy, validity, and reliability. These topics, as well as investigational strategies and experimental design, will be discussed later. In general, each strategy is associated with characteristic strengths and weaknesses, and knowing these enables a researcher to criticize papers more efficiently. For clinical research there is fairly widespread acceptance of the concept of a hierarchy of evidence. One example from the United States is given in Table 1-1.[29] British hierarchies place meta-analysis of RCTs at the highest level, and that system can be further divided according to the quality of the meta-analysis.[28]

Results

This section presents the results of the experiments, often in an order and a form that is designed to convince the reader of the truth of the paper's conclusions. The chapter on presentation of results (chapter 13) shows how data, figures, and tables may be manipulated to further the rhetorical purposes of an author.

Discussion

The discussion contains the logical arguments that link the data in the results section as well as the work of other investigators to the conclusions. This section puts the study in the context of the whole field of investigation. The discussion section is typically where rhetoric is most overtly practiced, as the importance of some observations is emphasized while the importance of others is downplayed or even ignored. An editorial in the *British Medical Journal* noted that the edi-

Table 1-1 Level of evidence for guideline recommendations of the United States Agency for Healthcare Research and Quality

Level	Type of Study	Grade of Recommendation
1	Supportive evidence from well-conducted RCTs that include 100 patients or more	A
2	Supportive evidence from well-conducted RCTs that include fewer than 100 patients	A
3	Supportive evidence from well-conducted cohort studies	A
4	Supportive evidence from well-conducted case-control studies	B
5	Supportive evidence from poorly controlled or uncontrolled studies	B
6	Conflicting evidence with the weight of evidence supporting the recommendation	B
7	Expert opinion	C

tors see many papers where the purpose of the discussion seems to be to "sell" the paper. They proposed a "structured discussion," analogous to the structured abstract, that follows the sequence (1) statement of principal findings; (2) strength and weaknesses of the study; (3) strengths and weaknesses in relation to other studies, discussing particularly any differences in results; (4) meaning of the study—possible mechanisms and implications for clinicians or policymakers; (5) unanswered questions and future research.[30]

Three general questions

A scientific paper is not necessarily an unbiased account of observations; it is more likely an attempt to convince the reader of the truth of a position. As noted by Ziman,[31] it is important to realize that much of the research literature of science is intended, rhetorically, to persuade other scientists of the validity of received opinions. Thus, a reader can expect an author to present his or her data in the most favorable light. Tables, figures, and even calculations may be done so that differences between groups are accentuated and the appearance of error is minimized. A reader's defense as a consumer of this information is an attitude of healthy skepticism. Three general questions a skeptical reader should ask are: Is it new? Is it true? Is it important?[32]

Is it *new?*

A minimum requirement for publication is that the information is new. However, *new* can be defined in various ways. If a paper using standard histologic techniques reporting the development of teeth in lynx were to be published tomorrow, it might well be new, because, as far as I am aware, the development of lynx teeth has not been described before. However, it probably would not be new in adding anything to our knowledge of tooth development in general. Such a paper would merely fill in the gaps, however small, in our knowledge. I think that journal editors are fairly lenient in their judgments on what constitutes new information. Kuhn[33] states that one of the reasons why normal puzzle-solving science seems to progress so rapidly is that its practitioners concentrate on problems that only their own lack of ingenuity keeps them from solving. Funding agencies are probably better gatekeepers of science in this regard, because an essential criterion for funding is originality.

The quality that often distinguishes good scientific papers from the mediocre is originality. Originality can appear in any component of the research process, including the questions being asked, the methods employed, the research design, or even the interpretation. Because science is a progressive business, approaches that were once original and sufficient can with time become derivative and deficient. Returning to the example, because scientists have been studying tooth development for decades using standard histologic techniques, there is not much hope that reworking the same approach would provide anything exciting; new methods would be required to bring new insights.

As a consequence of scientific progress, methods become outdated and standards change. Changing standards can be seen in biochemistry by examining the standards for publication of data using polyacrylamide gels. Early publications using the technique showed photographs of gels that did not have good resolution or uniformity and showed poor staining. The photographs of gels were often so uninformative that *Archives of Oral Biology* instructed authors to submit densitometric tracings of the gels. Currently, gel separations are done in two dimensions with superb resolution, and the proteins are stained with much greater sensitivity. A photograph of a gel that would have been acceptable 20 years ago would not be acceptable for publication today. In judging papers, therefore, a key question is whether the techniques and approach are up-to-date as well as whether the question is original.

This principle is so well accepted that investigators sometimes rush to apply new techniques to appear up-to-date. Fisher,[34] the pioneer statistician and author of the classic work on experimental design, warned, "any brilliant achievement . . . may give prestige to the method employed, or to some part of it, even in applications to which it has no special appropriateness."

Is it *true?*

Sound conclusions are the result of reliable observations combined with valid logic. Knowledge of measurement, types of observational errors, experimental design, and controls give some basis to assessments of the reliability of observations. Thus, sections of this book deal with these topics and the logic used to interpret the observations. But the ultimate test of any scientific observation is *reproducibility*, that is, the probability that any other scientist on reproducing the conditions of the observation would find the same result. A clue to the reproducibility of an observation is the consistency of the results within the body of the paper. Another means for evaluating the reliability of observations in a paper is to read what other scientists have written about the work, and citation analysis is an efficient means of uncovering that information.

A student might wonder whether it is necessary to learn such diverse concepts and examine the literature to such a detailed extent, particularly when it seems likely that the vast majority of publications are produced in good faith and come from institutions of higher learning. Ioannidis,[35] however, has argued that most published research findings are false. In his view, a research finding is less likely to be true when effect sizes are small, when there are a large number of tested hypotheses that have not been preselected, and when there are great flexibilities in designs, definitions, outcomes, and data analyses. Other problems impacting the truth of the conclusion are financial issues and other interests and prejudices as well as the number of teams in a field chasing statistical significance. I believe it is unlikely that most research findings are false, because if they were there would be more papers reporting failure to confirm results and many less confirming—albeit often indirectly—replication. Nevertheless, the considerations listed by Ioannidis serve to warn readers of the dental and medical literature that there is no shortage of well-documented threats to truth.

Is it important?

The importance of a paper cannot be tested in a completely objective manner. Maxwell[36] has argued—in my opinion, persuasively—that real progress in science is assessed in terms of the amount of valuable factual truth that is being discovered and that the accumulation of vast amounts of trivia (even if factually correct) does not amount to progress. The problem is that value judgments are highly subjective.

One can speculate about what qualities an ideal evaluator should have. Beveridge[37] has suggested the concept of scientific taste, which he described as a sense of beauty or esthetic sensibility. Beveridge explained scientific taste by stating that:

> The person who possesses the flair for choosing profitable lines of investigation is able to see further where the work is leading than are other people because he has the habit of using his imagination to look far ahead, instead of restricting his thinking to established knowledge and the immediate problem.

A person with scientific taste would be a good judge of the importance of a scientific paper. Traditionally, the skill of judgment is learned in the apprentice-master relationship formed between graduate student and supervisor. Techniques may come and go, but judging what is important and how it can be innovatively studied is the core business of scientists, and these skills are learned at the supervisor's knee. Thus, much importance is attached to the pedigree of a scientist, and some scientists take pride in tracing their scientific pedigrees to leading figures in a field of study.

Given the large variation in laboratory quality, there will always be significant differences in judgment. This diversity is evident in an extensive study of proposals submitted to the National Science Foundation. The study found that getting a research grant significantly depends on chance, because there is substantial disagreement among eligible reviewers, and the success of a proposal rests on which reviewers happen to be accepted.[38] Moreover, there is evidence that complete disagreement between pairs of referees assessing the same paper is common.[39] In biomedical science, the frequency of agreement between referees was not much better than that which would be expected by chance. Hence, it appears that objective and absolute criteria for the evaluation of a paper prior to publication are not available. Chapter 21 attempts to cultivate the skill of judgment by providing information on recognized sources of errors in judgments as well as citation analysis, a technique that can be used to access broadly based scientific assessments of published works.

References

1. Chargaff E. Triviality in science: A brief meditation on fashions. Perspect Biol Med 1976;19:324.
2. Norris SP. Synthesis of research on critical thinking. Education Leadership 1985;42:40–45.
3. Kurland DJ. I Know What It Says—What Does It Mean? Belmont, CA: Wadsworth, 1995:164.
4. Butler CB. Postmodernism: A Very Short Introduction. Oxford: Oxford Univ Press, 2002:37–42.
5. Bronowski J. The common sense of science. In: The Common Sense of Science. New York: Vintage, 1967:97–118.
6. Chambers DW. Lessons from badly behaved technology transfer to a professional context. Int J Technol Transfer Commercialisation 2005;4(1):63.
7. Chambers DW. Changing dental disease patterns. Contact Point 1985;63:1–17.
8. Fish W. Framing and testing hypotheses. In: Cohen B, Kramer IRH (eds). Scientific Foundations of Dentistry. Chicago: William Heinemann, 1976:669.

9. Perkins DN, Allen R, Hafner J. Difficulties in everyday reasoning. In: Maxwell W (ed). Thinking. Philadelphia: Franklin Institute Press, 1983:177.

10. Zipf GK. Human Behaviour and the Principle of Least Effort. Cambridge, MA: Addison-Wesley, 1949.

11. Pratkaris A, Aronson E. Age of Propaganda. The Everday Use and Abuse of Persuasion. New York: WH Freeman, 2001:38.

12. Garfield E. Current comments: Is the ratio between number of citations and publications cited a true constant? Curr Contents 1976;6:5–7.

13. Glenny A, Hooper L. Why are systematic reviews useful? In: Clarkson J, Harrison JE, Ismail A, et al (eds). Evidence Based Dentistry for Effective Practice. London: Martin Dunitz, 2003:59.

14. Garfield E. The literature of dental science vs the literature used by dental researchers. In: Garfield E. Essays of an Information Scientist, vol 5. Philadelphia: ISI Press, 1981–1982:373.

15. Relman AS. Journals. In: Warren KS (ed). Coping with the Biomedical Literature. New York: Praeger, 1981:67.

16. Worthington H, Clarkson J. Systematic reviews in dentistry: The role of the Cochrane oral health group. In: Clarkson J, Harrison JE, Ismail A, et al (eds). Evidence Based Dentistry for Effective Practice. London: Martin Dunitz, 2003:97.

17. Chambers DW. Habits of the reflective practitioner. Contact Point 1999;79:8–10.

18. Day RA. How to Write and Publish a Scientific Paper. Philadelphia: ISI Press, 1979:2.

19. DeBakey L. The Scientific Journal: Editorial Policies and Practices: Guidelines for Editors, Reviewers, and Authors. St Louis: Mosby, 1976:1–3.

20. Simonton DK. Creativity in Science. Cambridge: Cambridge Univ Press, 2004:85–86.

21. Goodman SN, Berlin JA, Fetcher SW, Fletcher RH. Manuscript quality before and after peer review and editing at Annals of Internal Medicine. Ann Intern Med 1994; 121(1):11.

22. Tacker MM. Parts of the research report: The title. Int J Prosthodont 1990;3(4):396.

23. Sackett DL. Evaluation: Requirement, for clinical application. In: Warren KS (ed). Coping with the Biomedical Literature. New York: Praeger, 1981:123.

24. Judson HF. Authorship, ownership: Problems of credit, plagiarism, and intellectual property. In: The Great Betrayal: Fraud in Science. Orlando: Harcourt, 2004:287.

25. Horton R. The hidden research paper. JAMA 2002;287: 2775–2778.

26. Tacker MM. Parts of the research report: The abstract. Int J Prosthodont 1990;3(5):499.

27. Fisher A. The Logic of Real Arguments. Cambridge: Cambridge Univ Press, 1988:22.

28. Fisher A. The Logic of Real Arguments. Cambridge: Cambridge Univ Press, 1988:27.

29. Kroke A, Boeing H, Rossnagel K, Willich SN. History of the concept of "levels of evidence" and their current status in relation to primary prevention through lifestyle interventions. Public Health Nutr 2004;7(2):279.

30. Docherty M, Smith R. The case for structuring the discussion of scientific papers. BMJ 1999;318(7193):1224–1225.

31. Ziman J. Reliable Knowledge: An Exploration of the Grounds for Belief in Science. Cambridge: Cambridge Univ Press, 1978:7.

32. DeBakey L. The Scientific Journal: Editorial Policies and Practices: Guidelines for Editors, Reviewers, and Authors. St Louis: Mosby, 1976:1.

33. Kuhn TS. The Structure of Scientific Revolutions, ed 2. Chicago: Chicago Univ Press, 1970:184.

34. Fisher RA. The Design of Experiments. Edinburgh: Oliver & Boyd, 1953:184.

35. Ioannidis JP. Why most published research findings are false. PLoS Med 2005;2:e124.

36. Maxwell N. Articulating the aims of science. Nature 1977; 265:2.

37. Beveridge WIB. The Art of Scientific Investigation. New York: Vintage, 1950:106.

38. Cole S, Cole JR, Simon GA. Chance and consensus in peer review. Science 1981;214:881.

39. Gordon M. Evaluating the evaluators. New Sci 1977;73:342.

2 | Scientific Method and the Behavior of Scientists

Thou hast made him a little less than angels.

—Hebrews 2:7

Because there is no one scientific method, any account of scientific method is bound to be incomplete or even inaccurate and misleading. Sir Peter Medawar, a Nobel laureate, has stated that "there is no such thing as a calculus of discovery or a schedule of rules which by following we are conducted to a truth."[1] Discoveries are made by individual scientists, who often have their own original and distinctive ways of thinking, and they do not necessarily follow any rigid protocol of scientific method.

The simple view advanced by Bronowski[2] is that scientific method is organized common sense, and indeed this concept is emphasized in this book. However, the inclusion of the term *organized* is not a small addition, for scientific method differs from common sense in the rigor with which matters are investigated. For example, precise operational definitions, procedures to quantify, and theories to explain relationships are often employed, and a great effort is made to avoid inconsistencies. Results should be subject to the systematic scrutiny of the investigator or other scientists, and limits on how far the results can be applied should be sought. Formal methods for describing scientific method are still the topic of philosophical examination. But philosophical speculation or practice do not greatly concern typical research scientists, who are largely occupied in puzzle solving[3] and who often seem too busy to consider how they got from A to B or how their investigational strategies relate to any philosophical concepts. There is increasing recognition that a key aspect in the development and acceptance of scientific facts and theories is the social interaction between scientists. Descriptions of an ideal

exist for both the scientific method and the behavior of scientists, but the ideal does not always correspond with reality. Nevertheless, as they are the norms they will be discussed here.

The Behavior of Scientists

The pioneer sociologist of science, Merton,[4] identified six guiding principles of behavior for scientists:

1. *Universalism* refers to the internationality and independence of scientific findings. There are no privileged sources of scientific knowledge[5]; scientific results should be analyzed objectively and should be verifiable or repeatable. In practice, this norm means that all statements are backed up by data or citations to published work. Internationalism is one of the characteristics of modern science that emphasizes collaboration; papers frequently have multiple authors from different institutions and countries.

2. *Organized skepticism* describes the interactions whereby scientists evaluate findings before accepting them. Ideally, scientists would check results by repeating the observations or experiments, but this approach is time consuming and expensive. At the very least, scientists try to determine whether reported results are consistent with other publications. An ironclad rule of science is that when you publish something, you are responsible for it. When

a finding is challenged, the investigator must take the criticism seriously and consider it carefully, regardless whether the investigator is a senior professor and the challenger the lowliest technician or graduate student.[6]

3. *Communalism* is the norm that enjoins scientists to share the results of their research. "Scientific knowledge is public knowledge, freely available to all."[5] One factor acting against the free exchange of information in a timely manner is the growing commercialization of scientific research. As both the institution and the principal investigator may benefit financially by obtaining rights to intellectual property, the time required to obtain patents results in delays in transmitting findings to the scientific community.

4. *Disinterestedness* is summed up by the dictum "Science for science's sake." At present, this norm appears to be honored more in breach than in observance. As noted above, many scientists patent their discoveries and form alliances with commercial interests. At one time, I served on a grants committee that dispersed funds for major equipment. It happened that two applications requested similar equipment, although there was not enough work to justify this duplication. One panel member wondered why the two groups did not combine and submit a single application. As it turned out, the two university-based principal investigators collaborated with different commercial interests. Ideally, scientists should not have any psychological or financial stake in the acceptance or rejection of their theories and findings.

5. *Humility* is derived from the precept that the whole of the scientific edifice is incomparably greater than any of its individual parts. This norm is in operation whenever scientists receive awards; they inevitably thank their coworkers in glowing terms. Scientists giving invited lectures in symposia are generally at pains to point out which graduate students or postdoctoral researchers actually did the work and include lab pictures in their presentations to share the glory (small though it may be).

Despite the norm of humility, clashes of egos still occur. Several rules of behavior govern the interaction of scientists in the case of a disagreement. Discussion should be detached; that is, the issues, and not the personalities, should be discussed. The question is not *who* is right but rather *what* is right. The debate should be constructive; for example, if a referee decides that a paper should be rejected, the referee's comments should indicate how the paper could be improved. Finally, scientists who disagree should be courteous; they can disagree without being disagreeable.

6. *Originality* is highly prized in science and features prominently in determining who wins awards and grants. Yet, originality is difficult to define precisely, and, as Merton[7] noted, there is a "gap between the enormous emphasis placed upon original discovery and the great difficulty a good many scientists experience in making one." The originality of a scientific work can reside in the novelty of the hypothesis being investigated, the methods used to investigate it, as well as in the results obtained. Perhaps the most common scientific strategy—the transfer method—involves applying methods and concepts from one field to the particular topics of an adjacent field. For example, one could test the effect of a drug in a rat macrophage cell line that already had been investigated in a mouse macrophage line. On such minor contributions has many a career been built.

Recognition is the "coin of science"

In the traditional description, scientists are portrayed as altruistic individuals, devoid of personal or selfish considerations and engaged in the objective search for truth. Scientists often adopt—or at least pay lip service to—this view. The *American Scientist*,[8] for example, published 75 case histories on "Why I became a scientist." Aside from two individuals, these scientists seemed to attach little importance to a good salary, an issue that greatly concerns many other professionals. Yet, anyone working with academics knows that this mundane matter is often hotly disputed.

In an anthropologic investigation into laboratory life, Latour and Woolgar[9] found that scientific activity is geared toward the publication of papers and, moreover, that personal motivations and interactions are prime factors in determining what gets done. High on the list of motivators is recognition. According to Cronin,[10] recognition is the exchange on which the social system of science hinges. Investigators insist that their work be cited where appropriate and dispute priority claims vigorously. A prominent example is the dispute between Robert Gallo and Luc Montagnier over priority in the discovery of HIV as the cause of AIDS. That conflict ended with the protagonists jointly writing a history of the discovery. Such disputes would be unlikely to occur between humble men. Thus, there seems to be considerable discrepancy between the ideals of scientific behavior and the way scientists actually behave.

High-impact research, collaboration, and the "shadow of the future"

Simonton[11] has reviewed the characteristics of highly creative scientists doing high-impact research. Great scientists tend to possess the ability to ask critical questions for a variety of topics. They do not work on just one project at a time but rather involve themselves with a number of independent projects simultaneously while employing a core set of themes, issues, perspectives, or metaphors. These projects may differ in their feasibility, intrinsic importance of the questions, interaction with other projects, specific type of research, progress, and amount of effort demanded of the investigator.

Increasingly, modern research scientists find collaboration worthwhile. Several studies have shown that the most prolific scientists tend to collaborate the most (briefly reviewed in Surowiecki[12]). Nobel laureates, for example, collaborate more frequently than their run-of-the-mill scientific colleagues.

Collaboration extends the range of topics that a scientist can investigate efficiently, because it provides a source of knowledge and technical competence not found in the investigator's laboratory. Moreover, in a collaborative project, work is almost automatically assigned to the laboratory where it most efficiently can be accomplished. Collaboration does come at the price of adding names to papers, which makes it seem that a scientist might lose some recognition by having to share it with others. I think, however, that for the important bodies of recognition of much research—namely, promotion, tenure, and grants committees—it is the number of papers that counts; the number of authors on a paper is most often not rigorously taken into account. That is, publishing four papers with three coauthors would be perceived more positively than publishing a single paper as a sole author. Collaboration seems to be most effective when done locally. Academic researchers were found in one study to spend only a third of their time with people not in their immediate work group; nevertheless, a quarter of their time was spent working with people outside their university.[12]

The political scientist Robert Axelrod[13] postulated that cooperation is the result of repeated interaction with the same people. Trust is not really required to form a collaborative partnership; the key to collaboration is "the shadow of the future." People in cooperative relationships should start off being nice, but they have to be willing to punish noncooperative behavior, with an approach of being "nice, forgiving, and retaliatory." I have seen this principle in operation in grants committees and for manuscripts submitted for publication in which there does seem to be an element of "you score my grant (or paper) highly and I will score yours highly." Thus old boys/girls networks are formed. Even professor-student relationships can be clouded by the shadow of the future. I know of one professor who distributed his course evaluation forms to his class with the trenchant proposition, "you give me a nice evaluation, I will give you a nice exam." It would take a brave student to ignore the dark cloud of a tough exam in the future—much safer to check all the boxes rating the forthright professor as excellent and hope that fellow students exhibit the same enlightened self-interest.

A case study of the effectiveness of retaliation is provided by Sir Cyril Burt, an influential British psychologist who was accused of falsifying data on the nature/nurture question of intelligence. Burt relished controversy and, according to Hearnshaw,[14] "never missed a chance to give back more than he got." Burt was not scrupulous in representing his opponents' arguments fairly and resorted to such devices as obfuscation, misrepresentation (eg, using fictitious names, he wrote and published letters to the editor in the journal that he edited himself), and making claims that were hard to verify.[15] As a high-handed editor of a prominent British journal, Burt was someone who you crossed at your peril. For a young scientist developing a career, cooperating with Burt would seem to be a much more attractive option than controverting with him.

Objectivity

Objectivity remains the cornerstone of scientific method. A scientist should be a disinterested observer interpreting data without personal bias or prejudice. Ideally, scientific observations should be objective, meaning that the same observation would be made by any qualified individual examining the same phenomenon. Conditions of observation should be arranged so that the observer's bias does not distort the observations. The personality of the scientist should be irrelevant to the observations. The mantra of practitioners of the new brand of scientific objectivity that emerged at the end of the 19th century was "let nature speak for itself."[16]

One indication of the attempt for objectivity is the pervasive use of the passive voice in scientific writing, as this seems to impart some distance between the observer and the observation. (I should note that the practice is changing in scientific writing; it is fair to say that current opinion favors the use of the active voice.) In any case, merely writing in the passive voice does not guarantee objectivity. It has been said that 17th-century epistemology aspired to the viewpoints of angels; 19th-century objectivity aspired to the self-discipline of saints.[16] These lofty goals are hard to obtain for 20th- and 21st-century mortals; increasingly, the objectivity of scientists has been called into question.

Aberrant behavior: Lack of objectivity (should the history of science be rated "X"?)

This attack has taken place on two fronts and involves two types of scientific soldiers: the generals of scientific history and the more humble common cannon fodder who fight for jobs, grants, and tenure.

Consider the following generals:

1. Claudius Ptolemy, generally regarded as the greatest astronomer of antiquity, appears to have altered his observations to fit his theories. Moreover, his writings appear to be a "cover up." One historian of science, Robert Newton, has dubbed Ptolemy "the most successful fraud in the history of science."[17]

2. There is good reason to think that Galileo was dishonest about some of his observations.[18]

3. Isaac Newton manufactured accuracy by taking rough measurements and producing calculations that claimed accuracy to six or seven decimal places. Moreover, Newton selected data to fit his hypothesis. Newton's correspondence with his publisher leaves little doubt about what he was up to; he adjusted values, one after another, so that his laws would appear to fit observational data. Newton termed these actions "mending the numbers." "No one," concluded Westfall[19] in his article "Newton and the Fudge Factor," "can manipulate the fudge factor so effectively as the master mathematician."

4. Einstein wrote ". . . it is quite wrong to try founding a theory on observable magnitudes alone. In reality

the very opposite happens. It is the theory which decides what we can observe."[18]

In all these instances, it appears that great scientists were subjective or at least considered observations to be secondary to theory. Kuhn[20] gives numerous examples of revolutionary scientists rising above the morass of observational data to construct their elegant theories, which at the time of their inception were no better than those of their predecessors. This heresy is not new; roughly 40 years ago Bondi[21] suggested that, in astronomy, observations had proven a less reliable arbiter of hypotheses than had theoretical considerations.

There is little danger that an intellect like Einstein's will be found in dental research, so you may be wondering what these stories have to do with this book. They simply show that the traditional explanation of scientific method does not provide an adequate description of how some outstanding scientists actually operate. Thus, it should come as no surprise that some of the lesser lights of science can also lack objectivity. This is particularly true when you consider that the rewards of science—grants, jobs, tenure, and even fame—go to the people who publish.

The pressure to publish has been invoked as one of the reasons for the increasing problem of scientific fraud. But dubious scientific practices have attracted critical comment for some time. Charles Babbage, famous for inventing the first mechanical computer, produced a typology in 1830.[22] Hoaxing, forging, trimming, and cooking formed the unholy quadrivium of Babbage's typology. The sins of forging and hoaxing are obvious enough, and Babbage viewed these as less serious problems for science, as forging was rare and hoaxes would eventually be discovered. *Trimming* consisted of making the reported precision of data appear better than it was by clipping off bits of data from high readings and adding them to low readings so that the reported average was not affected. *Cooking* comprised a range of practices that resulted in data agreeing with expectations. The term has considerable staying power; it was a common practice in my undergraduate days in physics labs to employ "Cook's Constant" to coax highly accurate values for physical properties (such as the gravitational constant "G") from antiquated and poorly maintained equipment.

Traditionalists argue that frauds eventually will be found out, because other researchers will be unable to repeat the fraudulent results. Nevertheless, scientific fraud has become an important issue. In *Betrayers of the Truth,* Broad and Wade[23] dissect some of the more widely known cases of scientific fraud, many of which concerned individuals in world-renowned institutions. In the instances reviewed by Broad and Wade, it was generally a coworker who blew the whistle; attempted replication of results by researchers in other laboratories played a minor role, if any, in the detection of fraud. Perhaps this is to be expected, because experimental systems often vary in detail from one investigator to another. If one investigator fails to confirm another's results, the variations can be attributed to differences in the experimental systems. To set up exact replications would be tedious, and there is little reward attached to confirming another's results. Thus, it is easier and more profitable for scientists to forge ahead with their own work rather than to confirm the work of others, and much data probably goes unchecked. Similarly, Kohn[24] in *False Prophets* and Judson[6] in *The Great Betrayal* examine instances of scientific fraud or suspected fraud in detail. Although there are abundant anecdotal reports of "bad apples," Mosteller,[25] a professor of statistics at Harvard and a former president of the American Association for the Advancement of Science, pointed out, perhaps with the statistician's penchant for using Ockham's razor, that: "Before appealing to fraud, it is well to keep in mind the old saying that most institutions have enough incompetence to explain almost anything."

Just how prevalent and significant the problem may be is difficult to determine. An early informal survey on scientific cheating concluded that intentional bias (a euphemism for cheating) may be widespread.[26] Objective data on such activities are obviously difficult to obtain because potential informants are reluctant to admit their failings. Nevertheless, a recent survey,[27] in which scientists were randomly selected from databases of the National Institute of Health's (NIH) Office of Extramural Research, incorporated mechanisms for confidentiality and obtained over 3,000 replies (a roughly 46% response rate). Misbehavior was broadly interpreted and included serious offenses, such as falsifying or cooking data, to the less serious, such as inadequate record keeping related to research projects. As many as one in three of the survey respondents admitted to committing at least one of the 10 most serious behaviors. The authors concluded that certain features of the research environment, such as perceived inequities in how resources are distributed, may have detrimental effects on the ethical dimensions of scientists' work. Thus, the approach toward scientific fraud may be changing from blaming aberrant "bad apples" to determining how the environment shapes scientists' behavior. The *British Medical Journal* devoted a special section to fraud in research in its issue of 6 June 1998 and

commissioned five answers to the question of how best to respond to research misconduct. The NIH has established an Office of Research Integrity that, among other duties, sponsors research on the topic.

It might be thought that cheating does not really affect scientific progress because in the long run errors will be corrected.[3] In my view, there can be no doubt that scientific fraud and related scientific misdemeanors do impair the efficiency of science, that is, the amount of useful information obtained per dollar invested. In my experience, granting agencies do a poor job of assessing how effectively their research funds are spent. Moreover, in universities and research institutions, credit is disproportionately given to those obtaining research money (which benefits the institution because of accompanying money to cover indirect costs), rather than those producing new information. Research funding can be readily and speedily measured; research impact may require a decade to determine. This allocation of recognition and rewards to the most grant productive may lead investigators to reason that the ends justify the means, or, to quote Doty's[28] assessment of scientific misconduct, "the validity of an action is decided by whether one can get away with it." The chances of getting away with the crime of obtaining research funds based on misleading data and unlikely promises are pretty good; granting panels or committees seldom reconvene to determine how good a job they did in funding significant research.

Unintentional bias

Perhaps more crippling to the cause of truth is unintentional bias, which occurs when an investigator unknowingly designs a study so that the information obtained is in some way biased. Unintentional bias is widespread and happens in social science, for example, when one group in the population is not considered. Piaget's classic studies on child development were based only on male children, and the work of renowned anthropologist Margaret Mead has been widely criticized for drawing conclusions about whole societies largely on the basis of interviews with teenaged girls.

An extreme form of unintentional bias is self-delusion, where scientists believe they are practicing appropriate scientific method but have lost objectivity. Dennis Rousseau[29] has proposed that errors in science created by a loss of objectivity consistently demonstrate a similar pattern. This "pathologic science" has three characteristics:

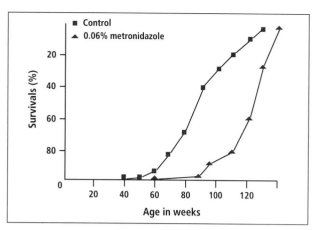

Fig 2-1 Survival vs age in controls and male rats receiving metronidazole. (Adapted from Rustia[31] with permission.)

1. The effect being studied is often at the limits of detectability, and increasing the strength of the causative agent may not increase the size of the effect.
2. The scientists are ready to dispose summarily of prevailing theories and to substitute revolutionary new ones.
3. The scientists avoid doing experiments that are critical tests of their theories or observations.

Two examples of pathologic science given by Rousseau[29] are the "cold fusion" process of generating energy and the "infinite dilution" process, whereby a biologically active solution is diluted so many times that no active molecules can be present, yet the solution continues to have an effect. A study on infinite dilution was published in *Nature*[30] and gave, in some people's eyes, some credence to the practice of homeopathy. It is noteworthy that in the instances of both cold fusion and infinite dilution, the traditional description of scientific method was operative; the aberrant results were checked by other investigators and found to be erroneous.

Objectivity can also be compromised by knowledge. It has often been said that what you see depends on how you look, but evidence suggests that what you see depends on what you know. For example, pathologists' judgments can be dramatically influenced by prior knowledge of the clinical features of a case. Hetherington[31] has reviewed several recent examples from astronomy in which the observations reflected personal biases rather than reality. In Hetherington's[31]

view, the fact that errors in observation are correlated with the expectations of observers has been demonstrated beyond reasonable doubt, and "the warping of judgment by knowledge, the influence on observational reports by preconceived opinion, is inevitable." The relationship of scientists to prevailing theories may be likened to that of fish to water; fish appear to be blissfully unaware of water even though the water must necessarily affect all their sensory inputs. Hetherington concludes, "the decline of theology followed from historical studies revealing that its supposedly divine sources were not absolute, but historically relative, subject to cultural forces. It remains to be seen whether historical studies of science may contribute to a strengthening of science's better features or to a weakening of confidence in modern science."[31]

The conclusion of this brief consideration of the behavior of scientists is that the reader must approach the literature with a critical and skeptical eye. For example, metronidazole, a chemotherapeutic agent against trichomonas infection, has proved useful in treating vaginitis and has been proposed for use in the treatment of periodontal disease. Two experienced cancer researchers tested the drug for carcinogenicity (Fig 2-1). They concluded, among other things, that the drug produced a significant incidence of pituitary and testicular neoplasms in male rats. However, the discussion paid little attention to the result that rats taking metronidazole lived longer. As cancer is more prevalent in elderly rats, as well as in elderly people, it is not surprising that there were more tumors in the metronidazole-treated group, because these rats lived long enough to develop tumors. It appears that the authors were so intent on looking for carcinogenic effects that they ignored the observation that they had discovered the "fountain of youth" for rats.[32]

The Storybook Version of Scientific Method

A traditional description of scientific method, sometimes called the *storybook scientific method*, incorporates several sequential steps.

1. Investigators must first decide what questions can be asked and whether the questions are worth asking.
2. They gather and organize the information pertaining to the problem.

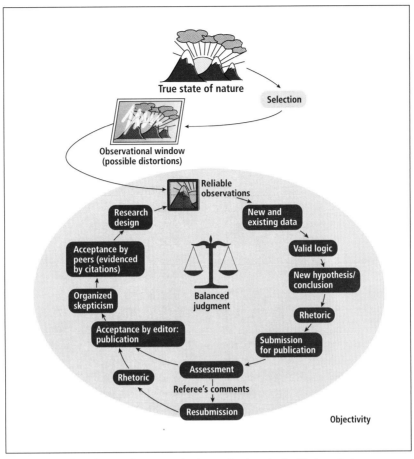

Fig 2-2 Typical products and processes in the production of scientific knowledge.

3. They form a working hypothesis that represents the most likely answer to the question.
4. They make observations that test the hypothesis. This stage involves choices about strategies and techniques.
5. If the results contradict the predictions of the hypothesis, the hypothesis is modified.
6. If the results agree with the hypothesis, the investigators devise other tests of the hypothesis in an attempt to prove themselves wrong.
7. If these subsequent tests support the hypothesis, the investigators accept the hypothesis and publish the results, which other scientists then attempt to replicate.
8. Successful replication as well as other tests of the hypothesis eventually lead to a consensus whereby another piece of information is added to the body of science.

One problem with storybook scientific method is that it contradicts what we know about how humans actually behave. People are reluctant to change their beliefs, even in the face of empirical evidence that proves them wrong (see chapter 21). The storybook scientific method gives scientists the duty to prove themselves wrong, contrary to people's natural inclination to prove themselves right. Moreover, the storybook version implies that replication of experiments should be the norm; the reward system of science is such that replication is unusual. Even if the storybook version does not accurately describe the actual practices of scientists, it is commonly used in presenting the results of research and in justifying conclusions. Another problem with the storybook scientific method is that it misses out on the cut and thrust of scientific dialogue, where typically scientists use all the rhetorical skills at their disposal to convince others of the truth of their conclusions. A somewhat more detailed and pragmatic approach to describing the production of scientific knowledge is given in Figure 2-2, and aspects of the process are described below.

Observation

An important limitation

Science is concerned with what can be observed, and observations are impressions made via the senses. The limitation of direct observation precludes certain important philosophical questions, such as the existence of God, from being answered by science. Medawar[33] notes that "it is not to science, but to metaphysics, imaginative literature, or religion that we must turn for answers to questions having to do with first and last things." Figure 2-2 posits that there is, in fact, a "true state of nature" that exists independent of any observers. In doing so, it ignores an ancient debate in philosophy between two opposing schools of thought: *realism* and *idealism*. Realists argue that the aim of science is to provide a true description of the world. Idealists hold that the physical world is in some way dependent on the conscious activity of humans.[34] An idealist might argue that an apple is not necessarily red in the dark (because no one can see it), or that a tree that falls in an isolated forest makes no sound (because there is no one to hear it). This metaphysical debate involving observable/unobservable distinctions, if it is relevant to any science at all, generally does not concern biomedical scientists.

A fundamental principle: Independence of the observer from the observation

Ziman[35] states that the fundamental principle of scientific observation is that all human beings are interchangeable as observers, and scientific information is restricted to those observations on which independent observers can agree. The assumption that all observers are equivalent is not merely a basic principle of Einstein's theory of special relativity; it is the foundation stone of all science.

But even this general rule seems to have an exception. Qualitative field research is the disciplined enquiry examining the personal meaning of individuals experiencing and acting in their social environments.[36] The researcher is more part of the phenomenon being investigated than a detached observer, and thus different observers might draw different conclusions. But even in qualitative field research, to attempt to ensure the reliability of the findings, scientists have developed strategies to minimize observer effects, such as *(1)* checking with the subjects if the observations are credible, *(2)* using prolonged times of observation, and *(3)* using triangulations in which data and theoretical interpretations are cross-checked between observers and studies.

Selection of observations

What is chosen to be observed depends on the immediate purpose of the investigation. In the December 2002 issue of the *Canadian Association of University Teachers*, Nobel laureate John Polanyi stated that for scientists, "the decision [of] what to investigate . . . is the most fateful of their lives."[37] Choosing what to observe is not just a matter of satisfying an idle curiosity. "For to obtain an answer of note one must ask a question of note, a question that is exquisitely phrased."[37] I always ask graduate students who are considering thesis topics, "what is the best possible outcome if everything goes right with the study you are planning? In particular, can the results be published and where?" Too often students plan studies that are doomed from the start by asking questions of insufficient importance or negligible novelty.

Until recently, funding agencies seemed to apply the cardinal rule that the observations must answer specific questions or test specific hypotheses. To label a proposal a "fishing expedition" was the kiss of death. The advent of genomic techniques has brought more acceptance of fishing expeditions, which are now fashionably called *exploratory research*. It remains true that asking specific questions is the best strategy for getting publishable answers.

Observations are made in the context of an overall research design. Typically, the design is based on the hypothetico-deductive model, whereby an investigator has a hypothesis (often based on previous studies), such as "substitution of sucrose in the diet by xylitol will reduce caries," and tests it. In designing the test, the researcher will have to determine a feasible investigative approach. If, for example, an experimental strategy is chosen, the investigator has to make decisions on such aspects as amounts of xylitol to be provided, population to which it is administered, ethics approval, measurement of sugar consumption, what teeth will be examined, how they will be examined, and when they will be examined. If the investigator decides on a case-control study, different issues arise, such as recruiting xylitol gum users and nonusers who are closely matched in relevant variables. The different designs will yield conclusions of varying certainty, and it may turn out that the most rigorous strategy is not feasible and compromises are necessary.

Issues in clinical studies

In clinical studies, the selection of observations often comes down to asking two principal questions: who and what?

Who

The ideal is that the sample of people studied is representative of the population to whom the conclusions will be applied. Nonrepresentative samples can lead to erroneous conclusions, and editorial guidelines for dealing with the problem have been established.[35] For example:

1. All participants in a study should be accounted for[38–40];
2. No more than 15% of the patients should be unavailable for follow-up;
3. The patients should be adequately described with clear eligibility (ie, inclusion/exclusion) criteria;
4. Details on randomization should be given.

What

Any clinical study must have an outcome variable or endpoint, ie, a measurement used to judge the effect of the intervention. A potential problem is the choice of an outcome variable. Sometimes investigators employ a surrogate end point (often a risk factor) that is related but not identical to the real variable of interest. For example, if the interest was in the effect of mouthrinse on dental caries, a researcher might measure the mouthrinse's effects on the accumulation of dental plaque or *Streptococcus mutans*. Because plaque, particularly the strain S *mutans,* has been implicated in the development of caries, the rationale follows that its reduction would result in the reduction of caries. This surrogate end point would enable an investigator to complete the study more quickly and cheaply than would be possible with a full-scale clinical trial using dental caries as the end point. But it might give misleading results if the mouthrinse removed plaque from surfaces that were not prone to caries but failed to remove it from pits and fissures. There might be an overall reduction of plaque but no change in tooth decay. The use of surrogate variables is particularly widespread in advertisements for dental products, because it is almost always cheaper and quicker to use surrogate end points than to perform a complete clinical study.

In medical research, the case of an inappropriate end point can be a life-or-death matter. In discussing this issue, Sackett[41] uses the example of clofibrate,[42] a drug that caused an almost 10% drop in serum cholesterol level (a key coronary risk factor) but increased the death rate by almost 20%.

Classification of observations

Classification of observations can be a complex process. The ideal is to group objects by some well-defined character or group of characters into classes that do not overlap. Much of pathology and classical biology is concerned with problems of classification, but classification can become an end in itself and sterile. Carolus Linnaeus devised methods for the classification of biologic materials that are still used today, but he also devised a method for classifying scientists according to military rank that is totally useless. (Needless to say Linnaeus was a general in his ranking system.[43])

Observational reactivity

A problem common to all observations is the probability that the act of observing alters what is being observed, just as television cameras covering a political event alter the actions of the participants.

Qualitative vs quantitative

Scientific observations may be qualitative or quantitative, with the latter being preferred. The chapters on measurement (chapter 11) and errors of measurement (chapter 12) address quantification in detail. However, qualitative observations can be valuable, particularly in sociologic studies. The most frequent techniques of qualitative research are in-depth interviews and participant observation. The information gathered may be used to produce hypotheses on topics on which there may be very little information, to describe social phenomena, and to gain greater insight into the mechanisms through which a known causal process works.[44]

Hypothesis

Hypotheses are provisional explanations of observations, conjectures on the nature of things that typically lead to predictions on what will be observed under specific conditions. Finding a well-stipulated hypothesis in some papers is difficult, but it is usually found in the introduction. The lack of a hypothesis often means that the author is adopting an unfocused and unproductive approach. In formulating a hypothesis, the scientist considers not only the data from the current study but the existing data in the scientific literature. Useful hypotheses are simple, remain internally consistent, explain all relevant facts, and, most importantly, are testable. The formation of hypotheses requires creative imagination. In the storybook description of scientific method, the investigator tests a hypothesis by trying to disprove it. Thus, scientists attempt to prove themselves wrong, an approach that differs from the natural tendency of people to prove themselves right. Moreover, at least in the storybook approach, scientists consider plausible alternative explanations for the data and show that these alternative hypotheses are incorrect. Typically, this is done in experimentation by the inclusion of appropriate controls. Only when all other hypotheses are exhausted do investigators reluctantly conclude that their own hypotheses are correct. Once they have done so, they have to convince other scientists.

Publication, repetition, consensus, and recognition

Publication

Academic science has been defined as a social institution devoted to the construction of a rational consensus of opinion over the widest possible field.[45] Observations must be published so that they can be considered by the scientific community. A paper's chances of acceptance for publication are best if the conclusion is well supported. But conclusions are supported not only by observations but also by logical argument and the style in which the information is presented. To obtain acceptance for their paper, authors become advocates for their conclusions rather than adopt the storybook role of the scientist as a detached observer who is reluctantly forced to accept the conclusion. In evaluating a scientific paper, the reader is forced to evaluate the rhetoric, that is, the persuasive devices used by an author. Rhetoric appears in many places in a scientific paper. In the introduction, the author outlines the importance of the problem; in the materials and methods section, an author might emphasize that the techniques are reliable and well accepted; in the results section, an author might present data to make the effects seen in the study look as significant or as precise as possible; in the discussion, an author might select references that support a particular viewpoint.

Unfortunately, scientific articles are written in a style featuring passive sentence construction and impersonal presentation of facts that readers find turgid and difficult to read.[46] Moreover, scientific articles may obscure the process by which conclusions were reached, as the intent is to distill the results into a co-

herent, interpretable story. Louis Pasteur advised students writing scientific papers to "make it look inevitable."[47] The process involved in arriving at the conclusions (the process of discovery) is often ignored; ordinary laboratory events such as mistakes, equipment breakdown, squabbles between workers, and going down blind alleys—details that would make the article longer but would not add anything to scientific knowledge—are not mentioned. Thus, publications emphasize the process of demonstration and the documentation of the findings.

A traditional problem in rhetoric concerns the issue of the order in which information is presented. As the process of demonstration requires a coherent story, the experiments may be presented in a different order in the paper than the sequence in which they were done in the laboratory. Likewise, the reasons given for doing an experiment in the paper may differ from the ones used in planning the study. Nobel laureate Peter Medawar[48,49] has argued that "the scientific paper is a fraud in the sense that it does give a totally misleading narrative of the process of thought that goes into the making of scientific discoveries."

Repetition, acceptance, and consensus

The agreement among scientists on the correctness of observations is obtained by repeating the observations. The ability of scientists to repeat an observation indicates a control over the conditions of observation, a situation often attained when the most relevant variables have been identified. A problem with the rapid growth of science is that many observations have not been checked, so researchers are unsure of the degree to which the data are trustworthy. Nevertheless, whether there is agreement can be determined only by publishing the results and observing other scientists' reactions to it.

The response of other scientists to published work has been described as "organized skepticism." Under ordinary circumstances, proponents—that is, the authors of the paper—accept the burden of proof. In theory, scientists remain skeptical unless they can reproduce the results. Contrary to the storybook version of science, the scientific community does not normally go out of its way to refute incorrect results. It seems to take less time and energy simply to bypass erroneous material and allow it to fade into obscurity.[50]

Perhaps the most generally accepted metric of agreement is the number of positive citations a paper receives from other authors. Citation analysis provides readers access to the views of the entire scientific community on a paper.[51] Thus, it captures what has been called the *widsom of crowds*—the phenomenon in which the average of a collection of diverse independent assessors yields a more accurate assessment than any individual expert's opinion.[52]

An important channel of communication that indicates acceptance, or lack thereof, is a letter to the editor. In theory, letters to the editor are important means for ensuring accountability of authors and editors; they might be considered to be a postpublication review process. A study of the response of authors of three randomized controlled trials to letters to the editor of *Lancet* indicated that more than half the criticisms made went unanswered by authors. Moreover, important weaknesses in these trials were ignored in subsequently published practice guidelines.[53] Acceptance, it seems, can occur even in the presence of known errors.

In general, the hypotheses that become accepted are those based not only on repeated studies but also on different kinds of studies that produce a converging line of evidence that leads to acceptance. Conversely, a single study that disagrees with a hypothesis may not be given much consideration; it is more likely that something is wrong in an isolated adverse study than in an army of confirming studies using diverse techniques. Unfortunately, accepting other scientists' work as correct can be difficult for scientists who are emotionally disposed to believe that others' contributions cannot be important. The geneticist Haldane[51] outlined four stages on the road to acceptance: *(1) this is worthless nonsense; (2) this is an interesting, but perverse, point of view; (3) this is true but quite unimportant; (4) I always said so.*

The observations and theories that remain are normally viewed as being correct and cumulative, each study adding— to use the cliche—another brick in humankind's great wall of knowledge. In this view, science can be distinguished from the humanities, because its products are cumulative. For example, a recent graduate with a BSc in genetics knows incomparably more genetics than Mendel, who founded a quantitative approach to the topic. But few would claim that any modern playwright is the equal of Shakespeare. Science, in this view, gets progressively closer to objective truth.

However, the view that science marches on guided by the logic of falsification and corroboration has been challenged in recent years, preeminently by Thomas Kuhn[20] in his book *The Structure of Scientific Revolutions.* In examining the history of science, Kuhn found that new theories are often inferior to the ones they re-

place in their ability to explain a wide range of phenomena. Thus, scientific theories are not necessarily a closer approximation to the truth, and scientific growth is not continuous. Another problem for the storybook scientific method is that scientists are reluctant to reject a theory when there is evidence that it cannot explain or in the event that it is wrong. One explanation for this reluctance is that a theory is not rejected when negative empirical evidence is discovered unless there is a better theory to take its place. Although Kuhn's views have received some degree of acceptance, working scientists—whom Kuhn regards as mere puzzle solvers—largely ignore his interpretation and continue to believe that as they attempt to falsify or corroborate theories, those unsupported by empirical data will be rejected. Cole[52] speculates that it even may be necessary for scientists to believe in the traditional view to proceed with the work of science.

Individually, scientists feel compelled to publish, because rewards in science are allotted to those who first arrive at a particular result. The preoccupation of some scientists with establishing priority is not new and has involved many great scientists, including Newton, Hooke, Huygens, Cavendish, Watt, Lavoisier, Jenner, Furlong, Laplace, and Gauss.[53] To establish his priority of observing the rings of Saturn for the first time, Galileo devised a scientific anagram that he included in a letter to Kepler: "Smaismrmilmepoetaleumibunenustlaviras," which could be decoded into "altissimum planetan tergeminum observali" (I have observed the uppermost planet triple).[54] Disputes over priority appear to be decreasing but, as witnessed by the Gallo-Montagnier dispute, are by no means dead. This may be due in part to the standard methods of publication, which record the date a paper is submitted. In some instances, such as the publication of the sequence of the human genome, scientists preempt priority disputes by coming to an agreement whereby the publications appear simultaneously.

After a scientist publishes a paper, the scientist awaits the collective judgment. Sometimes it never comes; a large proportion of papers are never cited. A few papers become classics, in that they are cited extensively over a long time or included in textbooks, which are repositories of accepted knowledge (and which are typically at least 2 years out-of-date on publication). But even textbooks contain errors; journals such as *Trends in Biochemical Sciences* and *Biochemical Education* have sections on "textbook errors," and readers must remain alert even when reading textbooks like this one.

References

1. Medawar PB. The Limits of Science. Oxford: Oxford Univ Press, 1984:16.

2. Bronowski J. The Common Sense of Science. New York: Random House Vintage, 1951:97–118.

3. Kuhn TS. Normal science as puzzle-solving. In: The Structure of Scientific Revolutions, ed 2. Chicago: Univ Chicago Press,1970:35–42.

4. Merton RK. Science and democratic social structure. In: Social Theory and Social Structure. Toronto: Collier Macmillan, 1968:604–615.

5. Ziman J. An Introduction to Science Studies: The Philosophical and Social Aspects of Science and Technology. Cambridge: Cambridge Univ Press, 1984:84.

6. Judson HF. The Great Betrayal: Fraud in Science. Orlando: Harcourt, 2004:242.

7. Merton RK. Reference groups, invisible colleges, and deviant behaviour in science. In: O'Gorman HJ (ed). Surveying Social Life: Papers in Honor of Herbert H. Hyman. Middletown, CT: Wesleyan Univ Press, 1988:174.

8. Seventy-five reasons to become a scientist. Am Sci 1988;76:450–463.

9. Latour B, Woolgar S. Laboratory Life: The Social Construction of Scientific Facts. Beverly Hills: Sage, 1979.

10. Cronin B. The Citation Process: The Role and Significance of Citations in Scientific Communication. London: Taylor Graham, 1984:20.

11. Simonton DK. Creativity in Science. Cambridge: Cambridge Univ Press, 2004:172–173.

12. Surowiecki J. The Wisdom of Crowds. New York: Doubleday, 2004:162–163.

13. Axelrod R. The Evolution of Cooperation. New York: Basic Books, 1984:174.

14. Hearnshaw LS. Cyril Burt, Psychologist. New York: Vintage Books, 1981:70.

15. Hearnshaw LS. Cyril Burt, Psychologist. New York: Vintage Books, 1981:288.

16. Wainer H. Graphic Discovery. Princeton: Princeton Univ Press, 2005:6.

17. Wade N. Scandal in the heavens: Renowned astronomer accused of fraud. Science 1977;198:707.

18. Brush SG. Should the history of science be rated X? Science 1974;183:1164.

19. Westfall RS. Newton and the fudge factor. Science 1973;179:751.

20. Kuhn TS. The Structure of Scientific Revolutions, ed 2. Chicago: Univ Chicago Press, 1970:144–159.

21. Bondi H. Fact and inference in theory and in observation. Vistas Astronomy 1955;1:155.

22. Judson HF. The Great Betrayal: Fraud in Science. Orlando: Harcourt, 2004:44–48.

23. Broad W, Wade N. Betrayers of the Truth: Fraud and Deceit in the Halls of Science. New York: Simon and Schuster, 1982.

24. Kohn A. False Prophets. Fraud and Error in Science and Medicine. Oxford: Blackwell, 1986.

25. Mosteller F. Evaluation: Requirements for scientific proof. In: Warner KS (ed). Coping with the Biomedical Literature. New York: Praeger, 1981:103–121.

26. Gordon M. Evaluating the evaluators. New Sci 10 February 1977:342.

27. Martinson BC, Anderson MS, de Vries R. Scientists behaving badly. Nature 2005;435:737–738.

28. Doty P. Cited by: Judson HF. The Great Betrayal: Fraud in Science. Orlando: Harcourt, 2004:224.

29. Rousseau DL. Case studies in pathological science. Am Sci 1992;80:54.

30. Davenas E, Beauvais F, Amara J. Human basophil degranulation triggered by very dilute antiserum against IgE. Nature 1988;333:816–818.

31. Hetherington NS. Just how objective is science? Nature 1983;306:727.

32. Rustia M, Shubik P. Experimental induction of hepatomas, mammary tumors, and other tumors with metronidazole in noninbred Sas:MRC(WI)BR rats. J Natl Cancer Inst 1979;63:863.

33. Medawar PB. The Limits of Science. Oxford: Oxford Univ Press, 1984:60.

34. Okasha S. Philosophy of Science: A Very Short Introduction. Oxford: Oxford Univ Press, 2002:58.

35. Ziman J. Reliable Knowledge: An Exploration of the Grounds for Belief in Science. Cambridge: Cambridge Univ Press, 1978:42.

36. Polgar S, Thomas SA. Introduction to Research in the Health Sciences, ed 2. Melbourne: Churchill Livingstone, 1991:97–98.

37. Polanyi JC. Free discovery from outside ties. Can Assoc Univ Teachers Bull 2002; 49(10):A3.

38. Simon R, Wittes RE. Methodologic guidelines for reports of clinical trials. Cancer Treat Rep 1985;69:1.

39. Bailar JC, Mosteller F. Guidelines for statistical reporting in articles for medical journals. Ann Intern Med 1988; 108:266.

40. Chilton NW, Barbano JP. Guidelines for reporting clinical trials. J Periodontal Res 1974;9(suppl 14):207.

41. Sackett DL. Evaluation: Requirements for clinical application. In: Warren KS (ed). Coping with the Biomedical Literature. New York: Praeger, 1981:123.

42. A co-operative trial in the primary prevention of ischaemic heart disease using clofibrate. Report from the Committee of Principal Investigators. Br Heart J 1978;40:1069.

43. Mason SF. A History of the Sciences. ed 2. New York: Abelard-Schuman, 1962:334.

44. Cole S. The Sociological Method: An Introduction to the Science of Sociology, ed 3. Boston: Houghton Mifflin, 1980:121.

45. Ziman J. An Introduction to Science Studies: The Philosophical and Social Aspects of Science and Technology. Cambridge: Cambridge Univ Press, 1984:10.

46. Gushee DE. Reading behavior of chemists. J Chem Doc 1968;8:191.

47. Holton G. Quanta, relativity, and rhetoric. In: Pera M, Shea WS (eds). Persuading Science. The Art of Scientific Rhetoric. Sagamore Beach, MA: Science History, 1991:174.

48. Medawar P. Is the scientific paper a fraud? In: The Strange Case of the Spotted Mice. Oxford: Oxford Univ Press, 1996.

49. Medawar P. Is the scientific paper a fraud? The Listener. BBC Third Programme. September 12, 1963.

50. Meadows AJ. Communication in Science. London: Butterworths, 1974:45.
51. Cronin B. The Citation Process: The Role and Significance of Citations in Scientific Communication. London: Taylor Graham, 1984:79.
52. Surowieki J. The Wisdom of Crowds. New York: Doubleday, 2004.
53. Horton R. Postpublication criticism and the shaping of clinical knowledge. JAMA 2002;287:2843.
54. Haldane JBS. The truth about death. J Genet 1963;58:464.
55. Cole S. The Sociological Method: An Introduction to the Science of Sociology, ed 3. Boston: Houghton Mifflin, 1980:129–130.
56. Merton RK. Priorities in scientific discovery: A chapter in the sociology of science. Am Sociol Rev 1957;22:635.
57. Meadows AJ. Communication in Science. London: Butterworths, 1974:57.

3 | Rhetoric

Science, then, necessarily involves rhetoric. And it also places scientists in what Burke calls "the human barnyard" where motives are never altogether pure and language must dramatize the inevitable ambiguity of motives.

—S. Michael Halloran[1]

Introduction

To publish in good journals, authors must convince referees and editors that their work is new, true, and important. To get work funded, investigators must persuade committees of their peers that the work is feasible, significant, and novel. Often, the criteria for such things as novelty and significance are not straightforward; the writer of the grant or paper must pose arguments for these qualities in the most persuasive way possible. *Rhetoric,* defined by Aristotle circa 323 BC as the faculty of discovering all the available means of persuasion in a given situation, doubtless has been practiced since before recorded time, but it played a particularly important role in ancient Greece and Rome. Two excellent texts on classical rhetoric that have been used extensively in preparing this section are those of Habinek[2] and Corbett and Connors.[3] Rhetoric was central to decision making in the classical world, and instructors in rhetorical techniques flourished. Indeed, handbooks of rhetoric are perhaps the best documented genre of ancient writings.[4] Civic discussion took place in public forums, and citizens voted on a wide variety of issues from state decisions, such as going to war or forming alliances, to criminal cases and property disputes. (Only male citizens participated in these discussions, while women, slaves, and outsiders were excluded; although this is discriminatory by present-day standards, it is important to remember that citizenship carried with it the duty of going to battle, if required.[5]) As these assemblies heard arguments, rhetoric focused to some degree on how the arguments sounded. Key elements of rhetoric were memorization and oration. Lists of rhetorical terms[6] include devices that add flourish to delivery rather than clarity to argument. When Vice President Spiro T. Agnew railed against the "nattering nabobs of negativism," he employed alliteration and onomatopoeia. A country-and-western singer might employ syncrisis when he croons, "pick me up on your way down." Such techniques find little application in scientific writing. Nevertheless, rhetoric plays a large, if sometimes subtle, role in science and has been the subject of close investigation.[7] As noted by an editor of *Lancet,* a scientific paper is an exercise in persuasion,[8] and it follows that readers of this literature should learn the tricks of the persuasive trade.

One problem with rhetoric for scientists, who are presumably interested in determining the true nature of things, was understood by Socrates and Plato; there is a fundamental dichotomy between the aims of the speaker and the aims of the audience. The speaker's goal is to persuade; the audience's goal is truth.[8] Plato, in particular, has been described as being no friend of rhetoric.[4] A platonic dialogue in *Gorgias* states, "the orator need have no knowledge of the truth about things; that it is enough for him to have discovered a knack of convincing the ignorant that he knows more than the experts."[9] Scientists have traditionally been wary of rhetoric even as they practice it. "Scientific heads are not turned by rhetoric" is the title of an article by a prominent proponent of evidence-based medicine.[10] However, rhetorical techniques and methods of influence abound in scientific articles and in the social interaction of scientists. The sensitive reader, particularly one who believes in the Merton norms for scientists and the storybook version of science, might be offended by some of the information that follows. My approach here is descriptive rather than prescriptive; I am not recommending any particular technique. The pragmatic point is that readers of the literature should know how to recognize rhetoric in practice and, on occasion, fight through the rhetoric to the underlying truth.

Some of the ancients' rhetorical techniques are employed commonly in science in what may be called "classical ways." One weakness in classical rhetoric, at least from a modern viewpoint, is the reliance on *commonplaces,* which were general arguments believed by many of the populace that could be used on many occasions. Examples include, "death is common to all" (used in praising fallen soldiers), "time flies" (when there is a need for urgency), or "death before dishonor" (when some might contemplate surrender). Modern persuasive techniques make less use of commonplaces, probably because modern audiences do not find them convincing.[11] Moreover, scientific arguments tend to be specific. Modern persuasive techniques have also been developed as a result of psychological and sociological scientific investigation, rather than the rough-and-ready empiricism of the ancients, who might judge the effectiveness of a speaker by the crowd he generated either at the door of the Senate or in the marketplace when it was his turn at the rostrum. Thus, persuasive techniques used in science are best considered against a background of the classical methods, as well as modern psychology.

Classical Rhetoric

Five canons of rhetoric

Aristotle proposed five canons of rhetoric, which are named here in Latin:

1. *inventio:* methods for discovering arguments
2. *dispositio:* methods for the effective and orderly arrangement of the parts
3. *elocutio:* style, "proper words in proper places"
4. *memoria:* memorizing speeches
5. *pronuntatio:* delivery of speeches

The latter two canons are not relevant to analyzing scientific papers.

Inventio

Inventio refers to a system for finding arguments. In theory, a well-trained orator could speak on any issue and on any side of an issue, but he needed raw material: the facts (or disputed facts) of the case, general principles applying to a situation, and convincing approaches to present the argument. Aristotle recognized two kinds of topics. The first—those useful in a special area of knowledge or arising from the particular circumstances—were called *idioi topoi* in Greek. In a judicial setting, for instance, Aristotle named five kinds of proofs: laws, witnesses, contracts, tortures, and oaths. Similarly, a scientific paper will have data specific to the investigation. A study in clinical periodontics might include data on the number and characteristics of the patients, the procedures used, and the outcomes of various measurements—such as attachment level—at various times. These types of topics constitute the raw material of the paper. Aristotle's second group of topics included those useful in arguments of all kinds—the so-called common topics (*koinoi topoi*). Aristotle named four common topics: *(1)* more or less (the topic of degree), as occurs in debates on any situation (eg, fluoride) where a recommended dosage is suggested; *(2)* possible and impossible, which can occur with respect to compliance with some theory; *(3)* past and future, as occurs in some epidemiological questions; and *(4)* greatness and smallness (the topic of size), which addresses the common concern of the size of a treatment effect.

Aristotle also listed 28 topics that might be considered as techniques to improve or support arguments.[6] An author may want to redefine a key term to support a contention or to define terms to favor the argument. (For example, in the field of dental implants, there is considerable debate over what criteria should be used to define a successful implant.) In making his list, Aristotle began the tradition of philosophers making lists of good or fallacious arguments. The gloomy philosopher Schopenhauer, prepared a list of 38 ways to win an argument,[12] of which some appear morally dubious and are the type of techniques that might be used by academic administrators who believe that the ends justify the means.

To make a scientific paper persuasive, however, authors have to employ persuasive techniques. Aristotle listed three main types of artificial proof.[6]

Logos or rational appeal

The arguments in a scientific paper could include both deductive and inductive logical approaches. Typically, *deduction* is certain and makes conclusions from statements, while *induction* makes inferences from verifiable phenomena. The deductive approach favored by Aristotle was the *enthymeme,* which can be considered a deductive syllogism in which a premise is missing. In a scientific paper, the deductive approach often occurs when the authors predict the consequences of their hypothesis. For inductive logic, Aristotle used the *example,* which leads to the probability of a statement being true, and can always be subject to challenge and refutation. In the periodontics example, if a difference were observed between two groups treated in different ways, the authors would be required to show through appropriate statistical testing that the difference could not be explained by chance. The rational appeal is central to all scientific papers.

Pathos or emotional appeal

Aristotle did not necessarily approve of the use of the emotional appeal, but he did know that it worked. Use of emotional arguments in scientific papers is rare; one of the norms of science is disinterestedness. But pathos does feature in discussions of science policy. Waddell[13] has written on the role of pathos in the decision-making process and has considered in detail the debate over the use of recombinant DNA in the early days of this technology in Cambridge, Massachusetts. The proponents' arguments included the use of the proposition, "if your child were suffering from these diseases [diseases that might be solved by advances in genetic knowledge], you would want help from those who could help." The opponents argued, "violating three billion years of evolution is dangerous." These views are a long way from dispassionate decision-making algorithms. Similarly, emotionally charged debates occur today on the issue of embryonic stem cells.

Emotion also surfaces in disputes over priority and funding. Multidisciplinary collaborative research has many virtues, but a vice is that the principal investigator, who controls the funds, may be tempted to direct funds disproportionately to his or her own projects. Funding decisions made in committees are supposed to be confidential, but sometimes information leaks out of the committees and supplies victims of bad reviews with motivation to inflict similar pain on their tormentors. In such cases, the motivation of pathos is not mentioned, and the criticisms are cloaked in the objective garments of logos.

Ethos or ethical appeal

Ethos or ethical appeal stems from the character of the speaker as shown in the speech (or paper) itself. Aristotle thought that this could be the most potent of the three modes of persuasion. The recommended procedure involved several steps: *(1)* ingratiate oneself to the audience to gain trust, *(2)* show intelligence, *(3)* demonstrate benevolence, and *(4)* exhibit probity.

In science, ethos is established primarily by conforming with the norms of scientific behavior outlined earlier: universalism, communalisim, humility, originality, organized skepticism, and disinterestedness. It has been said that scientific writing style capitalizes on the convenient myth that reason has subjugated the passions. Objectivity and disinterestedness is indicated by the use of the passive voice. Ethos is further established by the choice of methods and interpretive structure; choice of sound methods indicates a sound investigator. Finally, ethos is also indicated by the choice of literature citations. To a large degree, for negative citations are rare, the use of citation implicitly indicates that the cited work is accepted and is important to the current work—otherwise why cite it? As recognition is the coin of science, citations are like little gifts to the author and are, thus, part of the scientific reward system[14] Conversely, failure to cite someone could be construed as an insult and could be rhetorically damaging. A book on writing grant applications suggests that applicants find out the names of the grant committee members and cite them, provided such citations do not appear contrived.[15] Regardless of the motivation, citations to the work of others establish the author as a fair-minded person.

In everyday life, ethos or communicator credibility has less lofty aspirations. Credibility is seen as a combination of expertise and trustworthiness. Peripheral characteristics, such as skin color, are important. Arguing against their own self-interest, as scientists sometimes do in testing hypotheses, increases trustworthiness. The degree to which audience opinion can change depends on communicator credibility; a trusted communicator can achieve greater movement, while those with doubtful credibility can hope only for modest change.[16] Credibility in science is often judged informally by such things as number, source, and amount of grants, and papers published in leading journals as well as awards.

The Roman orator Cicero summed up the classical approach in his advice to orators, "Charm [ie, credibility, ethos], Teach [ie, sound message, logos], and Move [ie, call to action through emotion, pathos]." For many years, these steps have been effective.

Box 3-1 Medieval vs contemporary student rhetoric

Letter from rhetoric student B to his venerable master A, Oxford ca 1300[17]

"This is to inform you that I am studying at Oxford with the greatest diligence, but the matter of money stands greatly in the way of my promotion . . . the city is expensive and makes many demands, I have to rent lodgings, buy necessaries and provide for many other things which I cannot now specify. Wherefore I respectfully beg your paternity that by the promptings of divine pity you may assist me so that I may complete what I have well begun. For you must know that without Ceres [goddess of corn] and Bacchus [god of wine], Apollo [Sun god, poet] grows cold."

E-mail from law student Maxwell Brunette to his father, Saskatoon 2001

"If I maintain my average I will graduate with distinction . . . I have looked at my projected finances and debt position for the next 6 months and have realized that I will need help. . . . I will have a number of fairly large expenses to meet, such as rent deposits, rent, buying such necessities as a bed, microwave etc. . . . [please send] an extra $500 be included in the check that will pay for the repairs to the car."

As an example, we will consider two letters from students to their fathers asking for funds to continue their studies (see Box 3-1).

The first example comes from Oxford in the Late 13th century, that is, some 1,600 years after Aristotle. As background, the seven liberal arts of the middle ages were divided into two segments: the most basic required knowledge of the *trivium* (hence the word *trivial*), comprising grammar, rhetoric, and logic, and the more advanced requirements called for understanding the *quadrivium,* comprising arithmetic, astronomy, geometry, and music. It may seem strange that rhetoric precedes arithmetic in the curriculum, but, to continue their studies, students frequently had to convince their patrons to send money. Thus, most of the extant examples of medieval rhetoric are letters to parents or other sponsors requesting funds. These letters could show considerable sophistication; one exercise showed 22 ways to approach an archdeacon for funds. Thus, modern manuals for grant proposals come from an ancient line.

The letter from the medieval rhetoric student first establishes his ethos ("I am studying with the greatest diligence"); he then makes the rational appeal of logos by enumerating his expenses. Then he moves to the call to action through pathos, for, without anything to eat and drink, his intellectual work must fail.

My son Max's e-mail, some 700 years after the Oxford student and some 2,300 years after Aristotle, is remarkably similar. Ethos is established by the statement that if he maintains his average, he will graduate with distinction. Note that this ethos is specific to this communication. The reader, his father, is supposed to forget other times when his behavior was not so praiseworthy. (There is no need to mention, for exam-

ple, the grade school incident, in which he annoyed the French teacher by throwing his textbook out the window; such embarrassing events that might discredit the ethos of the current scholar are best left out of the discussion.) As did the Oxford student, logos is represented by the enumeration of expenses. Also, like the Oxford student who "must provide for other things that I cannot now specify," Max leaves himself some "wiggle room" by including the "etc." among the list of expenses. Neither student wants to specify costs too precisely. In Max's case, the motivational portion of Cicero's dictum—that is, the call to action—came in a supplementary telephone call that resulted in funds being dispatched from Vancouver to Saskatoon. (To be fair, the expenditure was worthwhile; Max did graduate from law with distinction.) This example indicates that the classical approach to persuasion continues to be effective.

Dispositio

Dispositio concerns the orderly and effective arrangement of arguments. Scientific writing tends to be logical; indeed, one authority believes that a scientific paper is primarily an exercise in organization. The format of the typical scientific paper,[18] IMRaD (Introduction, Methods, Results, and Discussion), is analogous to Aristotle's approach of introduction, narration, proof, and epilogue.[8]

While orators employ a number of organizational schemes,[19] the most common scheme used in scientific presentations is the *zoom-in . . . zoom-out* (zizo) approach, whereby the author reviews the general area of research in the introduction and "zooms-in" to the specific problem studied. In the discussion section, the author "zooms-out" to show how her research has advanced the field. The book *Dazzle 'Em with Style*[20]—intended as advice for young scientists—recommends only the zizo approach for giving seminars. However, a more detailed look at the rhetorical strategies used in the introductions of papers finds that scientists typically make four moves: *(1) create interest, (2) review history, (3) show a gap, and (4) introduce new research.*[21]

Nevertheless, the specific purposes of some papers are better served by other approaches, some of which are covered by Spicer.[19] A *chronological approach*, outlining how a procedure has developed over time, can be effective in reviewing a field. A *dialectic plan*, comparing two competing hypotheses and how they are to be resolved by the current study, can also be effective, particularly if one has been able to design a crucial experiment. The *facet approach*, whereby the author considers diverse aspects of a given problem, was applied to great effect in a seminar describing periodontal disease given by my former dean, Paul Robertson, when he applied for the Deanship of UBC. Robertson used the metaphor of a dragon to symbolize aspects of the diseases (eg, the fiery breath of the dragon represented the heat of inflamed tissues). That I remember that seminar given some 20 years ago demonstrates that the confidence to apply novel approaches can make a speaker stand out from the pedestrian crowd, who cling resolutely to the single organizational plan of zooming in and zooming out.

Elocutio

Elocutio is described as putting proper words in proper places, but communicator style involves more than word choice. Scientific authors attempt to imply their objectivity with word choice. Some of the issues of word choice in science are similar to those in writing generally; thus, the same principles found in reading critically apply to reading scientific writing.[21]

Accuracy is crucial in scientific word choice; terms used must conform with the rest of the scientific literature or must be defined explicitly. Precise language use avoids the problem in logic called the *fallacy of equivocation*. Moreover, scientists are typically conservative in their claims. Combined with the need for accuracy, this conservatism, as noted earlier, leads to conclusions that are qualified with hedge terms or phrases. Many authors finding that some factor X affects some biological activity Y but lacking any concrete evidence for the actual mechanism(s) will be hesitant to write, "X regulates Y." Rather, scientists will write something like, "X plays a role in regulating Y," a phrase that could be interpreted as, "I don't know how X works, but it is involved somehow."

The problem of presenting evidence and indicating its strength is of particular interest in science. Because all studies build on the foundation of other studies, citations play a key role. Latour and Woolgar[22] developed a scale to assess the strength of evidence by how it is cited. The strongest evidence, in their view, is so self-evident or well known that it needs no citation (eg, the formula for water is H_2O). Using an author's name to identify the study constitutes a stronger endorsement of the evidence than simply citing the study, and, of course, qualifying the findings of a study indicates the study's lack of strength or generalizability.

For scientific writers, however, the question of how much to qualify their own results is a particularly thorny problem. Claiming too much for findings invites referees to point out that the claims exceed the evidence, but claiming too little may lead them to ask, "So what? How has this paper advanced science?" An aggressive strategy is to state claims more strongly than the presented evidence supports and to cut them back in response to referees' criticisms. Consequently, readers of scientific papers should look closely at qualifying statements or hedges, which may reveal referees' concerns that likely are also the concerns of the reader. Serving on a grants panel, I was once the primary reviewer of an application that proposed the use of a model system to investigate a process that occurred in vivo. However, the proposed model system was an in vitro system, and one of the applicant's previous papers contained a qualifying sentence stating that the in vitro model system would be a very poor model of what would occur in vivo. Thus, this qualifying sentence undermined the premise of the proposed research program. Given the applicant's intention to build future research on this in vitro system, it is unlikely that the qualifying sentence was included in the paper initially, but rather that it was a hedge inserted to meet referees' concerns. A defensive strategy is to use the *modesty trope*, a conventional disclaimer to preempt criticism. Users of an in vitro system might write something like, "further experiments using animals are required to validate the mechanisms being proposed as a result of these in vitro studies."

Books on scientific writing often contain lists and rules for avoiding the most common lapses of style. According to these lists, wordiness and jargon are the chief problems, and they recommend replacing phrases like "a majority of" with "most" or rephrasing "in my opinion, it is not an unjustifiable assumption that" with "I think."

29

One of the most interesting and effective approaches to sentence construction is that of Gopen and Swan,[23] who advocate locating sentence elements according to common expectations of readers.

Audience

Most of the discussion of classical rhetoric presented above is given from the perspective of what the rhetor does; the audience has not been specifically considered. Classical rhetors knew the importance of tailoring their speeches to their listeners, but they lacked the scientific approach of controlling stimuli and quantifying responses that characterizes modern psychology. Moreover, modern studies of persuasion consider a broader range of influences, such as radio and television, than were considered by classical authorities. Scientific discourse occurs over a wide array of forums where persuasive techniques play a key role in decision making, including editorial boards for scientific publications, grants panels, science policy debates, and university committees. The formalism present in the IMRaD model used by scientific papers is absent in many of these situations. Scientists in these modern forums persuade and are persuaded by the approaches and techniques used in everyday reasoning.

Choosing the audience

One advantage of scientists is that they can, to a certain extent, choose their audiences by submitting their work to journals or granting agencies that they select themselves. Learning the names of editorial board or grants panel members helps scientists determine where to send their work. Even the most fairminded scientists would favor sending their work to places where it might be appreciated. To help this process, a scientist might suggest to the editor that certain reviewers are uniquely well qualified to review the work. Authors should refrain from being too obvious in advocating close friends and colleagues; referees should be at arm's length (sometimes interpreted as not having published with the author for at least 5 years). Conversely, the author can mention that certain persons would not be appropriate because of personal or professional differences, but this is best done before the fact; correcting such a situation afterwards

is exceedingly difficult (particularly as it is often difficult to be sure who the referees actually were). In his *Advice to a Young Scientist,* Medawar[24] notes:

> There are times when referees are inimical for personal reasons and enjoy causing the discomfiture that rejection brings with it; too strenuous an attempt to convince an editor that this is so may, however, convince him only that the author has paranoid tendencies.

Abelson's "MAGIC" Criteria for Persuasive Force

The social scientist Abelson[25] has proposed that several properties of data as well as their analysis and presentation govern their persuasive force. The first letters of these properties form the acronym *MAGIC*: magnitude, articulation, generality, interestingness, and credibility. I believe these criteria apply generally to all types of experimental research.

Magnitude refers to the size of the observed effect. Often investigators wish to compare two means. This comparison frequently is made by subtracting one mean from the other to give a statement such as, "pocket depth was reduced 1 mm by rinsing with chlorhexidene." Such a difference, however, must be interpreted in the context of the variability of the data, and effect-size indicators have been developed for various applications (see chapter 20). Magnitude is estimated by the ratio of means between the treated and control groups. This calculation gives rise to statements about the relative increase or decrease caused by a treatment, often described by such terms as "twofold increase" or "50% inhibition." Scientists' concern with magnitude is necessary to complement the other requirement for comparisons between groups—namely, that the difference is unlikely to be caused by chance. When the number in the groups is large, there may be statistically significant differences demonstrated for some factors, but the size of the differences are so small that the factors do not produce meaningful effects. It is evident that scientists find magnitude a convincing argument, given the widespread manipulation of magnification scales to produce larger apparent effects in figures. Because this problem is so prevalent, Tufte[26] has proposed an index called the *lie factor,* which is the ratio between the apparent visual effect seen in the figure and the actual numerical effect size (see chapter 13).

Abelson[25] defines *articulation* as the degree of comprehensible detail in which conclusions are phrased. A well-articulated publication, in Abelson's view, tells readers what they ought to know to understand the point of the study and what the results were. Many papers, to their detriment, fail to measure up to the criteria of articulation, because they end on a whimper, not a bang; they seem to end when the author runs out of words, rather than with a strong conclusion. I think articulation can also be considered as the degree to which claims are supported. Typically, papers in higher-impact journals offer more types of evidence to support their claims than those in lower-impact journals. In a study on cell signaling, one might consider publishing the results of immunostaining on one component of a signaling pathway, but that strategy likely would not be effective in getting the study published in a high-impact journal. Such a journal might require more types of evidence to support the claim, such as Western blots to show differences in specific protein levels, inhibitor studies, or immunostaining of other components in the relevant pathways.

Generality refers to the breadth of applicability of the conclusions. The conclusions of any research study are strictly limited to its particular conditions, but studies that can be applied widely, at least in theory, will have more impact. This happens quite naturally, because a prime reason for scientists reading the scientific literature is to apply concepts or techniques to their own studies. A study using conditions that are difficult to replicate or apply only to a very limited population will often have little impact, because other scientists cannot apply it to their own work.

Interestingness, Abelson[25] believes, indicates that the study has the potential to change what people believe about an important issue. An interesting result is often one that is surprising, and, because it unsettles previously held concepts, it makes the reader think about the topic. However, it can be risky to be too interesting. The *principle of least difference* holds that the master craftsman (or, in this case, scientist) demonstrates something that is sufficiently different from its predecessors to be considered distinctive, but the difference is sufficiently small that it does not imply criticism of what has preceded.[4]

Credibility refers to the overall believability of the conclusions, and it rests both on the soundness of the methodology and on how well the results agree with, or at least do not overtly contradict, other well-established studies in the same area. Abelson[25] states that a research claim or new theory that contradicts a prevailing theory or common sense can expect attacks on two fronts: methodologic issues, such as data analysis or technique, and coherence, that is, the question of whether a new theory can explain a range of interconnected findings. The burden of proof will rest with the proponent of the new theory.

The Persuasion Palette

The process of scientific persuasion is somewhat like a painter producing a painting. In painting, the artist uses a variety of colors to produce a unified whole. The particular colors chosen vary among paintings according to the desired effect; Mondrian's paintings blaze with primary colors, whereas Rembrandt's paintings are symphonies of blended earth tones, but both painters produced works that convinced critics to consider them masterpieces. Similarly, scientists employ various persuasive techniques depending on the situation. In choosing among rhetorical options, the scientist can be thought of as using a palette of persuasive techniques—the *persuasive palette*. The persuasive palette includes various theoretical principles and empirically based observations that can be mixed and matched to produce an overall persuasive effect. The components to be discussed include peripheral and central routes to persuasion, the principal principle, the theory of cognitive dissonance, the law of cognitive response, the cognitive miser concept, and Cialdini's seven principles of influence.

Two routes to persuasion

Excellent overviews of persuasion have been published by Pratkanis and Aronson,[16] Cialdini,[27] and Simons,[28] to which the reader is referred for more detailed information. The following sections are largely based on those sources, supplemented with more specific examples of how persuasive techniques are applied in the scientific community.

Modern psychology has determined that there are two routes to persuasion.[28]

1. In the *peripheral route*, the recipient extends little effort or attention. When the audience operates in

this mode, persuasive factors such as the attractiveness of the presenter and the presentation of any reason, however bogus, may actually work. Dental conferences, for example, typically have exhibitions directly or indirectly concerned with selling goods; the people working in the exhibitors' booths often possess more pulchritude than the attendees wandering the aisles. How much attention will a dentist pay to the selection of toys for his "treasure chest" for young clients? An attractive salesperson may tip the balance from one supplier to another.

2. In the *central route,* the recipient engages in careful consideration of the true merits of the case. The recipient may argue against the message, ask questions, and seek out other sources of information. For example, in buying a digital x-ray unit, a dentist might approach various companies, check with other dentists, and closely calculate the costs and the pros and cons of the various units. Thus, the dentist would adopt the more rigorous central route to investigate a major purchase. This approach to decision making mirrors the legal principle that the level of proof required increases with the seriousness of the case (as civil cases are decided on the balance of probabilities, and criminal cases adopt a beyond-reasonable-doubt standard). Therefore, expensive purchases warrant more consideration than inexpensive ones.

This example also illustrates that the choice of route depends on involvement. When a decision affects the decision maker personally, the tendency is to use the central route to develop counterarguments and seek out information. When the decision does not have a personal effect, the decision maker uses the peripheral route.

In Canada, there has been a recent tendency to markedly raise tuition to professional programs, such as law, medicine, and dentistry. The administrators' problem is that they at least must appear to have consulted the students about the matter. Students who will have to pay the increased fees will question whether the increase is justified; they will use the central route in evaluating the arguments for increases and will develop counterarguments. Administrators anticipating this problem use the following ruse: They consult the graduating class, that is, with students not subject to the increased fees. These students have only marginal interest, tend to adopt the peripheral route in evaluating the proposal, and, are generally easier to convince than those subject to the fee increase. I do not suggest that this is appropriate administrative behavior, but it is effective. In an article in the *National Post,* the situation was described as "about as bad an example of operating in bad faith as you'll see on campus."[29]

The principal principle

The selection of route of processing persuasive messages is an example of an overarching theme I call the *principal principle*: Never underestimate people's ability to identify their own self-interest and act accordingly. This principle is not a new insight. Aristotle taught that:

> In deliberations about the future the means are *exhortation* and *dissuasion* and the topics that figure most prominently are the *worthy* and the *worthless* or the *advantageous* and the *injurious* . . . when we are trying to persuade a person to do something we try to show that the recommended course of action is either a good in itself . . . or something that will benefit the person.[3]

The concept of benefiting the person should be interpreted very broadly. If, as noted earlier, recognition is the coin of science, then the common wisdom is to cite people who might be called upon to review your manuscript or grant. On the barnyard level of scientific interaction, another piece of advice to young investigators is never to submit an application to a panel that has a direct competitor among its members. Both rules simply state the obvious truth that a proposal, no matter how persuasively written, will have difficulty convincing a hostile audience.

A highbrow illustration of the principal principle can be seen in Ceccarelli's work *Shaping Science with Rhetoric.*[30] In brief, Ceccarelli examined three books (Dobzhansky's *Genetics and Origins of Species,* Schrödinger's *What is Life?,* and Wilson's *Consilience*) by prominent and distinguished authors who each addressed two groups with conflicting interests. The successful books (ie, influential in their scientific fields) promoted a conceptual shift that created possibilities of collaboration and furtherance of each group's interest. Moreover, the successful books used polysemy so that the two communities developed contradictory readings of the texts. Wilson's book failed because he favored one side's view over the other.

At various times in my career, I have had the opportunity to serve on panels that were preparing advice for guidelines on products or tests. Such panels had representatives from industry, academe, and regulatory bodies. Name tags were unnecessary to identify affiliations; the participants' arguments, analyzed through the lens of self-interest, located their positions. Manufacturers knew which guidelines would make their product appear best. Factions within the manufacturers knew which guidelines would best promote their own departments (such as microbiology). Independent testing laboratories knew which guidelines would bring them more business. Academics knew which recommendations would likely bring them grants. Each group furthered its own interest. Aristotle likely would have been disappointed but not surprised.

Theory of cognitive dissonance

Cognitive dissonance occurs when a person simultaneously holds two inconsistent beliefs or opinions. Such a state of inconsistency is so uncomfortable that people strive to reduce the conflict in the easiest way possible. Cognitive dissonance has been extensively used in propaganda. The main application is known as the *rationalization trap*.[31] First, the propagandist arouses feelings of dissonance by threatening the audience's self-esteem. Then the propagandist provides a solution, a way of reducing the dissonance by complying with a request.

The rationalization trap is common in sales pitches. At a continuing education course, I heard the following argument: Why should hardworking dentists have to reduce their fees and their income by accepting what the insurance company offers for various procedures? In doing so, the presenter argued, dentists not only reduce their income but rupture the sacred dentist-patient bond by involving a third party. The presenter suggested that the solution is to transfer the responsibility of collecting insurance payments (and accepting the shortfall between reimbursement levels and fees) to the patient. This approach, the presenter argued, maintains income, facilitates direct patient-dentist discussion, and makes patients value their dentists' work more because they know its cost. Moreover, this approach could be easily implemented by hiring the presenter's management team to train the dental office staff.

The law of cognitive response

The information-processing model of understanding persuasion views the audience as rational beings who sequentially process information. To persuade, this model argues, the persuader first has to attract people's attention, then have them understand the message, learn the arguments underlying it, and come to accept the arguments as true. Persuaders then should teach the audience the arguments so that they will come easily to mind.

The cognitive response approach to persuasion was developed in the late 1960s, in part because the information-processing model did not accurately predict people's response to the mass media. To summarize, investigators found that the mass media did not necessarily tell people what to think, but the media did tell them what to think about and how to do it. Moreover, it was found that a message could be persuasive even if it failed to accomplish some of the information-processing stages. Even more damaging to the concept of rational persuasion was that some messages could be persuasive even if their arguments were not understood.[32]

The *law of cognitive response* holds that the successful persuasion tactic is one that (a) directs and channels thoughts so that the audience thinks in a manner agreeable to the communicator's point of view; (b) disrupts any negative thoughts; and (c) promotes positive thoughts about the proposed course of action.

The law of cognitive response appears to be the principle used, almost instinctively, by authors in the introduction of a paper. The author selects which references will be used to frame the background of the research and emphasizes the particular aspect of the problem that will be studied. I use the term *problem* deliberately; the typical overall approach used in the introduction (at least in shorter scientific papers) is the problem-solution framework. To build interest, the introduction promotes the importance of the problem, emphasizes the novelty of the study (to disrupt the negative thought "Hasn't this been done before?"), and emphasizes the merits of the particular approach that has been adopted in the paper.

In fact, the law of cognitive response underlies the general principle of setting an agenda to implement the wishes of those in power. Years ago, the Medical Research Council (MRC) of Canada attempted to alter the composition of its grants committees to reflect the changing pattern of research. The attempt failed because in the consultation process, which mainly involved scientists who already had grants, the predominant emotion was fear; spreading the range of topics being studied posed the risk of reducing the funding for those who already had grants. If the funding pie were sliced into more pieces, the current grantees worried that most must get less and some might get nothing at all.

A second attempt at reorganization, however, was successful and resulted in the transformation of the MRC of Canada to the Canadian Institutes of Health Research (CIHR). The law of cognitive response was an unacknowledged but important participant in this transformation. First, the MRC hired a professional firm to manage the process. The background and agenda that they produced emphasized the positive possibility that the pie of research funding was going to get bigger and could support additional slices. The agenda was so arranged that discussion of negative aspects of forming CIHR never seemed to occur, but there was constant repetition of the benefits. The emotion aroused by the proposed transition was greed, and the proposal smoothly sailed to adoption.

Setting a positive framework for discussion also occurs in grant proposals and responses to reviewers. I was once involved in the assessment of proposals for the establishment of Materials Research in Science and Engineering Centers for the United States National Science Foundation. These centers are large and multidisciplinary, and the funding is considerable. The center directors and their staff are often eminent in their fields; indeed, some research teams numbered Nobel Prize winners among their members. Befitting such important and costly decisions, the reviewing process is intense and multistep, so that the final panel sees the reviews of the proposed centers from many scientists. Such intensive scrutiny, of course, produces many negative comments. Prior to the final assessment, the applicants can respond to the reviewers. From a rhetorical point of view, the interesting aspect was that each of these highly skilled grant-getters adopted the same approach. Rather than wading in and addressing the criticisms one by one, they first set the stage in a positive manner by noting the many positive comments made by the reviewers. Also true to the spirit of the law of cognitive response, the negative comments were downplayed and the benefits of funding the centers emphasized.

The soapbox effect and digressions

Two obvious and annoying ways of framing the climate of discussion are the soapbox effect and digres-sion. In the *soapbox effect*, one discussant repeatedly makes the same points, so he is said to be "on the soapbox," a reference to an era when politicians made improvised platforms of soapboxes from which to spew forth their views. The three key elements of the soapbox effect are (1) to prevent other discussants from voicing their views by hogging the discussion time; (2) to confuse audiences that message length equates message strength; and (3) to try to have the last word in a discussion, because audiences tend to think that the last words constitute the conclusion of a discussion. *Digression* is a related technique in which a discussant speaks on a matter unrelated or only marginally related to the topic of the discussion. As in the soapbox effect, the goals of digression are: (1) to prevent opponents from expressing their views simply because the digresser holds the floor; (2) to give the digresser a veneer of expertise, because he can digress on topics about which he actually knows something (or at least thinks he knows something); (3) to respond to a valid criticism by attempting to distract the audience. The latter stratagem is also known as the *red herring* method, which refers to the technique of drawing a red herring across the track of a hunted fox, thereby causing hounds to lose the scent.

The law of cognitive response as applied to clinical and academic dentistry

Although not emphasized in this text, persuasion plays a key role in clinical dentistry, because patients sometimes must be persuaded of a treatment plan's merits. In this context, the key principle recommended in such texts as *Tough Questions, Great Answers*[33] is similar to the advice in a popular song circa 1944 with lyrics by Johnny Mercer:

> You've got to accentuate the positive,
> Eliminate the negative,
> Latch on to the affirmative,
> And don't mess with Mr In-between.

Accentuating the positive is a prime principle of spin-doctoring. In clinical persuasion, this involves explaining not only *what* you do but *why*, with emphasis on the benefits to the listener (thus invoking the pathos element). Another rule is to keep the message brief but to develop positive points and themes (logos element).

Another key point of the law of cognitive response is never to repeat a negative allegation. For example, it once was alleged that the rapid rise in tuition costs at our faculty would reduce the quality of the dental students. The administrators responded that we had over 200 applicants that met our requirements—an answer that does not really address the concern, because the faculty wants not 200 qualified applicants, but a top 40 of the highest quality for the program. The response relates to the question, because, obviously, the faculty needs at least 40 warm bodies to fill the available spaces, but it does not address whether the quality of the students who enter the program is as good as it would be if a lower fee structure were in place.

Another spin-doctoring approach is to turn a negative point into a positive point. For example, if a department had problems arranging sufficient endodontic coverage in a student dental clinic, the students might complain. A spin-doctored response would be, "we are not satisfied if even one appointment is missed, and we are working hard to get more endodontic instructors."

Audience as "cognitive misers"

One rationale for the success of strategies such as the peripheral route to persuasion and the law of cognitive response is that people are "cognitive misers" and try to minimize the amount of energy used to solve problems. This concept is not new; it harkens back to the Zipf principle of least effort (see chapter 1) and to the view of Sir Johsua Reynolds, the 18th-century portrait painter, who is cited as saying, "There is no expedient to which a man will resort to avoid the real labor of thinking."[34]

One approach people use to simplify the task of making judgments is the use of *heuristics*, simple rules to solve complex problems. Using a simple rule rather than a complex calculation and assessment of factors reduces the cognitive load. Faced with a purchasing decision, one might use the rule "you only get what you pay for" as a rationale for choosing the more expensive model. Accepting a simple case study with n = 1 would conform with the heuristic principle of believing in low numbers and ignoring the difficulties of statistics. Judgment under uncertainty and the use of heuristics is covered in more detail in chapter 21.

The *snow job* is another example of using the cognitive miserliness of an audience for persuasive purposes. In this technique, more information is provided than realistically can be processed by the audience, which is evident in dental product advertisements packed with detail or grant applications supported by multiple appendices. Message-dense advertisements can present information faster than people can process it; advertisers present in 30 seconds a message that would take 35 seconds at a normal speaking rate.[32] One defense mechanism is the skill of developing counterarguments quickly.

The Cialdini principles of influence

Cialdini has reviewed the seven basic principles of influence in his best-selling book *Influence: Science and Practice*,[35] as well as in a review article in *Scientific American*.[36] The principles have wide application, but here I will concentrate on how they apply to persuasion in science.

1. *Contrast* means to make differences apparent. For example, prior to the popularization of tooth bleaching, some dentists told their patients that a sun tan was the solution to making teeth look whiter. In scientific literature, however, as the size of an effect is a factor in determining the impact of a study, authors develop the "art" of making favorable comparisons. The chapter on presenting results (chapter 13) details the common practice of making the differences between groups treated differently look as large as possible. Chapter 19, on experiment design, advocates developing conditions that maximize the difference between groups.

2. *Reciprocation* is the norm that obliges individuals to repay in kind what they receive. This tendency is so strong that it can even overcome dislike.[27] Often used in commerce (eg, free samples at food stores or "gifts," such as address labels from charities), it can be very effective. It has been shown that when a charity included a gift in its solicitation letter, the response rate almost doubled from 18% to 35%.[35]

Reciprocation also surfaces in concessions in negotiation. If a referee makes a comment on a manuscript, the authors typically modify their manuscript to reflect that concern. A troublesome aspect of reciprocation is illustrated by the finding that only 37% of authors who published conclusions that were critical of the safety of calcium channel blockers had received prior drug company support; however, 100% of authors supporting the drug's safety had received something (eg, from free trips to grants and employment).[37] It is hard to bite the hand that feeds you.

Reciprocation also happens in science where scientific groups routinely cite each other; the exchange of these coins of recognition can lead to mutual liking and call up another factor in producing influence.

3. *Consistency* is the tendency of people to behave in accordance with a previous commitment. A car salesman will ask the buyer for a deposit check to supposedly show the sales manager that the buyer is serious, but the real reason is to get the buyer to make a commitment to purchase the car, which the buyer will find psychologically difficult to reverse. In science, consistency is often invoked as a reason for policy. At a grants panel, a reviewer discussing a recommendation of a colleague might ask why funding for a technician for Dr X is not being recommended, when a technician was funded for Dr Y. This commitment to consistency is one of the ground rules of logic; reviewers have to treat like cases in the same way or be able to explain why not.

Authors often are at pains to show that their results agree with those of other workers.

4. *Social validation,* also known as the *principle of social proof,* refers to the finding that we view a behavior as correct in a given situation to the extent that we see others performing it.[27] This occurs in grants panel discussions when panelists jump on the bandwagon. One panelist might enunciate a principle, such as, "we have to give the young scientists a chance." Some will agree because they believe it to be true, but others will agree because it seems the right thing to do in this particular committee meeting.

Certainly, bandwagons feature in committee meetings. For a number of years, my own grants to the CIHR dental sciences committee were criticized for not being "molecular enough"; there were some on the committee who thought that it was more important to go "molecular" than to answer what were, in my own view, the most important questions. My response has been twofold; I have incorporated some experiments employing molecular biology (an example of reciprocation through concession), and, secondly, I have tried to emphasize why my suggested approaches were appropriate. It is easy to get bowled over by a bandwagon; by definition, bandwagons have a lot of momentum. It has proved effective, in my own case at least, to put at least one leg on a bandwagon even though I did not think the wagon was necessarily going in the right direction.

Sometimes bandwagons run off the road. Janis[38] describes *groupthink* as the phenomenon of mem-

bers of highly cohesive groups who, in striving for unanimity, override the realistic need to appraise alternative courses of action. Some years ago, I served on an MRC committee that gave fellowships to professionals who wanted to develop their research skills. When I first saw the information for each candidate that the committee was given to review, I believed that there was no way the committee could do the task well. The committee was given such things as undergraduate and professional marks, which—as they came from different universities with different marking systems and standards—were difficult to interpret; biased reference letters from referees the candidate had chosen; and a letter of support from the laboratory to which the candidate wished to go (the laboratory would get a "free pair of hands" if the application were approved). Nevertheless, the committee worked hard, and the senior members showed the junior ones, such as myself, how to complete the task. We learned from our teachers and achieved near consensus in our scores. We thought we had done well. Years later, however, a study found that the program was not successful in its objective, namely, that of identifying and supporting people who developed research careers. We were victims of groupthink, as identified by many of its salient characteristics: we shared stereotypes on what a successful candidate's record should look like; we believed in our inherent morality (as hardworking volunteers); we exhibited self-censorship in the group by not questioning the types of information we were given, though we all had private doubts; and we ended up with an illusion of unanimity.

5. *Liking* is important, because—as Cialdini posits—we most prefer to say *yes* to the requests of people we know and like. We tend to like people who are physically attractive and similar to us in their opinions, personality traits, background, and lifestyle. We also like people who like us; compliments are always appreciated, and flattery works even when we view it as untrue. Serving on grants committees in Canada is an unpaid and thankless task, but someone has to do it, and administrators must devise novel ways to convince people to do their duty. Years ago, I received a letter from the Deputy Director, Programs Branch, CIHR that stated:

> It is with great pleasure that I invite you to become Scientific Officer for the Multi-User Equipment and Maintenance Com-

mittee. Your ongoing achievements, the benefits of your expertise and your valuable contributions to previous committees have all been recognized and commended by your peers.

The flattery worked; I served on that committee and others.

Liking also is part of the formation of "old boys' networks" (these networks can also involve "old girls"). For the CIHR grants committee, it is customary that the committee goes out one evening to a splash-up dinner; everyone on the committee has worked hard, everyone is impressed with the scientific acumen of their committee colleagues, in vino veritas—all these factors contribute to liking. Everyone likes everyone else on the CIHR committee, in striking contrast to the usual academic milieu, where a few, at least, will be enemies or hostile competitors for scarce resources. Sometimes, a former committee member's application comes up for review. As will be seen in chapter 21, on judgment, it is difficult to revise a model. In this case, once a panelist thinks of a colleague as an able, hardworking scientist, it is difficult to envision a serious scientific blunder. Indeed, when a well-established colleague makes a mistake in a proposal that would prove damaging to a newcomer, it is interpreted simply as a minor slip.

6. *Authority* is a form of inductive argument, and its use in that context will be covered in chapter 6. Authority ranks rather low in the hierarchy of evidence in evidence-based dentistry or medicine, but it carries considerable clout in everyday life. I find it encouraging that the title of "Professor" makes strangers feel more accommodating toward me and causes them to perceive me as taller. One study found that the same man is perceived as 2 ½ inches taller when described as "Professor" than when described as "a student."[39] Juries, I have heard, believe male professors above all other types of witnesses. On such evidence, I am predisposed to believe that some principles of influence lead to real social good (at least for vertically challenged male professors).

The use of authority is common in science, because statements must be backed up by evidence, which is often given by a citation. Behind the citation are the data of the study, the authors, and the journal that published the study as well as, implicitly, the referees who reviewed the study. Sometimes, however, data are not available, and authority must serve as a substitute. This text, like many

others, is sprinkled with statements either based on my own experience or supported by the use of opinions of prestigious authorities, such as the Nobel Prize winner Medawar. Typically, authorities' statements are used when judgment is required and higher forms of evidence are not available on the topic. As Medawar[24] stated in the preface of *Advice to a Young Scientist,* "These are my opinions and this is me giving them . . . my judgments are not validated by systematic sociological research and are not hypotheses that have stood up to repeated critical assaults."

Another use of authority occurs in grant applications. Modern work is often multidisciplinary, and a typical applicant may wish to use techniques for which he or she lacks experience. To fill this gap, an investigator will recruit a collaborator who has an established publication record in the particular area.

7. *Scarcity* surfaces because resources are always limited in scientific research, as are awards. Thus, those who garner the resources or awards garner recognition, and, of course, recognition is the coin of science. Scarcity motivates authors to publish in high-impact journals. Those who publish in such journals must beat back stiff competition, and their work is viewed as more interesting or important than those who publish in lower-impact journals.

Summary

The preceding examples demonstrate that rhetoric plays a large role in scientific discourse. Scientists must persuade to publish and to get grants and recognition. They persuade and are persuaded by rhetorical techniques from everyday discourse. Because they fall into some of the same traps as the naive and unwary public, it is necessary for scientists to become familiar with techniques to separate the grains of truth from the rhetorical chaff.

References

1. Halloran SM. Technical writing and the rhetoric of science. J Tech Writing Commun 1978;8(2):77–88.
2. Habinek T. Ancient Rhetoric and Oratory. Oxford: Blackwell, 2004.

3. Corbett EPJ, Connors RJ. Classical Rhetoric for the Modern Student, ed 4. New York: Oxford Univ Press, 1999.

4. Habinek T. The craft of rhetoric. In: Ancient Rhetoric and Oratory. Oxford: Blackwell, 2004:38–59.

5. Habinek T. Rhetoric and the state. In: Ancient Rhetoric and Oratory. Oxford: Blackwell, 2004:1–15.

6. Lanham RA. A Handlist of Rhetorical Terms. Berkeley: Univ of California Press, 1969.

7. Gross AG. The Rhetoric of Science. Cambridge, MA: Harvard Univ Press, 1990.

8. Horton R. The rhetoric of research. BMJ 1995;310:985–987.

9. Newman S. Aristotelian rhetorical theory as a framework for teaching scientific and technical communication. J Tech Writing Commun 1999;29:325–334.

10. Greenhalgh T. Commentary: Scientific heads are not turned by rhetoric. BMJ 1995;310:987–988.

11. Habinek T. Ancient Rhetoric and Oratory. Oxford: Blackwell, 2004:49

12. Boswell J, Starer D. Five Rings, Six Crises, Seven Dwarfs, and 38 Ways to Win an Argument. New York: Penguin, 1990.

13. Waddell C. The role of pathos in the decision-making process: A study of the rhetoric of science policy. In: Harris RA (ed). Landmark Essays on Rhetoric of Science: Case Studies. Mahwah, NJ: Hermagoras Press, 1997:127–150.

14. Paul D. In citing chaos: A study of the rhetorical use of citations. J Business Tech Commun 2000;14:185–222.

15. Reif-Lehrer L. Grant Application Writer's Workbook. Boston: Jones & Bartlett, 1999:17.

16. Pratkanis A, Aronson E. The credible communicator. In: The Age of Propaganda: The Everyday Use and Abuse of Persuasion. New York: Freeman, 2000:121–132.

17. Haskins CH. The Rise of Universities. Ithaca: Cornell Univ Press, 1923:77–78.

18. Sollaci LB, Pereira MG. The introduction methods, results, and discussion (IMRaD) structure: A 50 year survey. S Med Libr Assoc 2004; 92:364–367.

19. Spicer K. Think on Your Feet: How to Organize Ideas to Persuade Any Audience. Toronto: Doubleday, 1986.

20. Anholt RRH. Dazzle 'Em with Style: The Art of Oral Scientific Presentation. New York: Freeman, 1994.

21. Kurland DJ. I Know What It Says—What Does It Mean? Belmont, CA: Wadsworth, 1995.

22. Latour B, Woolgar S. Laboratory Life: The Construction of Scientific Facts. Princeton: Princeton Univ Press, 1986.

23. Gopen GD, Swan JA. The science of scientific writing. Am Sci 1990;78:550–558.

24. Medawar PB. Advice to a Young Scientist. New York: Basic Books, 1979:67.

25. Abelson RP. Statistics as Principled Argument. Hillsdale NJ: Erlbaum Associates, 1998:11–14.

26. Tufte ER. The visual display of quantitative information. Cheshire, CT: Graphic Press, 1983:161–169.

27. Cialdini RB. Influence: Science and Practice, ed 4. Boston: Allyn & Bacon, 2001.

28. Simons HW. Persuasion in Society. Thousand Oaks, CA: Sage, 2001.

29. Perreaux L. Law students vote to double tuition for incoming class. National Post, February 6, 2003.

30. Ceccarelli L. Shaping Science with Rhetoric: The Cases of Dobzhansky, Schrödinger, and Wilson. Chicago: Univ of Chicago Press, 2001.

31. Pratkanis A, Aronson E. The rationalizing animal. In: Age of Propaganda: The Everyday Use and Abuse of Persuasion. New York: Freeman, 2000:40–47.

32. Pratkanis A, Aronson E. Mindless propaganda, thoughtful persuasion. In: Age of Propaganda: The Everyday Use and Abuse of Persuasion. New York: Freeman, 2000:33–40.

33. Wright R. Tough Questions, Great Answers: Responding to Patient Concerns about Today's Dentistry. Chicago: Quintessence, 1997.

34. The quintessential innovator. Time 1979; 114(17).

35. Cialdini RB. Reciprocation: the old give and take. In: Influence: Science and Practice, ed 4. Boston: Allyn & Bacon, 2001:19–51.

36. Cialdini RB. The science of persuasion. Sci Am 2001;284: 76–81.

37. Yaphe J, Edman R, Knishkowy B, Herman J. The association between funding by commercial interests and study outcome in randomized controlled drug trials. Fam Pract 2001;18:565–568.

38. Janis I. Victims of Groupthink. Boston: Houghton Mifflin, 1972.

39. Wilson PR. The perceptual distortion of height as a function of ascribed academic status. J Soc Psychol 1968;74: 97–102.

4 | Searching the Dental Literature

Kathryn Hornby, MLS, DMD
Donald M. Brunette, PhD

Computers and the Internet make finding information seem easy; however, finding the *right* information can be difficult. Additionally, keeping up-to-date with the literature is a challenge because of the rapid increase in scientific information. Not only does the number of scholarly journals continue to increase, but so do the number of articles per journal, as well as the length of the articles.[1] In addition, the emergence of genomic and proteomic technologies is adding to the rapid information growth.[2]

Although the Internet has made more information accessible, it can be difficult to determine whether this information is valid, reliable, and scientifically sound. Therefore, health professionals need to understand the flow of scientific information and the tools and techniques available to them to get the right information at the right time. Other factors may influence a person's ability to find information, eg, perhaps no one has studied the question being asked, and therefore the information may not even exist. And, although the Internet makes a vast amount of data available, some information is still only available in print. Understanding a few things about publishing and search techniques can make the information-finding process more efficient and effective.

Information Resources

An integral part of the research process is the dissemination of results, which may involve presenting results at conferences, publishing results in peer-reviewed journals, or writing a book on a subject. Traditionally, published information has been categorized as *primary, secondary,* or *tertiary* information. The use of these categories differs somewhat between disciplines, but, in general, primary literature consists of original work and research.[3] In the sciences, a *primary source* usually means a journal article or possibly a conference proceeding with the original research results. The Council of Biology Editors defines a primary scientific paper as follows:

> An acceptable primary scientific publication must be the first disclosure containing sufficient information to enable peers (1) to assess observations; (2) to repeat experiments; and (3) to evaluate intellectual processes; moreover, it must be sensible to sensory perception, essentially permanent, available to the scientific community without restriction, and available for regular screening by one or more of the major recognized secondary services.[4]

These secondary services include indexing services such as PubMed, Biosis, and EMBASE.

Secondary sources, including most books, review articles, and indexes to the literature, usually summarize, review, or organize information. Reference books, such as an encyclopedias, handbooks, or dictionaries are often considered *tertiary sources* of information.[5]

Many of the information resources referred to in this chapter are available through libraries, in particular academic or organizational libraries.

Box 4-1 Example outline of a Cochrane Systematic Review

- Abstract
- Plain language summary
- Background
- Objectives
- Criteria for considering studies for this review
  Types of studies
  Types of participants
  Types of interventions
  Types of outcome measures
- Search methods for identification of studies
- Methods of the review
- Description of studies
- Methodological quality
- Results
- Discussion
- Authors' conclusions
  Implications for practice
  Implications for research
- Potential conflict of interest
- Acknowledgments
- Characteristics of included studies
- Characteristics of excluded studies
- Additional tables
- Analyses
- Sources of support
- Index terms
- Cover sheet
- References

Books

Books can cover a significant amount of material, serving as comprehensive sources of information on topics both broad and narrow in scope. Often an author of a nonfiction book has examined evidence and current knowledge in a subject area, compiling information into a comprehensive in-depth overview of a topic. However, a drawback of books is their lack of currency; publication of information in book format is usually a lengthy process. Traditionally, the material first goes through the journal-publishing cycle then the book-writing and -publishing cycles; in fact, by the time a book is newly published, some of the information may already be several years old, and new editions usually are made available only once every few years. The exception would be books that are published electronically (ie, eBooks), for which different models of updating are possible; for example, portions of a book may be updated on a regular basis.

Review articles

Another secondary information source is the review article, of which there are different types. The traditional review article uses a narrative approach, usually giving an overview of a topic, summarizing developments, and possibly discussing future directions. The author may or may not cover the topic in depth and rarely describes the methods and criteria used to evaluate the information presented. Review articles often have extensive references and can be good sources for directing a researcher to other articles on a topic.

A different type of review article is a *systematic review*. Authors of systematic reviews describe their methodology for conducting the review. The reader can judge the depth of the review by considering how exhaustively the existing research on the topic was covered, how inclusive or exclusive were criteria for including studies, and how the information was extracted and analyzed. This level of disclosure enables readers to decide whether the process was sufficiently rigorous and, therefore, how much weight to give the results. Systematic reviews may or may not include *meta-analyses*. In a meta-analysis, the results of several studies are pooled and statistically analyzed.

As the amount of information available continues to grow, there has been an increased emphasis on resources containing syntheses of evidence on specific questions or topics. An important example of this type of resource is the Cochrane Database of Systematic Reviews (CDSR). The reviews and database are produced through an organization called the Cochrane Collaboration (www.cochrane.org), an international nonprofit organization comprising more than 50 centers that facilitate the process of conducting systematic reviews. The CDSR is part of the Cochrane Library, which is available through Wiley Interscience. Many university libraries and other organizations provide access to CDSR; for example, the Canadian Dental Association makes it available to its members. Following a structured methodology, the reviews examine and provide analyses of research results on specific topics in a variety of health areas. Box 4-1 provides an example of typical components of a systematic review.

Fig 4-1 Partial results of a "Cited Reference Search" on the author, DM Brunette, in the Web of Science (accessed November 2006).

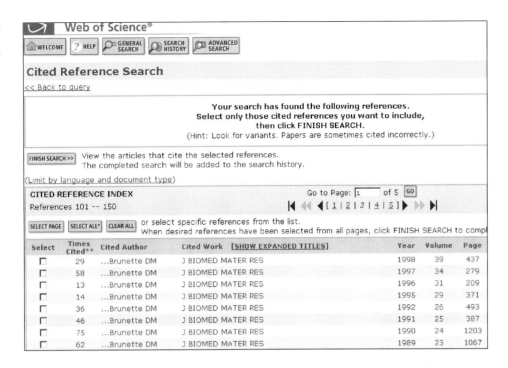

Indexes

For very current or specific information, a research study is the ideal resource. Journal articles are good sources of primary research information, and the most efficient way to find peer-reviewed articles is to use an appropriate article index.

For articles on dental research, MEDLINE is one of the most used indexes in North America today. MEDLINE is an index to journal articles in the life sciences. It is produced by the US National Library of Medicine (NLM) and contains more than 15 million records. MEDLINE can be searched using several different interfaces, including PubMed (www.pubmed.gov), which is the NLM's own search tool, or OVID. MEDLINE includes citations and abstracts from over 5,000 (primarily scholarly) journals.[6]

Many other journal indexes are available, and many, like MEDLINE, are subject based. Other such indexes include EMBASE (Elsevier), CINAHL (EBSCO), and PsycInfo (American Psychological Association). EMBASE is a biomedical and pharmacological index; CINAHL is an index to nursing and allied health literature; and PsycInfo indexes the literature in the field of psychology. Some indexes are multidisciplinary; Academic Search Premier (EBSCO), for example, indexes scholarly journal articles as well as newspapers and popular magazines from many different disciplines. Thomson Scientific's Web of Science, in addi-

tion to providing citation analysis (discussed below), is another large multidisciplinary index. Because of the vast number of indexes in existence, it is often helpful to enlist the help of a librarian when attempting to locate an index related to a specific area of interest.

Citation analysis

Citation analysis is a method of tracking the evolution of research as one author's idea is accessed and built upon by another. It also can be used to track controversy in science as works are cited in scholarly discussions and disputes. Resources for citation tracking include the Web of Science, Google Scholar (scholar.google.com), and Scopus (Elsevier). The Web of Science is the most long-standing source providing this type of information.

For an example of citation analysis, see Fig 4-1, which presents a small selection of the 203 references retrieved from a search on "DM Brunette" (the book's author) using the Web of Science "Cited Reference Search" feature. Selecting a specific record reveals the works in which Dr Brunette's material was cited, and the research thread can be followed forward from there.

A search on Google Scholar for "Author: DM Brunette" retrieved 142 records—fewer than the 203 found in the Web of Science search. Some results overlapped, but each search revealed unique citations. Not only were different articles retrieved, but a look at the citation analyses for articles common to both searches revealed that the subsequent citation information also differed. For example, Web of Science showed the 1992 article published in the *Journal of Biomedical Materials Research* (shown in Fig 4-1) as being cited 36 times, while Google Scholar reported it as being cited only 27 times. Therefore, for this author, Web of Science contains more information; however, because the information from each source differs, a search of both databases would be required to complete an exhaustive search. Scopus, a large citation and abstract database, also reports forward citing of articles, which would doubtlessly differ from both Web of Science and Google Scholar. The use of citation analysis in the evaluation of papers is addressed in chapter 21.

Although this structure of information flow (eg, journals, books, indexes) is valid, it is shifting as the need to cope with vast amounts of new information demands different resources and new technologies, and as the Internet presents opportunities not previously available.

The Internet

The Internet is affecting both the traditional sources and flow of information. Conference proceedings and peer-reviewed journals are still sources of primary literature, and indexes such as MEDLINE classify information to make it searchable. However, there are now more and different information resources. The number of resources that provide evaluated information and present the results of evaluated research in clinical contexts, such as the Cochrane Database of Systematic Reviews, is increasing. These resources are often referred to as *evidence-based* or *filtered* databases. Examples of such information sources include InfoPOEMs (Wiley InterScience), UpToDate (UpToDate), and FirstCONSULT (Elsevier), to name a few. An example of an evidence-based resource in dentistry is the journal *Evidence-based Dentistry*, which publishes evaluated current evidence in dentistry through summaries and expert commentaries.

The Internet is a valuable source of information and a vehicle for providing access to information, including library catalogs, indexes, and books and journals themselves. However, because anyone can create a website and publish information, it is definitely a "buyer beware" situation.

Searching the Internet with general online search tools such as Google, Yahoo, or Windows Live can be effective, but these tools find information only on websites that allow free access to their information; therefore, they do not search all available online sources. Some websites (eg, commercially available eBooks or indexes or databases like individual library catalogs) require subscriptions or passwords; in such cases, the search engines will bring you no further than the entry page. General Internet search engines often miss information available in the "deep" or "invisible" web.

Search engines facilitate searching information published on the Internet by individuals, associations, and many other organizations—information that, in the past, was difficult to obtain. Exemplifying this is "grey literature," which is information produced by organizations but not available through commercial publishers. For example, organizations often publish reports, guidelines, policy statements, consumer information, and other valuable resources that are not commercially available, but that have been made easily available through organization websites.

The Internet has also made possible new initiatives in publishing such as open access publishing, providing free access to scholarly publishing. Examples of such initiatives are the Public Library of Science (www.plos.org) and BioMed Central (www.biomedcentral.com).

Another open access initiative is the development of institutional repositories (IR). IRs facilitate the archiving of an institution's "intellectual output." For a university, this output will comprise many different types of information, including administrative documents and, of course, scholarly work. The digitization and organization of papers, images, and data sets—to name a few possible information formats—will facilitate access to these resources in the long term.

Another type of resource available through the Internet is the preprint database, repositories of research articles that may not have gone through the peer-review process but are available online. The theory behind this type of resource is that it facilitates sharing of information between researchers at a more rapid pace than traditional peer-reviewed publishing. An example of a preprint repository in the health field is NetPrints—Clinical Medicine and Health Research (clinmed.netprints.org), which is sponsored by the BMJ Publishing Group. NetPrints has the following warning on their site: "Articles posted on this site have not yet been accepted for publication by a peer reviewed journal. They are presented here mainly for the benefit of fellow researchers. Casual readers should not act on

---

Box 4-2 Information resources with free access

Databases

Medline (PubMed)	http://www.ncbi.nlm.nih.gov/sites/entrez/
Google Scholar	http://scholar.google.com/
Windows Live Academic	http://academic.live.com
Scirius	http://www.scirus.com/srsapp/

Journals

BioMed Central	http://www.biomedcentral.com/
Journal of the Canadian Dental Association	http://www.cda-adc.ca/jcda/index.html
Free Medical Journals	http://freemedicaljournals.com/
HighWire Press	http://highwire.stanford.edu/lists/freeart.dtl
Public Library of Science (PloS)	http://www.plos.org/journals/index.html
PubMed Central	http://www.pubmedcentral.nih.gov/

---

their findings, and journalists should be wary of reporting them."[7]

Search engines continue to evolve, with some being referred to as *second generation search services*. An online tutorial describes what criteria search engines such as Google, Ask.com, and Clusty use to order results by relevancy: "Google ranks by the number of links from the highest number of pages ranked high by the service," and "Clusty organizes its clustered results by keyword and/or concept."[8]

At present, using these tools is not usually the most effective method of finding primary literature, but this assessment may change with the development of tools like Google Scholar and Windows Live Academic. The specialized sources mentioned earlier, such as MEDLINE, organize information about articles published in the life sciences for effective searching, making the task of finding primary literature much easier (Box 4-2).

Evaluating Information Resources

Peer-reviewed vs trade journals

One approach to finding valid information is to use reliable information sources. When an article is submitted to a *peer-reviewed (or refereed)* journal, it goes through an evaluation process; the editor sends the article to experts (referees) in the field for critical review before deciding whether to accept it for publication. The peer-review process (a key characteristic of scholarly publishing) is a form of quality control, and the articles published in refereed journals should be of high quality because of this process. However, there are no guarantees; the review process is not infallible and depends heavily on how well the reviewers are versed in critical appraisal techniques themselves. Therefore, it is always necessary to read the peer-reviewed literature using the critical appraisal skills described in this book.

Some indexes allow you to limit the retrieved articles to those appearing in refereed journals (Box 4-3). Another way to determine whether a journal is refereed, or to find a refereed journal, is Ulrich's Periodicals Directory (ProQuest CSA), now available online. However, the directory lists more than 1,000 publications (refereed and not refereed) under the subject "dentistry," which makes it difficult to ascertain which of these are the key journals for a specific area of interest. One method of making this determination is to use the *impact factor* (IF), which is a measure of a particular journal's impact based on how often that journal's articles are cited. The formula used to calculate a journal's IF is:

$$IF = \frac{\text{Total no. of citations in the year}}{\text{Total no. of articles published in the previous 2 years}}$$

For example, the journal *Critical Reviews in Oral Biology and Medicine* has an IF of 3.933 (Box 4-4), which means that in the last 1 or 2 years, it would have been cited 3.9 times on average. A journal's IF can be found online in the Journal Citation Reports available

Box 4-3 Refereed dentistry journals from the subject categories dentistry, oral surgery, and medicine (publication start year)[9,10]

Acta Odontologica Scandinavica (1939)
American Journal of Dentistry (1988)
American Journal of Orthodontics and Dentofacial Orthopedics (1915)
Angle Orthodontist (1931)
Archives of Oral Biology (1959)
Australian Dental Journal (1956)
British Dental Journal (1880)
British Journal of Oral and Maxillofacial Surgery (1963)
Caries Research (1967)
Cleft Palate-Craniofacial Journal (1964)
Clinical Oral Implants Research (1990)
Community Dentistry and Oral Epidemiology (1973)
Cranio—The Journal of Craniomandibular Practice (1982)
Critical Reviews in Oral Biology and Medicine (1990) (incorporated into Journal of Dental Research)
Dental Materials (1985)
Dental Materials Journal (1982)
Dental Traumatology (1985)
Dentomaxillofacial Radiology (1971)
European Journal of Oral Sciences (1893)
European Journal of Orthodontics (1979)
International Dental Journal (1951)
International Endodontic Journal (1981)
International Journal of Oral and Maxillofacial Implants (1986)
International Journal of Oral and Maxillofacial Surgery (1972)

International Journal of Periodontics and Restorative Dentistry (1981)
International Journal of Prosthodontics (1988)
Journal of Adhesive Dentistry (1999)
Journal of the American Dental Association (1913)
Journal of Clinical Periodontology (1974)
Journal of Cranio-Maxillo-Facial Surgery (1973)
Journal of Dental Research (1913)
Journal of Dentistry (1972)
Journal of Endodontics (1975)
Journal of Oral and Maxillofacial Surgery (1943)
Journal of Oral Pathology and Medicine (1972)
Journal of Oral Rehabilitation (1974)
Journal of Orofacial Pain (1987)
Journal of Periodontal Research (1966)
Journal of Periodontology (1930)
Journal of Prosthetic Dentistry (1951)
Journal of Public Health Dentistry (1966)
Operative Dentistry (1976)
Oral Diseases (1995)
Oral Microbiology and Immunology (1987)
Oral Oncology (1965)
Oral Surgery Oral Medicine Oral Pathology Oral Radiology and Endodontics (1915)
Periodontology 2000 (1993)
Quintessence International (1970)
Swedish Dental Journal (1979) (formerly Odontologisk Revy, 1908)

through Thomson Scientific's ISI Web of Knowledge and is just one of many measures used to determine a journal's influence. In some situations, such as if the subject area is very specialized or if a journal title is very new, a journal may still be influential, yet not have one of the highest IFs.

Quality assurance is the goal of peer review, and using information from a peer-reviewed source is intended to provide more reliable and valid information. Health professionals may also receive many trade journals, which do not have a peer-review process and often contain articles that are clinically focused. Although it is always important to view information critically no matter the source, because of the lack of peer review in trade journals, it is especially important to view this information critically. There are several differences between scholarly and trade journals. Scholarly journals have a peer-review process, and the arti-

cles include the author's contacts and institutional affiliation. The content in scholarly journals is intended for expert and professional audiences. In addition, the scholarly article has a recognized format; for a scientific study, this consists of an introduction and methods, results, discussion, conclusion, and references sections. The article also often includes tables, graphs, and figures to present its results. A very important part of a scholarly publication is the referencing of other scholarly work, listed in the reference section and/or bibliography. Trade journals, on the other hand, do not have a peer-review process. They do not follow a specific format, and their articles are often shorter and may contain glossy illustrations and images. References are not usually included in trade journal articles, and these journals may present the point of view of a particular manufacturer or clinician.[11]

Box 4-4 Dental journals ranked by 2005 impact factor[9]

Critical Reviews in Oral Biology and Medicine	3.933	Oral Surgery Oral Medicine Oral Pathology	1.193
Journal of Dental Research	3.192	American Journal of Dentistry	1.186
Periodontology 2000	2.377	International Journal of Oral and Maxillofacial Surgery	1.123
Oral Oncology	2.266		
Journal of Clinical Periodontology	2.225	Journal of Cranio-Maxillo-Facial Surgery	1.017
Dental Materials Journal	2.219	International Journal of Periodontal Research	0.963
Journal of Adhesive Dentistry	2.216	Journal of the American Dental Association	0.935
Oral Microbiology and Immunology	2.210	American Journal of Orthodontics and Dentofacial Orthopedics	0.916
Dental Materials	2.060		
Journal of Periodontal Research	1.947	International Dental Journal	0.908
Journal of Endodontics	1.933	Journal of Public Health Dentistry	0.854
Journal of Orofacial Pain	1.932	Acta Odontologica Scandinavica	0.783
Clinical Oral Implants Research	1.897	Angle Orthodontist	0.778
European Journal of Oral Sciences	1.784	Journal of Prosthetic Dentistry	0.748
Journal of Periodontology	1.784	Australian Dental Journal	0.735
Caries Research	1.721	Journal of Oral Rehabilitation	0.717
Operative Dentistry	1.678	Dental Traumatology	0.716
Journal of Oral Pathology and Medicine	1.661	British Dental Journal	0.658
Journal of Dentistry	1.636	European Journal of Orthodontics	0.651
Community Dentistry and Oral Epidemiology	1.631	Dentomaxillofacial Radiology	0.640
International Endodontic Journal	1.606	Cleft Palate-Craniofacial Journal	0.574
Oral Disease	1.445	British Journal of Oral and Maxillofacial Surgery	0.573
International Journal of Oral and Maxillofacial Implants	1.412	Swedish Dental Journal	0.568
		Quintessence International	0.540
International Journal of Prosthodontics	1.346	Cranio—The Journal of Craniomandibular Practice	0.522
Archives of Oral Biology	1.288		
Journal of Oral and Maxillofacial Surgery	1.246		

The Internet

Although the Internet is a powerful tool in its ability to present information and make it accessible, it is often difficult to determine the quality of the information retrieved, because high-quality and poor-quality information may not look different initially. Therefore, as an important step in forming an effective search strategy, it is important to understand different types of information sources.

The following is a summary of the University of British Columbia Library's web page on criteria for evaluating Internet resources.[12]

- *Author:* Is the author clearly identified? Does the author have credentials for writing on this subject? Is the author affiliated with any organization(s)? Is there contact information for the person or organi-

zation sponsoring the site? Who creates and maintains the information?

- *Accuracy:* Does it state whether there is a peer-review process and what that process is? Does the publication provide references to the information it presents so the information can be verified? Is statistical information clearly presented and referenced?

- *Currency:* Is the creation of the document or page clearly dated? Is it clear when or if the information has been updated and/or revised? Does it state how often the information is updated or reviewed?

- *Objectivity:* Is there advertising on the page and/or site? If so, is it clear that it is advertising and not content? Is the perspective of the information presented clear?

- *Coverage:* If there is a print version of the same information, does the web source indicate whether it is the same as or different than the print source—for example, is it an abridged version, or does it have additional content?

- *Purpose:* Does the site indicate its purpose? Is it to sell something, to make a political point, to educate, or to entertain?

Conducting a Search

Defining the question

The first and probably most difficult step in finding information is to define the question. Asking a good question is not easy. Many people find that initially they only have a vague idea of what they are looking for, which often results in hours spent looking on the Internet and finding thousands of results—none of which provides the appropriate answer. Moreover, clarifying the question is an important step, because different types of questions require different resources, as discussed below.

Sackett et al[13] have developed a useful approach to asking answerable clinical questions. The question is composed of three to four components and is commonly referred to as *PICO*:

P = Patient or Problem
I = Intervention
C = Comparison (if relevant)
O = Outcome(s)

For example, if someone wanted to know whether soft drinks consumed by schoolchildren increase their tooth decay, using PICO to identify the key concepts in the question would look like this:

P = schoolchildren
I = soft drinks
C = not applicable
O = rate of tooth decay

Providing the following question: Does consumption of soft drinks increase the rate of tooth decay in schoolchildren?

Where should the researcher look first to find the answer to this question? A website sponsored by soft drink manufacturers? Probably not. Looking for a systematic review of the literature on this question or for research articles on this topic would be more effective.

Choosing a resource

As mentioned above, defining the question guides the choice of resources. For finding information on the question "What is the blood supply to the mandible?" a book or atlas on anatomy (electronic or print) will be most useful, whereas a question about antibiotic prophylaxis may be addressed well in a practice guideline. Researchers with a specific patient-focused question might need to consult the journal literature to find out whether any studies that address the question have been conducted.

If a book is the best source of information on the topic, searching a library catalog is a good approach. The library catalog will indicate whether the library owns the book and where it is located. Because books are becoming available electronically, access to the book may entail either physically locating it in the library or simply linking to an electronic version through the catalog.

Finding an article requires different tools. A researcher who already has identified an article and just wants to read it can look in the library's catalog to see if it owns or provides access to electronic versions of that journal. (It is important to remember to look up the journal title, rather than the article title, in the catalog.) Finding an article based on a question is usually a two-step process of, first, searching an index for an article on the topic, and, second, finding the actual article. However, this two-step process is becoming increasingly seamless as libraries link users from indexes directly to full-text electronic journal articles.

Keyword searching vs classification systems

Once the question is defined and the resource selected, how does a researcher actually perform the search? Unfortunately, there is very little standardization among resources, and each resource requires slightly different search techniques. The good news is that these can be simplified to two basic approaches, and once they are understood, it is not difficult to apply them to a given resource.

The *keyword* (sometimes called *textword*) approach assumes that all or some of the text in the database is searchable. The computer simply scans the database looking for the word or words entered. Keyword searching is a very powerful method, but it does have drawbacks. First, it is a very literal way of searching;

the computer is not aware of what is *meant* but will only look for what is *entered*. Therefore, it is necessary to think of all of the different forms (eg, different expressions and synonyms) in which the search item may appear. A keyword search for something as seemingly straightforward as *teeth* would need to include not only the word *teeth* but also the words *tooth*, *incisor*, *incisors*, *premolar*, *premolars*, *molar*, *molars*, etc. Searching for *teeth* as a keyword will return only results that have that precise word. Thus it is important to include all the terms that make up the concept—as well as singular and plurals—and any different spellings (for example, *pediatric/paediatric*). For some topics, it can be time consuming to form a list of all possible relevant terms. Another drawback is that, because the search retrieves anything with the term(s) entered, many results may contain the term(s) but may not be relevant. For example, a keyword search for information on *aspirin* would retrieve articles authored by John Aspirin, even though such articles may have nothing to do with the subject *aspirin*. Therefore, keyword searching often turns up many irrelevant results. To reduce this problem, Internet search engines such as Google have developed complex algorithms designed to return the most relevant results at the top of the retrieval list.

The second approach to searching is to use a *classification system*. The best example of this in the health-related journal literature is the Medical Subject Headings (MeSH) produced by the US NLM and used for indexing journal articles in MEDLINE. EMBASE, CINAHL, and PsycInfo all have subject headings as well, and, of course, they are all different.

Using a system such as MeSH differs from keyword searching in that it is a conceptual approach to searching. For MEDLINE, the indexers look at each article and apply subject headings appropriate to the article's content. This means that under the subject heading *myocardial infarction*, all the articles under that heading will be about myocardial infarction, even if the author has used the term *heart attack* or *MI* instead.

Other familiar classification systems are those used by libraries: the Library of Congress system, used by academic libraries; the NLM's classification, used by medical libraries; and the Dewey Decimal System, used by public libraries. These systems group materials on the same topic so they will be in one location, permitting browsing for books in the library. Dentistry books are in the WU section (see appendix 1).

Both keyword searching and subject heading searching have strengths and weaknesses. The power of a keyword approach is its ability to comb through databases, looking for the occurrences of words, while the benefit of using a subject heading approach is that the search results are highly relevant. The keyword approach's weakness is that it can be complex to develop and may return many irrelevant results; a drawback of the subject heading approach is that there may not be a term suitable for a specific search. A strength and weakness of subject heading searching is that people perform the indexing (conceptual work); this allows the classification to be more intuitive, but also leaves it open to human error.

Search techniques

There are techniques for searching by keyword or subject headings that allow a researcher to manage and combine results. Some common techniques, such as Boolean operators, truncation, and phrases, are described below.

Boolean operators

The Boolean operators *OR*, *AND*, and *NOT* may be familiar to many readers. These simple words are powerful tools in the search for information.

The term *OR* is commonly used to combine synonyms. As mentioned above, finding information about a particular concept using a keyword approach would require combining several terms in order to capture all the relevant information. For the question in the PICO example above (Does consumption of soft drinks increase the rate of tooth decay in schoolchildren?), which includes more than one concept, each concept is built by including all synonyms and forms of the words. For the concept *tooth decay*, the keyword search might look something like this:

Concept A = decay OR decayed OR decays OR caries OR carious ...

This retrieves results with any of these terms (Fig 4-2).

The concept of *soft drinks* also must be developed when using keywords, possibly looking something like this:

Concept B = soft drink OR soft drinks OR carbonated drink OR carbonated drinks OR carbonated beverages OR carbonated beverage OR pop OR cola OR colas OR ...

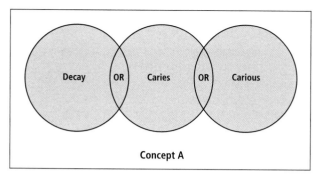

Fig 4-2 Keyword searches using *OR* will retrieve sources that have any of the search terms.

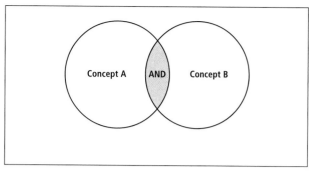

Fig 4-3 Keyword searches using *AND* will retrieve sources that contain both search terms.

Once the major concepts are built, they must be combined with the operator *AND*. Using *AND* will tell the search engine to only return results that have a term from each of your concepts, ie, both concepts in one article:

Concept A (tooth decay, etc) AND Concept B (soft drinks, etc.)

This search will retrieve results that contain both concepts (Fig 4-3).

NOT is a term used to exclude results containing a specified term. This operator should be used with caution, because it is easy to inadvertently exclude relevant information.

Truncation

In the above examples, both Concept A and Concept B are unwieldy, due to the inclusion of singular, plural, and other word endings. Many search engines allow you to place a symbol at the end of a word, which tells the search engine to retrieve the word stem with different endings. A common symbol used for truncation is the asterisk (*), although this is not universal. Most search engines have a "help" or "search tips" link that explains which symbols the system uses. So, for Concept A (*tooth decay*), the search might look like this:

Concept A = decay* OR caries OR carious

Note that enough of the word must be used to make the results meaningful; a search on *cari** would return too many unrelated terms, such as *Caribbean* or *caring*.

Concept B's search might look like this:

Concept B = soft drink* OR carbonated drink* OR carbonated beverage* OR pop OR cola OR colas OR...

Phrases

If, in the above example, the researcher prefers to search for *tooth decay,* it may be necessary to enclose the words in quotation marks ("*tooth decay*") to instruct the search engine to search this as a phrase. (Exact functionality depends on how the particular search engine operates.) The use of quotation marks will limit the results of the search to sources that contain the exact phrase. For example, if the search engine searches *tooth decay* as a phrase with quotation marks, this search will not retrieve articles that state, "the tooth was decayed."

Parentheses

Finally, parentheses are used to appropriately group the terms and operators to control the order of the search.

(Concept A) AND (Concept B)
(decay* OR caries OR carious) AND (soft drink* OR carbonated drink* OR carbonated beverage* OR pop OR cola OR colas)

Explode

The above examples used a keyword approach. If the search were performed in MEDLINE, which uses MeSH, it might look like this:

explode beverages AND explode dental caries

Fig 4-4a The screen shot illustrates a search for two terms, *soft drinks* and *tooth decay*. The search has retrieved 65 items.

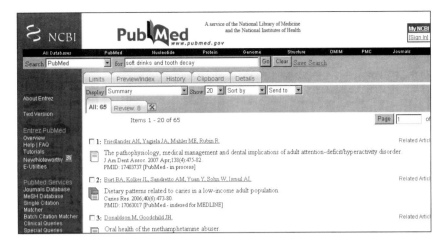

Fig 4-4b Clicking the "Details" tab under the search box will reveal how the search was performed. In the above example, the term *soft drink* was searched as two separate keywords, then combined with *AND*. Adding quotation marks would allow *soft drinks* to be searched as a phrase. *Dental caries* has been searched both as a MeSH term and as a keyword phrase. This is an example of mapping: the keyword *tooth decay* has been mapped to the MeSH term *dental caries*.

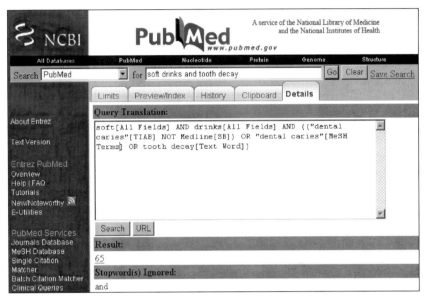

MeSH is a hierarchical classification system with broad subject headings that are broken down into narrower headings. *Explode* is a term used in MEDLINE to express the function of including narrower subject headings in the search. The following example shows how the subject heading *beverage* is broken down further into narrower subject headings:

Beverage
    Alcoholic beverages
    Carbonated beverages
    Coffee
    Milk
    Milk substitutes
    Mineral waters
    Tea

The explode function instructs the search engine to retrieve the information filed under the *beverage* heading as well as all of the narrower subject headings. At this time, PubMed automatically explodes terms; if researchers do not want to use this feature, they must turn it off. The opposite is true with OVID: if researchers want to include articles filed under the narrower headings, they must select the explode function while searching.

Figure 4-4 provides an example of a MEDLINE search using the PubMed interface. PubMed allows the user to enter terms, then the system attempts to map the terms to MeSH. In addition to the MeSH search, PubMed also searches the entered terms as keywords. This system is effective but can have drawbacks, including large result sets (due to the keyword search) or too few

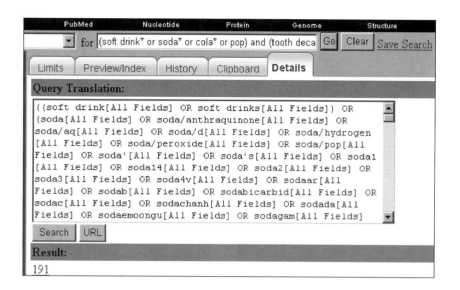

Fig 4-4c To increase results, more terms (synonyms) were added to the search, and the extensive search performed by the engine is evident. Adding terms increased the retrieval to 191 results; however, because there are so many keywords, the additional terms might also increase the number of irrelevant results.

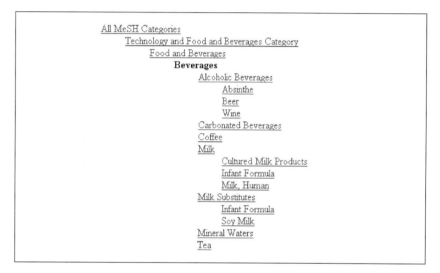

Fig 4-4d There is no subject heading for *soft drinks*, so it may be necessary to use a broader term, such as *beverages*. This excerpt from the MeSH browser (which can be accessed through the "MeSH Database" link on the left menu bar under "PubMed Services") shows that narrower headings for beverages include the term *carbonated beverages*, which would include soft drinks.

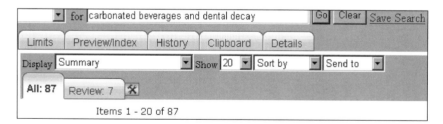

Fig 4-4e Searching for *carbonated beverages AND dental decay* retrieves 87 results. This is likely due to retrieving fewer irrelevant records.

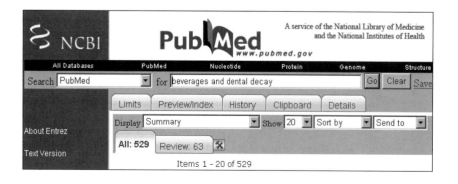

Fig 4-4f Searching the broad term *beverages AND dental decay* retrieves many more results because PubMed automatically searches the narrower terms under the broad heading.

relevant results if the term does not get mapped to an appropriate subject heading. PubMed also provides the option of building a search using MeSH (see Fig 4-4d) and other features available in MEDLINE. For more information, see the tutorials on the PubMed website (www.nlm.nih.gov/bsd/disted/pubmed.html).

Understanding the difference between using a classification system or keyword approach and how to use the various search techniques facilitates searching, but practice is the only way to become a truly effective searcher.

Summary

- Define the question first. This guides the choice of which information resource to use.
- Understanding how information is organized helps in the selection of appropriate resources.
- The Internet is a good source of information, yet it heightens the need to understand how to evaluate information.
- Rapid advances in technology are changing how information is managed. Search engines are using linking and concept-clustering techniques to improve relevance ranking of information.

The day when there is one resource to meet all our information needs is not yet here. We still have many resources to choose from, and more are being developed. These resources offer different yet overlapping results. On the surface, it seems as though the world of information is getting easier to access, but, in fact, it is becoming very complex as technology changes how we organize, retrieve, and manage information. Understanding how scientific information flows, what types of information resources are available in a specific field, and how to use information search tools greatly assists in finding and using information effectively.

References

1. Tenopir C, King DW. Towards electronic journals: Realities for scientists, librarians, and publishers. Psycoloquy [electronic journal] 2000;11(84):1. Available at: http://psycprints. ecs.soton.ac.uk/archive/ 00000084/. Accessed 24 November 2006.
2. Cockerill MJ, Tracz V. Open access and the future of the scientific research article. J Neurosci 2006;26:10079–10081.
3. Primary, Secondary & Tertiary Sources. Available at: http://www.library.jcu.edu.au/LibraryGuides/primsrcs.shtml. Accessed 11 October 2005.
4. Council of Biology Editors. Cited by: Day RA. How to Write and Publish a Scientific Paper. Phoenix: Oxyx Press, 1988:9.
5. Library research skills for biologists. Available at: https://www.webct.ubc.ca/public/library_biol_skills/index.html. Accessed 10 November 2005.
6. MEDLINE Fact Sheet. Available at: http://www.nlm.nih.gov/pubs/factsheets/medline.html. Accessed 26 November 2005.
7. NetPrints Clinical Medicine & Health Research website. Available at: http://clinmed.netprints.org/. Accessed 7 July 2006.
8. Second Generation Searching on the Web. Available at: http://www.internettutorials.net/second.html. Accessed 24 July 2007.
9. Journal Citation Reports. Science edition. Accessed through: Web of Science. Philadelphia: Thompson Scientific, 2005. Available at: http://portal.isiknowledge.com/.
10. Ulrich's Periodical Directory. Bethesda, MD: ProQuest, 2006. Available at: http://www.ulrichsweb.com/ulrichsweb/.
11. Academic and popular journals. Available at: http://www.library.auckland.ac.nz/subjects/bus/topicguides/academic_popularjnls.htm. Accessed 20 August 2006.
12. Criteria for evaluating Internet resources. Available at: http://www.library.ubc.ca/home/evaluating/. Accessed 7 July 2006.
13. Sackett DL, Richardson WS, Rosenberg W, Haynes RB. Evidence-Based Medicine: How to Practice and Teach EBM. New York: Churchill Livingstone, 1997.

5 | Logic: The Basics

The Reverend Sydney Smith, a famous wit, was walking with a friend through the extremely narrow streets of old Edinburgh when they heard a furious altercation between two housewives from high-up windows across the street. "They can never agree," said Smith to his companion, "for they are arguing from different premises."

—Peter B. Medawar[1]

Logical analysis concerns the relationship between a conclusion and the evidence used to support it[2] and has obvious relevance to the evaluation of scientific papers. An *argument* is the expression of logical analysis and consists of both a conclusion and supporting evidence. The statements of evidence are *premises*, which are ideally statements of *fact* (ie, a datum of experience known to be true, because it can be verified by others). Typically, however, because of the paucity of well-established facts, a less stringent criterion for the premises is used, namely, that they at least be plausible. Often in deductive arguments, the statements may be principles or ideals, such as "All men are created equal." Premises may not support the conclusion in one of two ways: (1) the facts are implausible or not true, or (2) the facts are not appropriately related to the conclusion. The relationship between the premises and the conclusion is the domain of logic.

Some Basic Standards and Ground Rules

In assessing an argument several ground rules apply.

1. *Rationality*: Those making an argument are expected to have reasons for their beliefs.

2. *Consistency*: Where two cases are similar, a reason for not treating them the same way must be offered.
3. *Open-mindedness*: The evaluator must be open-minded, that is, prepared to consider other points of view and, when evaluating logic, prepared to reason from premises with which one disagrees.
4. *Balance*: The evaluator should be concerned only with defects in proportion to the degree that they affect the conclusions. If the major conclusions are sound, there is little point in nitpicking a paper with minor criticisms.

In analyzing logic, it is often necessary to clarify the issues and to analyze the arguments underlying the positions, which may be complex, having several arguments linked together. For each argument, it is important to identify the conclusions and the premises. This task is sometimes made difficult because of the convolutions of scientific writing. In addition, the terms of an argument must be used precisely. The measure of the completeness of an analysis depends on the number of valid and significant distinctions contained in the works being compared.[3] The number of distinct terms is related to the number of distinctions. For example, early work in connective tissue spoke of *fibers*; subsequently, some of the fibers were called *collagen*; today no less than 17 types of collagen are distinguished. Thus, as the analysis of fibers has become more complete, the descriptive terms have multiplied.

Fallacy of no evidence: Assertions

Fallacies are mistakes in reasoning, and they are made in various ways. A common fallacy is the fallacy of no evidence, where some statements are not supported by evidence. Statements not supported by evidence are called *assertions*. Surprisingly, the simple technique of repeating a statement often causes people to believe the statement, particularly when the speaker has an air of authority. Although many simple assertions are obvious (eg, those made in radio or television commercials) others are more insidious. Statements of belief, apparently unsupported by evidence, are found in the discussion section of scientific papers. The best way to deal with assertions is simply to challenge them by asking what evidence supports them. This strategy risks making the questioner appear ignorant, but the risk may be smaller than anticipated, for it is not unusual for the evidence of even widely accepted conclusions to be weak. Reasonable people have grounds for their beliefs, but often these can be discovered only by questioning.

Fallacy of insufficient or inappropriate evidence

Sometimes evidence presented for a conclusion does not seem to bear directly on the conclusion but, nevertheless, is related to the conclusion. For example, an advertisement directed at dentists for a toothpaste formulated for children states that the abrasiveness of the product has been reduced. Included in the advertisement is a figure showing that children's dentin is softer than adult dentin, implying that use of the toothpaste will reduce abrasion on children's teeth and that dentists should recommend it to their pediatric patients. The data are correct; children's dentin is softer than adults' dentin, so the issue is not the truth of the data; rather, the problem is how the data relate to the implied conclusion. In my view, to make the conclusion that children need the specially formulated toothpaste sound, three additional pieces of evidence are needed:

1. Evidence that erosion caused by abrasive toothpastes is a significant problem; that is, there are children who required clinical treatment or who suffered pain because of erosion caused by standard toothpastes. Establishing this premise would require an epidemiologic study. However, some would argue that just the chance of reducing erosion on children's teeth is sufficient reason to recommend a less-abrasive toothpaste.

2. Evidence that use of the children's toothpaste actually reduces erosion. This might be demonstrated most convincingly by a clinical study in which users exhibit less abrasion than users of a standard toothpaste. However, it might be argued that a laboratory study could also demonstrate that the special formulation causes less erosion of children's teeth. Extracted primary teeth could be assessed for erosion after being brushed with the new toothpaste or a standard brand for specified periods of time, using an apparatus that applied a known pressure on the brush.

3. Evidence that the new toothpaste is as effective as standard toothpastes in plaque removal and reduction in caries, because these are the principle reasons for toothpaste use.

This simple example illustrates that what constitutes relevant or sufficient evidence can depend, as noted in points 1 and 2, on individual judgment. On other issues, such as point 3, there probably would be widespread agreement. Nevertheless, accepting any conclusion and implementing action involves applying appropriate standards. Setting standards requires judgment, which in turn requires justification and is open to criticism. If too high a standard is set, it will seem that nothing can be known with certainty. For example, although the philosopher Descartes concluded that certainty is the impossibility of doubt, Fisher[4] has argued that Cartesian skepticism is an inappropriate standard in normal circumstances. Excessively high standards for accepting conclusions lead to inaction; aging professors sometimes suffer from masterly inactivity, for if nothing can be established with certainty, why bother doing research? On the other hand, setting low standards for accepting conclusions leads to the tolerance of error and a condition of gullibility or naivete.

The assertability question

In *The Logic of Real Arguments,* Fisher[5] advocates the assessment of conclusions by the use of the assertability question (AQ): What argument or evidence would justify the assertion of the conclusion, or, expressed slightly differently, what evidence would I require before I believed the conclusion?

The AQ can be an efficient tool for analyzing scientific articles, because it leads the questioner to focus on the critical issue of whether the data presented as evidence for a conclusion are relevant and sufficient. The answer to this question often can be found by scanning a paper's abstract or summary and identifying the main conclusions. If the data in the paper are identified as relevant by the AQ, then the paper may deserve a closer look; otherwise, it may be a better use of time to look at other articles. For example, my answer to the AQ for the conclusion of the children's toothpaste advertisement comprises the three points given earlier. When these points are not answered, I do not feel compelled to look more closely at other aspects of the advertisement (such as exactly how hardness of dentin was measured or the taste of the toothpaste).

The AQ also forces the questioners to consider explicitly the appropriateness of the standards of evidence that they employed.[6] In some fields of research, the standards of evidence may relate to the particular techniques used. In biochemical research, the standards for declaring a preparation of a particular protein pure have undergone continuous revision upwards as new methods of analysis (which reveal contamination) or preparation (which lower the possibility of contamination) are developed.

An Introduction to Deductive Logic

A valid deductive argument is one in which the premises provide conclusive grounds for the truth of the conclusion. Deductive logic is valuable, because it establishes new relationships between different terms. Although most people consider themselves logical, a test of university students' ability to solve simple problems in deductive logic found that, on average, they scored only 20%![7] If deductive logic is helpful in evaluating experimental research, it likely must be studied, since most people do not acquire logic naturally. Because certain errors and weaknesses in logic appear more frequently than others, learning the most common errors makes them easier to spot. The deductive logic section of this chapter intends not only to summarize the rules of fundamental deductive logic but also to indicate effective approaches to critique scientific presentations on the basis of logic. This is by no means a complete presentation; more detailed information on logic can be found in sources devoted to the topic.[8-12]

Formal deductive arguments are most frequently encountered in the discussion section of scientific papers. Scientists use deductive logic when they believe that they have established certain facts and wish to relate their findings to other information.

The use of deductive logic in science has a checkered history. Ancient Greek as well as medieval philosophers were more concerned with what *should be*, rather than with what actually *was*, and made no distinction among science, philosophy, and religion. Such speculative philosophers relied on a maximum of reasoning and hypotheses and a minimum of observation, particularly observations that verified the truth of the deductions. Observation was connected to practical work, which was believed to be inferior to contemplation. The modern term for this approach is *armchair science*. In the medieval world, it was thought that truth about the physical world could be arrived at by the exercise of reason upon a few observed facts. Deductions, although valid, were sometimes based on false (or speculative) premises and thus were not sound. Consequently, deductive logic fell into disrepute as the primary means of scientific inquiry.[13]

The use of deductive logic is most productive when the axioms are well established, as in Mendelian genetics, but it also can work well in less-established schemes. Watson and Crick proposed that, on the basis of x-ray diffraction patterns, DNA comprised two strands linked by hydrogen bonds.[14] Others deduced that this model could be tested by exposing DNA to conditions that rupture hydrogen bonds and seeing if single strands of DNA could be obtained. Such deduction requires expert knowledge. In this example, the scientists who deduced the consequences of the Watson-Crick model were familiar with physical chemistry. Similarly, some dental research also tests the deduced consequences of hypotheses. However, there is not, in many instances, a firm knowledge of underlying mechanisms, and the tests are not as rigorous as would be desired.

A second use of deductive logic in scientific articles occurs in the discussion section. Although philosophers might argue that inductive logic is never certain, scientists often will treat the results of their research as established facts. They combine these newly discovered facts with previously reported data to arrive at new conclusions or hypotheses. In some instances, it is the new relationship between the facts that is discussed, and the logic used to arrive at the conclusions is deductive.

Table 5-1 Categorical statements						
Code	Quantity	Quality	Quantifier	Subject	Copula	Predicate
A	Universal	Affirmative	All	Canadians (D)	Are	Brave people (U)
E	Universal	Negative	No	Canadians (D)	Are	Brave people (D)
I	Particular	Affirmative	Some	Canadians (U)	Are	Brave people (U)
O	Particular	Negative	Some	Canadians (U)	Are not	Brave people (D)

Syllogisms

Aristotle postulated that arguments could be cast into a basic pattern called the *syllogism*. A categorical syllogism consists of two premises and a conclusion. An example of a valid syllogism in a standard form is the following: All scientists are dishonest; Einstein was a scientist; therefore, Einstein was dishonest. This is a valid syllogism. If the premises are true, then the conclusion is true. The conclusion, however, would not be sound if either premise were false.

An example of an invalid syllogism follows: Some men are philosophers; some men are Greeks; therefore, some Greeks are philosophers. Although probable, the argument is invalid, because the truth of the premises does not guarantee the truth of the conclusion.

Testing the validity of syllogisms is not necessarily obvious, which is evident by the example of the probable but invalid argument. However, testing can be done rigorously and relatively simply, as will be discussed; there are, however, some problems. The first problem is identifying the structure of the argument, which requires the recognition that an appeal to reason rather than observation is being made. Second, the reader must determine which parts of the argument are premises and which are conclusions. The premises often can be identified by words such as *since, for, on account of,* and *because.* Conclusions are often preceded by indicators such as *therefore, thus, hence, so, it follows that, consequently,* and *we may infer that.* Authors can either state the premises before giving the conclusion or start from the conclusion and work backward.

Imprecise terms pose another problem in analyzing arguments. Words can have emotional or evaluative overtones and take on different meanings, depending on the context. For example, the word *or* can be used in an exclusive sense, as in the phrase "take it or leave it," in which *or* means *either one; not both. Or* is used in a weak or inclusive sense in the sentence, "If it is snowing or raining the game will be canceled." Pre-

sumably the game would be canceled if a mixture of snow and rain were falling. *Or* in this inclusive sense means *either; possibly both.* In symbolic logic, the symbol for the inclusive sense of *or* is *v.* For an equivalent meaning to *or* in the exclusive sense, the symbol *v* must be used with two additional symbols in a particular combination. Although this sounds complex, it results in clarity. Unfortunately, ambiguity exists when arguments are stated in everyday language. Scientific arguments are made in everyday, although somewhat stilted, language and are not framed in the precise but abstract terms of the symbolic logician. A compromise that helps clear up ambiguity, but still enables the analysis to be conducted in everyday language, is translating the arguments into a standard form to obtain statements in the form of precise propositions.

Categorical statements

The traditional four statements and their properties and representations are given in Table 5-1. The A and I statements are affirmative in quality, while the E and O (from *nego,* meaning *I deny*) are negative in quality.

The quantity of a statement is *universal* if it refers to all members of a class, and *particular* if it refers only to some. A subject (and/or predicate) is *distributed* (indicated by the letter *D* in Table 5-1) if it refers to the whole class it names. Obviously, the subject of A and E statements are distributed. A trickier problem is the distribution of the predicate terms. The predicate of the A statement (all Canadians are brave people) is not distributed (marked *U* in Table 5-1 for *undistributed*). Not all brave people are Canadians. The predicate of an E statement (no Canadians are brave people) is distributed, because, in asserting that the whole class of brave people is excluded from the whole class of Canadians, this statement asserts that each and every brave person is not a Canadian. Another convention is that a statement referring to a specified individual (eg, Socrates is mortal) is treated as a universal statement, because it refers to the whole of the subject (in this case, all of Socrates).

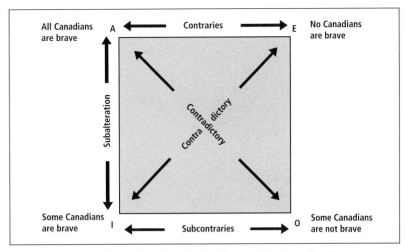

Fig 5-1 The square of opposition. (Reprinted with permission from Copi.[8])

Many categorical statements lack the standard form shown in our examples. The statement, "Some enzymes denature at high temperatures," does not contain a form of the verb *to be*, but it can be altered with no change in meaning to "Some enzymes are heat-labile substances." The altered statement has the standard form. Some common but nonstandard quantities easily can be translated to standard form. Terms such as *every, any, everything, anything, everyone,* and *anyone* usually can be interpreted as *all. A, an,* and *the* can mean either *all* or *some,* depending on the context. Phrases using *only* or *none but* generally imply that the predicate applies exclusively to the subject. These can be altered with no change in meaning to A statements (eg, "Only proteins are enzymes" becomes "All enzymes are proteins.")

The relationships between categorical statements are summed up in the traditional square of opposition (Fig 5-1). Any arguments that depend on numerical or probabilistic information for their validity are asyllogistic and cannot be analyzed by the following methods. Two statements are *contradictory* if one is the denial of the other. They cannot both be true, and they cannot both be false. Statements that differ in both quantity and quality are contradictory (eg, A contradicts O; E contradicts I). Two propositions are said to be *contraries* if they cannot both be true, although they might both be false. Two propositions are *subcontraries* if they both cannot be false though they might both be true.

Categorical syllogisms

A *syllogism* is a deductive argument in which a conclusion is derived from two premises. In a valid syllogism, if both premises are true, the conclusion must be true.

Categorical syllogisms contain three categorical statements, which use three terms twice. An example of a valid syllogism is the following:

premise 1	All dentists are crooks.
premise 2	Doug is a *dentist*.
conclusion	Therefore, *Doug* is a *crook*.

The *major term* (crook) appears as the predicate of the conclusion. The *minor term* (Doug) appears as the subject of the conclusion. The *middle term* (dentist) appears in both premises but not the conclusion. While this syllogism is valid, the conclusion is unsound, because one of the premises (all dentists are crooks) is false.

Rules for valid categorical syllogisms

The syllogism examples on Greeks and philosophers and dentists and crooks have similar form, but one is valid and the other is invalid. An argument is invalid when its conclusion is not justified by its premises; it is still possible for the conclusion to be found factual in subsequent investigation. For an argument to be considered as *valid*, it must follow four rules.

1. A valid categorical syllogism contains just three terms, which must be used in the same way throughout the argument. If a term is used in different senses, the fallacy of equivocation is committed. This fallacy is particularly easy to commit if a term is used imprecisely.

   Consider the syllogism:

premise 1	The causative agent of periodontal disease is plaque.

premise 2   Plaque is the causative agent of dental caries.
conclusion   The causative agent of periodontal disease is the causative agent for dental caries.

This syllogism has a valid form. However, if the plaque mentioned in the first premise is subgingival plaque while the plaque specified in the second term is supragingival plaque, the syllogism is invalid. Rule 1 is violated, because there are really four terms, not three, used. The middle term, *plaque*, has been used in two different senses.

2. In a valid standard-form categorical syllogism, the middle term must be distributed in at least one premise. This is the rule most often violated in everyday reasoning. In the example of an invalid syllogism involving Greeks and philosophers, the middle term, *men,* is not distributed. Despite being invalid, such conclusions may have a high probability.

3. A term that is distributed in the conclusion must be distributed in the premises. Frequently, this rule is used when evaluating arguments that contain premises starting with the word *some*.
(a) If either premise starts with *some*, then the conclusion must also start with *some*.
(b) No deductively valid conclusion can be made when both premises start with the word *some*.

But other arguments that do not contain premises starting with *some* can also commit this error as shown below:

premise 1   All Canadians are brave people.
premise 2   No Americans are Canadians.
conclusion   Therefore, no Americans are brave people.

The term *brave people* is distributed in the conclusion but not in the premises.

4. (a) If there is a negative premise, there must be a negative conclusion.
(b) If there are two negative premises, the argument is automatically invalid.

This rule is particularly important when interpreting negative results, for to show that a thing lacks one property does not necessarily prove that it has another.

As an example of testing a categorical syllogism, consider the argument made by Iversen[15] on chalones. It is not acceptable logic to say: Chalones cause proliferation delay and thus tumor regression; cancer cure is always associated with tumor regression; ergo, chalones cure cancer.

First, we can identify whether this is a logical argument, for Iversen states that it is not acceptable logic. The general form of the argument looks like a categorical syllogism, but we must translate it to standard form. The first premise is complex, as there is a causal link between proliferation delay and tumor regression as well as between chalones and tumor regression. However, inspection of the premises and the conclusion indicates that the three principal terms are *chalone, tumor regression,* and *cancer cure.* For the moment, we can ignore *proliferation delay* and concentrate on *tumor regression.* The argument recast in standard form becomes:

premise 1   All chalones are tumor regressors.
premise 2   All cancer cures are tumor regressors.
conclusion   Therefore, all chalones are cancer cures.

In applying rule 1, the syllogism passes, because there are just three terms. However, rule 2 dictates that the middle term, *tumor regressors,* be distributed in at least one premise. The term *tumor regressor* is not distributed, so the syllogism is invalid. Iversen is correct when he states it is not acceptable logic.

The fallacy of existential assumption
The chalone example illustrates another problem of scientific logic: reification or misplaced concreteness. The concept of chalones is that of tissue-specific growth inhibitors, but, unlike various other growth regulators, chalones have not been purified; you cannot order a bottle of chalones from Sigma Chemical (which has almost every known biochemical). Thus, in a practical sense, chalones do not exist, and the argument commits the fallacy of existential assumption. However, the general concept of growth inhibitors exists, and the term *chalone* can be used in literature searches.

The mixed hypothetical syllogism

Conditional propositions take the form: If P then Q (P is the *antecedent*, and Q is the *consequent*). There are two valid forms of the mixed hypothetical syllogism that employ conditional propositions. The first, in the affirmative mood, is called *modus ponens*:

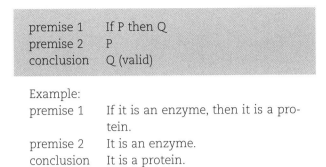

premise 1	If P then Q
premise 2	P
conclusion	Q (valid)

Example:
premise 1	If it is an enzyme, then it is a protein.
premise 2	It is an enzyme.
conclusion	It is a protein.

Notice that the second premise affirms the antecedent of the conditional proposition, not the consequent. If the consequent is affirmed, then the argument is invalid (the fallacy of affirming the consequent; see chapter 7).

The other valid mixed hypothetical syllogism is in the negative form. Called *modus tollens,* it is given below:

premise 1	If P then Q
premise 2	Not Q
conclusion	Not P (valid)

Example:
premise 1	If it is an enzyme, then it is a protein.
premise 2	It is not a protein.
conclusion	It is not an enzyme.

The fallacy associated with *modus tollens* is the fallacy of denying the antecedent:

If it is an enzyme, then it is a protein.
It is not an enzyme.
It is not a protein (invalid).

The pure hypothetical syllogism

A pure hypothetical syllogism has the following structure:

premise 1	If P then Q
premise 2	If Q then R
conclusion	If P then R

Example:
premise 1	If it is an enzyme, then it is a protein.
premise 2	If it is a protein, then it contains amino acids.
conclusion	If it is an enzyme, then it contains amino acids (valid).

The disjunctive (alternative) syllogism

A valid disjunctive syllogism takes the form:

premise 1	Either P or Q
premise 2	Not Q
conclusion	P

Example:
premise 1	Either Jones is a boy, or Jones is a girl (a disjunctive premise).
premise 2	Jones is not a girl (a categorical premise).
conclusion	Therefore, Jones is a boy.

The disjunctive (either/or) proposition states that at least one (and possibly both) of its components is true. The disjunctive syllogism is valid only where the categorical premises (eg, Jones is not a girl) contradict one part of the disjunctive premise, and the conclusion affirms the other part.

The disjunctive syllogism is widely used in scientific reasoning. For example, should several plausible hypotheses be tested and all but one found not to be true, they would be eliminated, and the remaining hypothesis would be accepted. In statistical hypothesis testing, it is assumed that there are only two hypotheses: the null hypothesis and the alternative hypothesis. The null hypothesis is tested so that it can be rejected and the alternative hypothesis accepted. The major fallacy associated with the use of the disjunctive syllogism is the *UFO fallacy* (see chapter 8), where the list of possible alternatives is not exhausted in the premises.

Chains

Arguments can be linked together so that the conclusion of one syllogism is a premise of a subsequent syllogism. Clearly, the chain is only as strong as its weakest link.

Suppressed premises

Some arguments contain only two terms: a premise and a conclusion. For example, since all enzymes are proteins (premise), they are interesting to study (conclusion). To make this conclusion valid, a second premise must be true; namely, all proteins are interesting to study.

Suppressed premises occur frequently in scientific papers, and in everyday reasoning, because many people do not like to belabor obvious truths. However, a good strategy for hiding a weak point in an argument is to use a suppressed premise, simply because a weakness not stated directly is difficult to detect. Suppressed premises can occur in scientific papers as additional information that is needed, but is not supplied, to correctly interpret a statement. In most cases, the author believes that the information is so widely known there is no need to state it directly. For example, the most widely quoted paper in biomedical research is the method by Lowry et al[16] for the determination of protein. The authors note that the amount of color obtained with the method varies with different proteins. The suppressed premise of those who have used the method is that the color-producing qualities of their protein sample are the same as those of the protein (normally bovine serum albumin) used in the calibration of a standard curve. In some situations (eg, in solutions containing collagen) it would be unlikely for this assumption to be true.

A major problem of an argument with a suspected suppressed premise is determining what the suppressed premise is. For the argument to be sound, the suppressed premise, together with the expressed premise, must yield a valid conclusion. But there may be several ways for an argument to be framed.

Before accusing an author (or speaker) of any particular suppressed premise or error in logic, the lack of precision of logical form in everyday language prescribes trying various forms of statement (ie, categorical, hypothetical, disjunctive syllogisms) to test for more than one way of expressing the missing premise so that a valid argument still results.[8]

Occurrence and sources of error in deductive logic

Deductive logic is sufficiently complex that it is easy to make errors. When subjects were asked to evaluate deductive arguments, the following kinds of errors were distinguished[17,18]:

1. Failure to accept the logical task. Many people fail to distinguish between a conclusion that is logically valid and one that is factually correct. These people evaluated the conclusion and not the logical form of the argument.
2. Restatement of a premise or conclusion so that the intended meaning is changed. Many subjects interpret propositions (such as, all As are Bs) to mean that the converse is true (all Bs are As).
3. Omission or addition of a premise.
4. Misinterpretation of a statement of the form no As are Bs (E statement) to mean that nothing has been proved.
5. Probabilistic inference (ie, reasoning that things with common qualities or effects are likely to be the same) accounted for many errors. This error can occur when rule 2 for valid syllogisms (ie, the middle term must be distributed at least once) is violated.

Most of these errors are errors in the validity of the logic, not the truth of the premises. A second group of fallacies argue from a false premise (see chapter 8). These arguments are so common and have persisted for so long that they may be viewed as being traditional fallacies.

The Value of a Formal Analysis of Arguments

Having worked through this chapter, the reader may be wondering whether it was worth the effort. Although truth tables and Venn diagrams figure highly in logic textbooks, they are not normally found in the *Journal of Dental Research*. Moreover, it might be argued, deductive logic will not tell us anything new; that is, it will not tell us anything that was not already contained in the premises. While true, these considerations overlook the value of the process. In analyzing an argument, a researcher must determine the premises and the conclusions and consider carefully how terms are used. Formal analysis of arguments enables the researcher to see if premises are missing and, by setting the premises apart, forces the researcher to consider whether they are plausible. Finally, the validity of the logic can be assessed in a straightforward manner to determine when the premises are true if the conclusions are binding.

References

1. Medawar PB. Induction and Intuition in Scientific Thought. London: Methuen, 1969:48.
2. Salmon WC. Logic. Englewood Cliffs, NJ: Prentice Hall, 1963:1.
3. Adler MJ, Van Doren C. How to Read a Book. New York: Simon and Schuster, 1963:162.
4. Fisher A. The Logic of Real Arguments. Cambridge: Cambridge Univ Press, 1988:136–138.
5. Fisher A. The Logic of Real Arguments. Cambridge: Cambridge Univ Press, 1988:22.
6. Fisher A. The Logic of Real Arguments. Cambridge: Cambridge Univ Press, 1988:27.
7. Chapman LJ, Chapman JP. Atmosphere effect re-examined. In: Wason PC, Johnson Laird PN (eds). Thinking and Reasoning. Harmondsworth: Penguin, 1959:83.
8. Copi IM. Introduction to Logic, ed 4. New York: MacMillan, 1972.
9. Salmon WC. Logic. Englewood Cliffs, NJ: Prentice Hall, 1963.
10. Capaldi N. The Art of Deception. New York: Brown, 1971.
11. Beardsley MC. Writing with Reason. Englewood Cliffs, NJ: Prentice Hall, 1976.
12. Gilbert MA. How to Win an Argument. New York: McGraw Hill, 1979:28–39.
13. Fowler WS. The Development of Scientific Method. Oxford: Pergamon, 1967:17–36.
14. Watson JD, Frick FHC. Molecular structure of nucleic acids: A structure for dexyribose nucleic acid. Nature 1953;248:765.
15. Iversen OH. Comments on "chalones and cancer." Mech Ageing Dev 1980;12:211.
16. Lowry OH, Rosebrough NJ, Farr AL, Randall RJ. Protein measurement with the Folin reagent. J Biol Chem 1951;193:265.
17. Henle M. On the relation between logic and thinking. Psychol Rev 1962;69:366.
18. Chapman LJ, Chapman JP. Atmosphere effect re-examined. J Exp Psychol 1959;58:220.

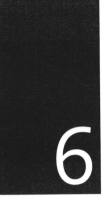

6 Introduction to Abductive and Inductive Logic: Analogy, Models, and Authority

"Did you observe his knuckles?. . . Thick and horny in a way which is quite new in my experience. Always look at the hands first, Watson. Then cuffs, trouserknees, and boots. Very curious knuckles which can only be explained by the mode of progression observed by—" Holmes paused and suddenly clapped his hand to his forehead. "Oh, Watson, Watson, what a fool I have been! It seems incredible, and yet it must be true. All points in one direction. How could I miss seeing the connection of ideas? Those knuckles how could I have passed those knuckles?"

—Sir Arthur Conan Doyle[1]
From *The Adventure of the Creeping Man*

The purpose of studying logic for the analysis of scientific papers is to evaluate the strength of the conclusions in relation to the evidence offered for their support. Deductive logic makes explicit the content of the premises and clarifies the relationship between the terms, but it does not yield anything new. Inductive and abductive arguments have conclusions whose content exceeds that of the premises and, for that reason, are never certain.

Abduction and Scientific Discovery

Abduction is defined as reasoning that accepts a conclusion on the grounds that it explains the evidence.[2] The term was proposed by Charles Sanders Peirce, the originator of pragmatism, who described himself as a "laboratory professor" and whom some consider the greatest American philosopher. He used the word *abduction* to address a variety of issues from the logic of discovery to the economics of research.[2] In essence, abduction as a logic of discovery posits that when an unfamiliar natural phenomenon is observed, a scientific investigator typically hypothesizes an explanation out of all the theoretically possible explanations. In general, scientists make choices with some valid basis;

otherwise, the task of formulating and testing hypotheses would be endless.[3]

Abduction can be considered a form of inference, like deduction and induction, but if the best available evidence is weak, it is a weak form of inference. Weinreb[3] distinguishes *abduction* from *deduction* and *induction* as follows:

> The truth of the premises combined with valid or correct form make deductive and inductive arguments certain or probable, respectively; whereas the truth of the premises of an abductive argument makes the truth of the conclusion *possible*.

In *The Adventure of the Creeping Man*,[1] Sherlock Holmes observes that 61-year-old Professor Presbury has taken on apelike abilities and behaviors. Using abduction, Holmes reasons that the apelike behavior was produced by monkey-gland extracts, for Holmes had discovered that Presbury had obtained monkey-gland serum in an attempt to rejuvenate himself. The motive for his treatment was that Presbury had become engaged to Miss Morphy, a young woman perfect in both mind and body. Holmes notes that her father (Professor Morphy) had not objected to the engagement, as Presbury was rich. To modern readers, the conclusion that monkey-gland serum could produce apelike behavior is pure science fiction,[4] but, in that era, gland extracts were viewed as a possible means of rejuvenescence. Sherlock Holmes' name is often associated with deduction, but many of his "deductions" were actually instances of creative abduction.[3,5,6] In such instances, his conclusions were by no means certain. Based on this story—in which one professor injects himself with mysterious serum to become virile and apelike, and another allows his daughter to be engaged to a rich man very much her senior—the reader might conclude through abduction that Doyle did not think highly of professors.

Induction

This section considers some common forms of inductive reasoning and some of the fallacies associated with them. In evaluating inductive logic, the term *acceptable* or *correct* is used in place of the term *valid*. *Valid* implies that the truth of the premises guarantees the truth of the conclusion, which is never the case for inductive logic. There are three rules that may be applied to test the acceptability of the conclusion of an inductive argument.[7]

1. The premises are true.
2. The argument has correct form.
3. The premises of the argument embody all available relevant evidence.

The role of additional evidence in inductive logic

In contrast with deductive arguments, which are self-contained, additional evidence is relevant to inductive arguments. Consider Doug, who is a dentist enrolled in a PhD program.

Argument A:
premises
1. 90% of dentists earn over $20,000 per year.
2. Doug is a dentist.
inductive conclusion Doug probably earns over $20,000 per year.

Argument B:
premises
1. 90% of graduate students earn less than $20,000 per year.
2. Doug is a graduate student.
inductive conclusion Doug probably earns less than $20,000 per year.

Arguments A and B both have correct inductive form and true premises, but they contradict one another. The difficulty is that neither A nor B uses all of the relevant evidence on Doug's income. Hence, we must weigh the available evidence, or recombine it into a more suitable form, so that all the information is used.

An important aspect of the role additional evidence plays in interpreting scientific papers is an *aberration of logic*, which can be described as *proof by selected instances*.[8] In this form of deceit, an argument is claimed to be supported by certain facts that are, in fact, true. But while an argument may contain nothing but facts, it does not necessarily contain all the facts. If facts that are damaging to the conclusion are omitted, then the inductive logic used to arrive at the conclusion is flawed.

Proof by selected instances is used in clinical presentations with selected cases. Clinicians seldom present their failures but often emphasize their successes. In the absence of good experiment design, which includes such factors as method of patient selection, elimination of bias, objective criteria, and comparison groups, such demonstrations of success mean little. Moreover, physicians do not process the absence of cues as efficiently as they process the presence of cues.[9] That is, they are more struck by data in which two markers are correlated positively and may not look for situations where one marker is present and the other is absent.

The data presented in Table 6-1 are taken from a study involving 112 infants.[10] At first glance, these data appear to support the hypothesis that children run a greater risk of caries and infection with *Streptococcus mutans* (the bacteria associated with dental caries) when the mother is infected with *S mutans*. The missing information, however, is the scores of the other 104 children and their mothers. If there were high scores among the mothers whose children did not have caries, the hypothesis would be weakened. If this information were to be omitted, the authors would be telling only part of the story, and the conclusions would be suspect. (Brown et al[10] did report on the *S mutans* scores of all 112 participants in another table.)

Proof by selected instances is also practiced by biomedical scientists. As noted by Trinkhaus,[11] micrographs taken from the ultrathin sections used for electron microscopy show great variability. In consequence, it is easy to find the expected and to disregard the rest. If microscopists publish only pictures that support their conclusions, they are guilty of proof by selected instances. However, proof by selected instances is re-

Table 6-1 Example of incomplete evidence*

Child (< 2 years) with caries	Teeth (no.)	Decayed teeth (no.)	*S mutans* score Infant	Mother
1	6	4	High	Moderate
2	6	4	Moderate	High
3	4	2	High	High
4	10	8	High	High
5	12	2	High	High
6	16	3	High	High
7	16	13	Low	Moderate
8	12	2	Low	High

*Data taken from Brown et al.[10]

ally the practical application of the *law of cognitive response* (see chapter 3), a rhetorical device that advises would-be persuaders to focus attention on data that support one's position.

The requirement to use all available evidence explains the importance attached to the date of an article. As a general rule, a more recently published article is better. Authors writing in 1965 have less evidence available to them than authors writing in 2007. Thus, all other things being equal, the earlier authors are less likely to be correct. It is not necessarily illogical to change your mind. As available evidence changes, so must the conclusions.

Forms of inductive argument

Analogy

A common form of inductive argument is analogy, which has the following form:

premises   1. A (the source) has the properties P_1, P_2, P_3.
2. B (the target) has properties P_1, P_2, P_3.
3. A (the source) also has P_x.
conclusion by analogy   B (the target) also has P_x.

An analogy becomes stronger as the two classes of objects become more similar. For example, it would be better to test drugs intended for human use on monkeys rather than on insects. In general, to whatever extent there are relevant similarities (ie, to the point of the argument), the analogy is strengthened. Relevant differences weaken the argument.

As might be expected of any inductive argument, analogy is not certain, for similarity is not identity. There is always some point at which the analogy will break down. This does not invalidate the argument form, because it is only important that the similarity holds in the respects that are relevant to the argument. Scientific theories have been constructed by analogy. An example of this is the Bohr theory of the atom, originally modeled on the solar system. Murphy[12] has stated that the soundness of an analogy depends on how faithfully the terms of the discussion are translated into symbols, and how faithfully the conclusion from the manipulation of symbols is translated back. In the Bohr model, the symbol represented by an electron as an entity with a discrete locale did not adequately explain some of its properties, and, although useful, the Bohr model has been superceded.

Although it likely appears that analogy is a weak method of inference, it forms the basis of a considerable portion of our legal decisions. A *judicial precedent* has been defined by a former Lord Chancellor as "a judgment or decision of a court of law cited as an authority for deciding a similar state of facts in the same manner, or on the same principle by analogy."[13] Because legal judgments are assumed to be reasonable decisions made by reasonable people, we can conclude that analogy is a useful form of argument. However, like all inductive arguments, analogies must be evaluated in the presence of all available information. It is clear why the rules of evidence are so important to the legal process. If, for instance, relevant information was suppressed, the reasoning process used to arrive at a decision would be unacceptable.

Despite the widespread use of analogy in law, there is an active debate among legal theorists on the soundness of arguments based on analogy, and attempts have been made to transform analogies into frameworks of deduction.[3]

Analogy and scientific discovery

Analogy is frequently used in proposing models to guide investigations, perhaps the most cited example being the Bohr model of the atom, mentioned earlier. As noted by Bell and Staines,[14] analogies are easy to find but difficult to justify. A proponent must show in detail how the phenomena are alike and that the similarity does not derive from an arbitrary choice of a descriptive term. Like any explanation of phenomena, the analogy should make some testable predictions based on independent evidence, in other words, evidence that was not taken into consideration in forming the analogy.

Scientists use analogies frequently in problem solving (3 to 15 analogies in a 1-hour lab meeting); often these analogies are based on superficial features in common.[15] Moreover, scientists use structural analogies when formulating hypotheses, such as comparing gene structure and function between species.[15]

In a paper on treatment of temporomandibular joint disorders, Lous[16] argued as follows:

> Joint stretching is a method of treatment frequently used in physical medicine. In 1955 Bang and Sury described a new principle in the treatment of intervertebral disc lesions. A traction splint . . . was used, and extension of the vertebral column could be demonstrated radiographically. About 50% of the patient group experienced relief of pain and increased range of movement. . . . A similar effect on the temporomandibular joint (TMJ) can be obtained by using spring mechanisms placed between the maxillae and the mandible.

This is a clear case of proposing an experiment based on reasoning by analogy. The analogy suggests that what works for intervertebral disc lesions will work for the TMJ.

Models

Reasoning by analogy in experimental science occurs through the use of models. In principle, a model represents and demonstrates the fundamental principles of the system of interest. Mice carrying the lymphoproliferation (lpr) mutation demonstrate many similarities to people with systemic lupus erythromatosus. It would be reasonable to test the effects of drugs or various immunotherapies on the affected mice, but the fruitfulness of such an approach would depend on how closely the disease of mice resembled that of humans. Other models can be more abstract. Physiologists model systems by writing equations for well-established processes that might be occurring in a system, performing the necessary calculations, and comparing the calculated results to the observed results. A close correspondence between the observations and calculations suggests—but certainly does not prove—that the processes are operating.

All models are simplifications of reality, but the degree of simplicity varies. A conceptual model may be only a basic approximation of what processes might be operative. Physical models are widely used in science; the force distribution of implant designs has been studied by embedding the implants in plastic and using polarized light to observe stress patterns. Ideally, as in the physical sciences and engineering, modeling can comprise writing equations for well-established processes from prior theoretical knowledge. Models can often provide an explanation for a vast range of observed facts; in some instances, the explanatory scheme is so realistic that it can be called a *mechanism*. Additionally, an empirical approach to represent cause-effect relationships from experimental data sometimes is used in modeling. Where there is a lack of understanding about mechanisms or processes, a common approach is the black-box model, which does not rely on any intuitive interpretation in terms of the actual processes occurring in the black box; it merely relates input to output. Often, relating the input to output is done mathematically by the use of transfer functions, such as those devised by Laplace and Fourier.[17] This model is valuable, because it enables scientists to make accurate predictions in the absence of total understanding.

There are sophisticated statistical means to test hypotheses and validate quantitative models. In periodontics, there has been much discussion of whether attachment-level changes occur in bursts or gradually. The decision of which model is operative is important, because it has implications for how a clinician should treat the disease. There are generally two criteria for model selection: (1) hypothesis testing, and (2) cross-validation.[17–19] In the hypothesis-testing approach, the model with the greater prevalence is put forward as the null hypothesis, and other models are tested as alternative hypotheses. The advantage of this method is that there is only a small chance to accept a more complex or less prevalent model; the disadvantage is that it favors the prevalent models. In the cross-validation approach, all models are considered equal, and the best model is the one that produces the minimum-error least-squares fit to the data when each data point is excluded sequentially and fitted with the model and the remaining data. In a study using the cross-validation technique, Yang et al[18] found that neither the burst nor the gradual-loss models were good predictors of change in attachment level of subjects with moderate-to-severe periodontal disease. Yang et al[18] also used the black-box approach, where the operator inside the black box was an autoregressive time-series model—that is, the past behavior of the site was used to predict its future. Sadly, they found that a model that fits well to past data cannot be accurately extended into the future. Thus, their findings illustrate the principle familiar to economists that "he who lives by the crystal ball will often have to eat shattered glass." A problem with models is that particular assumptions that underlie a model's use may not be valid. In the periodontics black-box study, like many economic forecasts, the assumption was that the processes that operated in the past would continue to operate in the future. Such an assumption may well be valid for brief periods, but could be unreliable over extended periods.

Argument from authority

In the discussion section of scientific papers, it is not unusual to see a statement such as, "Jones concluded that . . ."—usually an attempt to support a conclusion by virtue of the reliability of the person (or institution) making the statement. This is not necessarily good proof. Lord Kelvin, although widely acknowledged as a great scientist in his own time, pronounced shortly after their discovery that x-rays were an elaborate hoax,[20] illustrating that in science the best appeal is not to *authority* but to *observation*. The ultimate test of any statement must be observation. However, an appeal to authority is not necessarily wrong simply because it is not necessarily sound. Reasonable people make reasonable conclusions. If an authority has based judgment on objective evidence that could be examined and verified by any competent person, then such an authority is considered reliable. The format for the legitimate use of the argument from authority is given below.

premises	1. A is a reliable authority on subject X (that is, the vast majority of statements made by A on subject X are true).
	2. S is a statement made by A on subject X.

conclusion	S is probably true.

The most common ways that the argument from authority is misused are listed below[21]:

1. The authority may be misquoted or misinterpreted, or a statement may be used out of context. For this reason, when an appeal to authority is made, the source should be documented.

2. The authority may have no special competence in the subject under discussion. This misuse of appeal to authority often occurs in advertisements. Mickey Mantle, who was a great athlete, used to promote treatments for athlete's foot, but, as far as I know, he had no special knowledge of mycology. In 1970, Linus Pauling, a two-time Nobel Prize winner, strongly advocated the use of vitamin C to cure the common cold. Many people believed that such an eminent scientist must be right. By 1979, however, numerous tests had demonstrated that vitamin C does not significantly affect the course of the common cold.[22] Pauling was an expert, but an expert in chemistry, not nutrition or pharmacology.

3. Authorities may express opinions about matters that have no available evidence. This is not legitimate, for one attribute of a reliable authority is that such an authority is evaluating objective evidence.

4. Authorities can disagree. If scientists quote only the authorities with whom they agree, they bias the evidence, and the appeal to authority is not legitimate. It is difficult to pick up this type of misuse unless a reader knows the literature well. In legal cases involving expert witnesses, a good strategy is for a lawyer to employ an expert who holds an opposing view to the expert employed by the opponent. If authorities disagree, the appeal to authority is weakened. A reliable authority is one who holds views that are representative of her field; if there is controversy, it is proper to cite the arguments for both sides of the issue.

5. An authority may have an axe to grind. Chapter 3, on rhetoric, illustrated that communicator credibility is enhanced by appearing to argue against self-interest, but the converse is also true. It is reasonable to be skeptical if an authority stands to gain something by having a view accepted. A common tactic for a lawyer questioning an opponent's expert witness is to inquire whether the expert is being paid, as this self-interest will reduce credibility.

6. The authority must be current. I once knew a very engaging and articulate dentist who made a decent living as an expert witness. His reputation was based

on a paper he had published 40 years earlier. Armed with this paper and an academic position, he was able to convince judges of his expertise, yet his knowledge (and presumably his testimony) could not be authoritative, as he had little knowledge of current developments in his field.

The book *Eat to Win* by Haas achieved considerable popularity, a fact that is not surprising, as most people like to eat and like to win. The book's popularity was further enhanced, when tennis star Martina Navratilova credited her success to Haas's program. Haas's credentials, however, include a PhD from Columbia Pacific University, an unaccredited institution that offers nonresident doctoral degrees in 1 year or less by receiving credit for "life, work, and all learning experiences."[23] Knowledgeable reviewers of Haas's work do not recommend the book, as it contains many basic errors and misconceptions.[23] Other books on health or nutrition depend for their credibility on the MD after the author's name. Remember the old joke:

Q: If the person who graduates at the bottom of the West Point class is called the *goat,* what do they call the person who graduates at the bottom of the medical class?
A: *Doctor.*

Despite these problems with the use of authority, scientists regularly defer to the knowledge of experts.[24] Biochemists, for example, may rely on the findings of crystallographers, even though they do not understand the principles and practices of that discipline. A problem with the spread of a multidisciplinary approach is that no single author of a paper may be able to justify intellectually the entire contents of an article—a desideratum, if not a requirement, for authorship. A Nobel laureate involved in a case involving a colleague's fraud lamented, "one has to trust one's collaborators"[25]; such trust may be required, because the expertise to assess the data may not be present in some of the authors. Argument by authority, then, appears to be a sort of necessary evil in the complex world of modern science.

References

1. Doyle AC. The Adventure of the Creeping Man. Available at: http://sherlock-holmes.classic-literature. co.uk/the-adventure-of-the-creeping-man/. Accessed May 31, 2007.
2. Hookway CJ. Peirce, Charles Sanders. In: Honderich T (ed). The Oxford Companion to Philosophy. Oxford: Oxford Univ Press, 1995, 648–651.
3. Weinreb LL. Legal Reason: The Use of Analogy in Legal Argument. New York: Cambridge Univ Press, 2005:21–23.
4. Van Liere EJ. The physiological Doctor Watson. Physiol 1958;1(2):53–57.
5. Harrowitz N. The body of the detective model: Charles S Peirce and Edgar Allan Poe. In: Eco V, Sebok TE. The Sign of Three: Dupin, Holmes, and Peirce. Bloomington, IN: Univ of Indiana Press, 1988:179–197.
6. Eco V. Horns, hooves, insteps. Some hypotheses on three types of abduction. In: Eco V, Sebok TE. The Sign of Three: Dupin, Holmes, and Peirce. Bloomington, IN: Univ of Indiana Press, 1988:198–230.
7. Salmon WC. Inductive logic. In: Logic. Englewood Cliffs, NJ: Prentice Hall, 1963:53–58.
8. Thouless RH. Straight and Crooked Thinking. London: Pan, 1974:32.
9. Christensen-Szalanski JJ, Bushyhead JB. Physician's use of probabilistic information in a real clinical setting. J Exp Psychol Hum Percept Perform 1981;7:928.
10. Brown JP, Junner C, Liew V. A study of *Streptococcus mutans* levels in both infants with bottle caries and their mothers. Aust Dent J 1985;30:96–98.
11. Trinkhaus JP. Cells into Organs. Englewood Cliffs, NJ: Prentice Hall, 1984:7.
12. Murphy EA. A Companion to Medical Statistics. Baltimore: Johns Hopkins Univ Press, 1985:25.
13. Jowitt WA. Dictionary of English Law. London: Sweet and Maxwell, 1959:1385.
14. Bell PB, Staines PJ. Reasoning and Argument in Psychology. London: Routledge and Kegan, 1979:104.
15. Dunbar K, Blanchette I. The in vivo/in vitro approach to cognition: The case of analogy. Trends Cogn Sci 2001;5:334.
16. Lous I. Treatment of TMJ syndrome by pivots. J Prosthet Dent 1978;40:179–182.
17. Hall CW. Errors in Experimentation. Champaign, IL: Matrix, 1977.
18. Yang MC, Marks RH, Clark WB, Magnusson I. Predictive power of various models for longitudinal attachment level change. J Clin Periodontol 1992;19:77–83.
19. Spilker B. Guide to Clinical Interpretation of Data. New York: Raven Press, 1986.
20. Kuhn TS. The Structure of Scientific Revolutions, ed 2. Chicago: Univ of Chicago Press, 1970:59.
21. Salmon WC. Logic. Englewood Cliffs, NJ: Prentice Hall, 1963:63–67.
22. Coulehan JL. Ascorbic acid and the common cold: Reviewing the evidence. Postgrad Med 1979;66:153.
23. Barr SI. Eat to win: An opinion. BC Runner 1985;2:3.
24. Koslowski B. Theroy and Evidence of the Development of Scientific Reasoning. Cambridge, MA: MIT Press, 1996:82.
25. Cited in Judson, HF. The Great Betrayal: Fraud in Science. Orlando: Harcourt, 2004:292.

7 | Inductive Logic: Hypothesis and Causation

Hypothetical Inference

The conclusions of scientific research can be regarded as provisional explanations or *hypotheses*. It is worth discussing the logic of hypothetical inference in detail, because formal hypotheses play a central role in descriptions of scientific method. Moreover, the most common means of criticizing scientific papers is by formulating alternative explanations of the data. Understanding the structure of the underlying reasoning shows why this approach is so effective. An excellent discussion of this topic can be found in Hempel,[1] on which much of this chapter is based.

For the purposes of logical analysis, the testing of hypotheses can be expressed using conditional statements. Conditional statements have the form: Let there be a hypothesis H, which implies a certain event E. If H then E, where H is called the *antecedent* and E the *consequent*.

premise 1	If H then E.
premise 2	E is true.
conclusion	It becomes more credible that H is true.

Example:
premise 1	If Emil killed the cat, then it has stopped breathing.
premise 2	The cat has stopped breathing.
conclusion	It becomes more credible that Emil killed the cat.

The fact that the cat has stopped breathing makes the statement "Emil killed the cat" possible, and hence more credible, than if the cat were alive. But other explanations are possible: the animal could have died of natural causes, some other person could have killed it, etc. In this reasoning, note that the consequent (the cat has stopped breathing) is affirmed and is used to infer the truth of the antecedent. By deductive reasoning, this argument is fallacious, because the conclusion is not necessarily true even when the premises are true. Thus, in logic textbooks, this type of argument, which is a fallacy, is sufficiently common that it has been given a name: the *fallacy of affirming the consequent*.

You can reduce the uncertainty of the inductive reasoning process by gathering more information. It is particularly effective if the hypothesis H implies other events.

Example:
event 1	If Emil killed the cat, then he will look guilty.
event 2	If Emil killed the cat, then he will have cat fur on his hands.

If each of these events in turn is found to be true, then the hypothesis becomes progressively more credible, although an absolute magnitude of its credibility is not determined.

The example of Emil and the cat was chosen to illustrate the uncertainty of this form of inductive reasoning, but often it is difficult to see the uncertainty of the logic because of the high probability of the statements. Consider the following:

premise 1	If this is a fair die, the ace will appear one sixth of the time.
premise 2	The ace has appeared one sixth of the time.
conclusion	It becomes more credible that this die is a fair die.

On the surface, this appears to be a legitimate argument, but a statistician would not be satisfied. An expert would want to know how many times the die had been thrown, for if premise 2 were based on just six throws of the die, the evidence that it was fair (or for that matter unfair) would be weak. The argument could then be attacked by constructing an alternative argument that would also fit the information: "If this die is loaded, then it is not unlikely that (if only a few tosses of the die were made) the ace might turn up one sixth of the time." This example illustrates the role of specialized knowledge in the criticism of scientific work; it enables alternative explanations to be suggested for a given phenomenon.

Disproving hypotheses

Although we cannot prove that a hypothesis is true, we can prove rigorously that it is false.

Consider the following:

premise 1	If H is true, then so is E.
premise 2	Not E.
conclusion	H is not true.

This is a deductively valid argument called *modus tollens*, in which the conclusion is sound if the premises are true (see chapter 5). Hence, it is possible to disprove a hypothesis rigorously. To return to our example:

premise 1	If Emil killed the cat, then it has stopped breathing.
premise 2	The cat has not stopped breathing.
conclusion	Emil has not killed the cat.

Although the disproof of a hypothesis can be logically rigorous, another problem remains. When you state that an event (E) has not occurred, you can only do this within the limits of detection that are set by the observational conditions. That is, the statement *Not E* is susceptible to two interpretations: *(1)* E did not occur and the conclusion is sound, or *(2)* E occurred but could not be detected by the observational conditions used, in which case the conclusion is not sound.

Investigations in dental science sometimes report that there was no difference between treated patients and control subjects. But an observed result of no difference between treated and control groups could mean many different things, including:

1. There really is no difference.
2. There is a difference, but the measurement techniques used were too insensitive to detect the difference.
3. There was no difference in the particular patients used in the study, but selection of a different type of patient may yield a different result.
4. The treatment was not applied properly.

The list could continue. Because failure to observe something can be explained in many ways, some journals refuse to publish papers based entirely on negative findings.

Auxiliary hypotheses

People do not like being wrong. When the available evidence indicates that their favored hypothesis is wrong, scientists often devise ingenious explanations. Such explanations may be possible, because the hypothesis was not tested directly but was tested by a method that required another hypothesis to be true as well. Suppose that a researcher had a belief that recurrent caries were more common under composite fillings than under amalgam. To test this hypothesis, the researcher examined the radiographs of patients who had received the two types of filling but found no difference. At first glance, it appears that the hypothesis must be rejected; however, there is a way out, which can be seen by putting the arguments into a standard format:

premise 1	If both H and H-1 are true, then so is A.
premise 2	A is not true.
conclusion	H and H-1 are both not true.

Example:

premise 1	If there is an effect of restorative material on recurrent caries (H) and all recurrent caries can be detected on radiographs (H-1), then we will see more caries under some materials.
premise 2	No effect was seen; ie, there was no statistical difference in the number of caries found under different types of restoration.
conclusion	It is not possible that there is both an effect of restorative material and that all recurrent caries are detected on radiographs.

It still can be maintained that there is a difference between the materials (ie, H is true), because it is possible that not all recurrent caries are detected on radiographs (that is, H-1 is false). H-1 (in this case, the hypothesis that your measuring technique is valid) is called an *auxiliary hypothesis*. The initial hypothesis can be defended by denying the truth of the auxiliary hypothesis. Thus, by adding auxiliary hypotheses, a favorite hypothesis can be protected from rejection. However, the overuse of this method weakens the credibility of the original hypothesis. Hypotheses of this kind, called *ad hoc hypotheses*, are particularly bad if they are arranged only to explain particular results and lead to no additional test implications.

Hypotheses relating to cause and effect

Common sense and David Hume

The poet e. e. Cummings wrote that "All causes are lost causes; otherwise they would be effects." But science is pragmatic, and scientists are pragmatists who must identify cause-effect relationships. Many experiments are designed to find out the causes, or at least the conditions, that will bring about a certain effect. Francis Bacon is often quoted in this regard as saying, "Knowledge is power and the aim of science is the production of the means." The belief underlying many experiments is what might be called the *commonsense view of causality*, which rests on the faith of the regularity or uniformity of nature. It has two tenets:

1. An identical cause will always produce an identical effect; thus, experiments can be repeated.
2. There is a reason for any change; events do not occur at the whim of the gods. For example, the appearance of disease must be caused by some change in either the internal milieu of the body or the environment.

The British empirical philosopher David Hume clearly defined why people attach cause-effect relationships to a series of events (although he denied that there could be any logical validity in our conception of cause and effect).[2,3] In his *Treatise on Human Nature*, Hume listed eight principles often used to establish causes for effects. Hume's treatise even included such concepts as a dose-response relationship, using an example of the amount of heat and the response of pain or pleasure. For simple situations, however, Hume's principles can be condensed to three rules for investigating cause-effect relationships:

1. The cause preceded the effect in time.
2. The cause and effect are contiguous in time and place, that is, a connection must exist between the two events that explains how they are connected causally.

3. Repeated conjunction; ie, there is a history of regularity in the relationship of the cause and the effect.

The third condition is often the most decisive. It foreshadowed the use of probability theory and associated measures by modern epidemiologists, which to a large extent have replaced the simple cause-effect conception.

Necessary vs sufficient conditions

In discussing cause-effect relationships, different types of causes have been noted:

1. A *necessary condition* is a condition that must be present to obtain an effect. One of the necessary conditions for dental caries is the presence of bacteria. If the necessary conditions of an event are known, it can be prevented from happening, simply by removing one condition. To prevent caries, we attempt to remove bacteria.
2. A *sufficient condition* is a condition that automatically leads to another event. The difference between the necessary and the sufficient condition is that although a necessary condition must be present, it alone will not necessarily produce the effect; a sufficient condition is sufficient to produce the effect by itself. In some cases, a sufficient condition is really a set of necessary conditions, all of which must be present at the same time and place. Dental caries, for example, are the result of the interaction of diet and bacteria in a suitable host.

Causal factors/contributory causes

Conditions that may be neither necessary nor sufficient conditions, but which, nevertheless, stand in a causal relationship to the phenomenon, are called *causal factors* or *contributory causes*. Consider the relationship between cigarette smoking and lung cancer. Both retrospective and prospective studies have demonstrated a statistical link between smoking and lung cancer. However, as noted by Stone[4]:

1. Many people who smoke do not contract lung cancer; therefore, smoking is not a sufficient cause.
2. Some people who do not smoke do contract lung cancer; therefore, smoking is not a necessary cause.

However, it remains possible that:

1. Smoking is one of a group of causal factors that is sufficient for lung cancer.

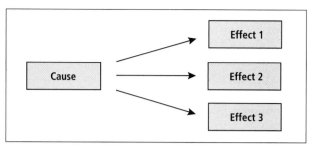

Fig 7-1 Pleiotropy. A single cause produces multiple effects.

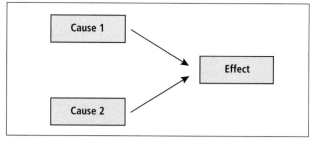

Fig 7-2 Conjunction/interaction. Two or more causes occur together to produce an effect.

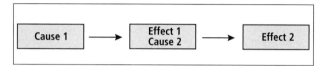

Fig 7-3 Causal chain effect.

2. In some instances, smoking introduces a factor X that may be a necessary and/or sufficient cause.

3. A hidden factor Y exists that may cause both smoking and lung cancer. One might argue that, although improbable, some factor, such as stress, may cause an immediate tendency to smoke cigarettes and a later one to develop cancer.

Patterns of Causation

The concept of causal factors leads us to consider different patterns of causation (discussed in greater detail by Spilker[5]). Various patterns are possible, but only the most common are discussed here.

Direct

A single direct cause produces a single effect. In biology and medicine, *direct causes* are defined as those that act on the same level of organization (eg, cellular, organ, organism) as the effect being measured.[5] Causes that act at different levels of organization are by definition *indirect*. In the clearest instances, the effect occurs immediately. It is common sense that for many phenomena, the longer the interval between the cause and the effect, the less the correlation between

them, because the intervening time presents the opportunity for other events to exert an influence.

Pleiotropy

When a single cause produces multiple effects, it is called *pleiotropy* (Fig 7-1). The triple response of physiology illustrates a single stimulus of pressure producing redness, swelling, and heat. An example of pleiotropy is found in genetic diseases that affect many physiologic systems. If the nature of the genetic disease is unknown, researchers might postulate that a secondary effect is the primary malfunction.[6]

Conjunction/interaction

Two or more causes that necessarily occur together to produce an effect are called *conjunctions* or *interactions* (Fig 7-2). Dental caries form in a susceptible host only if certain bacteria and dietary conditions are present. Conjunctions can also lead to multiple effects.

Chains

In a causal chain, the first cause (C1) leads to the first effect (E1), which in turn leads to a second effect (E2) (Fig 7-3). E1 may be considered an intervening variable and E2 the outcome variable. C1 might not have any

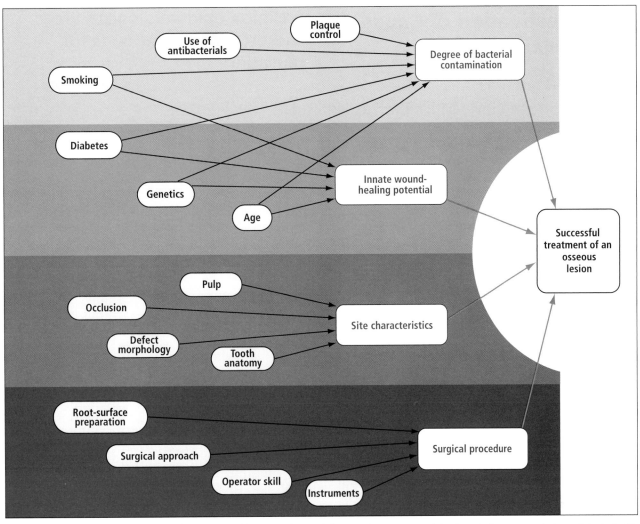

Fig 7-4 Example of a complex cause-effect relationship. Many factors influence the outcome of treatments for osseous lesions. Adapted with permission from Kornman et al.[7]

effect if the link between E1/C2 and E2 were destroyed. An inflamed tooth would activate the trigeminal nerve ganglion, which would lead to the perception of pain. If the ganglion were inactivated—for example, by local anesthetic—there would be no perception of pain.

One problem with chains is that they may branch; that is, sometimes changes in the intervening variable (E1) do not necessarily cause a change in the outcome variable (E2), as was illustrated in the clofibrate example (see chapter 2).

Complex etiology

Complex etiology occurs when multiple direct and indirect causes occur together and, according to Spilker,[5] operates in almost all clinical situations (Fig 7-4). The practical ability to study and effectively interpret a particular phenomenon limits consideration to the major direct cause(s) and few (if any) indirect causes.

The direct investigation of cause-effect relationships is possible, when one causal factor is dominant in the particular situation being investigated. The effect of an antibiotic on a microbial infection may be studied, even though the immune system may also be active against the infection, because, over a short time, the effect of the antibiotic is much greater than the effect of the immune system. In some studies, however, the phenomena under investigation are complex, and possibly have various operative causal factors. In these circumstances, a statistical model may be developed; the adequacy of the model is judged by the proportion of the variance that is explained.

The Investigation of Cause-Effect Relationships

A philosopher's view: Mill's methods

John Stuart Mill developed a number of methods called *canons of induction* for the analysis of causes and effects in certain situations, including the method of agreement, the method of difference, the joint method of agreement and difference, the principle of concomitant variation, and the method of residues. In practice, the canons of induction boil down to one simple rule: Vary one factor at a time, and observe the result.[8] Various means used in an attempt to achieve this ideal will be given in chapter 19, on experiment design.

A microbiologist's view: Koch's postulates

Of continuing interest in periodontology is the traditional method developed by Robert Koch in the late 19th century, which is used to prove that a microorganism has caused a disease. The proof is provided if the following criteria exist:

1. The microorganism must be regularly isolated from cases of the illness.
2. It must be grown in pure culture in vitro.
3. When such a pure culture is inoculated into a susceptible animal species, the typical disease must result.
4. The microorganism again must be isolated from such experimentally induced disease.

Koch's postulates fulfill Hume's criteria. Postulate 1 deals with regularity (Hume's principle 3). Postulate 3 establishes a time sequence (Hume's principle 1) and, at the same time, provides a reason for believing that there is a mechanism whereby the organism can produce the disease (Hume's principle 2). The other two postulates ensure the validity of the microbiologic techniques. Interestingly, Postulate 3 has been criticized as being a tautology, for a susceptible animal is one that is identified by the presence of the disease.[9]

A clinical epidemiologist's view: Sackett's diagnostic tests for causation

The establishment of cause-effect relationships is an exercise in inductive reasoning and can never be certain. Different authorities, then, may require different degrees of certainty. Some members of the cigarette industry might reject medical authorities' conclusions that establish a link between smoking and lung cancer. Technically, they would be correct, because stringent proof of a link would require true experiments in humans, demonstrating the effects of smoking on lung cancer. Such an experiment could not be done ethically, but, using less stringent criteria, reliable authorities have concluded that a link between cancer and smoking exists. Causation is often discussed in relation to the etiology of disease; however, cause-effect reasoning also applies to treatments. A successful treatment, after all, is one in which the treatment caused the success. In the discussion below, the term *outcome of interest* refers to effects that may be desired (as in clinical treatments) or undesired (as in disease). Sackett[10] has proposed and ranked the following nine diagnostic tests for establishing causation. The relative importance of each test is indicated here by the number of stars.

Four-star criterion

1. There should be evidence from true experiments in humans. In true experiments, identical groups of individuals, generated through random allocation, are and are not exposed to the putative causal factor and are observed for the outcome of interest.

Three-star criteria

2. The strength of the association must be determined. In other words, what are the odds favoring the outcome of interest with, as contrasted to without, exposure to the putative cause? The calculation of the strength of association is covered in chapter 17.
3. There must be consistency. Similar studies must have similar findings, as has occurred in the smoking–lung cancer investigations.

Two-star criteria

4. There must be a consistent sequence of events of exposure to the putative cause, followed by the outcome of interest.

5. There must be a gradient of increasing chance of the outcome of interest associated with an increase in dose or exposure to the putative cause.

6. The cause-effect association must make epidemiologic sense. There should be agreement with the current distributions of causes and outcomes.

One-star criteria

7. The cause-effect association should make biologic sense. There should be some mechanism that explains the effects.

8. The cause-effect relationship should be specific. There should be a single cause related to a single effect. (Sackett admits that this criterion is a weak one.)

9. The last and least of Sackett's tests is analogy, the similarity to another previously demonstrated causal relationship.

Sackett's criteria pass Hume's test: criterion 1 deals with temporality; many of Sackett's other criteria relate to Hume's criteria of a history of regularity, and the diagnostic tests of biologic and epidemiologic sense satisfy Hume's criterion 2. In addition, Sackett's criterion 5 is similar to Mill's principle of concomitant variation.

Others might weigh differently the relative importance of the various tests. Nevertheless, I think most would agree that these diagnostic tests can be used to increase the efficiency of a literature review, because they focus the reader's attention on the papers that will shed the strongest light on the causal question.

A pharmacologist's view: Venning's five types of convincing evidence

The criteria for establishing convincing evidence can vary between disciplines. Drug testing has received considerable attention, and criteria have been clearly thought out. Venning[11] proposed five types of convincing evidence for establishing a cause-effect relationship between a drug (cause) and an adverse reaction (effect): (1) rechallenge data, (2) dose-response data, (3) data from controlled studies, (4) experimental data on mechanisms of pathogenesis, and (5) close association in time and space. In his view, strong evidence for an adverse effect comes from (1) uniqueness of the adverse event, (2) extreme rarity of the adverse event

in the absence of drug usage, and (3) improvement after withdrawal without rechallenge. Like Koch's postulates, these criteria incorporate elements specific to the discipline; for pharmacologists, dose-response curves are important. But the criteria also require more elaborate kinds of evidence than the simple time course considered by Hume. As always, the evidence becomes stronger when different techniques or approaches corroborate each other.

Ends and Means

Once a cause-effect relationship is established, the cause can be introduced as a means to acquiring an end that is the cause's effect. For example, the discovery that replacing sucrose with an artificial sweetener in rat diets reduces caries suggests that various products for human consumption might be modified. Sucrose reduction by replacement with artificial sweeteners then might be considered a means to a desirable end (caries reduction).

The first rule in considering whether to introduce a means to obtain an end is to consider the other consequences before adopting the means.[12] In the case of sweeteners, side effects may be a concern; some link saccharin to cancer. Replacing sucrose with saccharin in some products might not be possible, because it requires less bulk to produce the same amount of sweetness. There might be problems in obtaining enough saccharin or finding new jobs for sugar workers. This list of possibilities could continue, but only after considering all the possible consequences can a wise decision be made.

The second rule of contemplating ends and means is to consider the alternative means to attaining the desired end. In the example, different artificial sweeteners, such as aspartame or sorbitol, or different methods of reducing sucrose intake, might be examined.

A commonsense view of explanation

Insofar as hypotheses represent provisional explanations of observations, it is worth examining *explanation*. Beardsley[12] has outlined the process of explanation. In brief, there are three essential ingredients:

1. Something to be explained, termed the *explainee*; eg, pain in a tooth.
2. Something that does the explaining, termed the *explainer*; eg, presence of deep decay and pulpal irritation.
3. A conditional bridge that links the explainee and the explainer; eg, if there is deep decay and pulpal irritation, the tooth will be painful.

Selecting the right explanation depends on systematically ruling out the various alternatives. In our example, there are explainers besides decay, such as gingival recession, which could produce sensitivity in the tooth in appropriate circumstances. Some explainers are simply not possible, and some could be ruled out by direct examination. If explainers contradict the facts, they could be rejected (eg, if no decay were found on the tooth). Other explanations might fail because the conditional bridge is weak. Explaining the pain in the tooth by means of the phase of the moon would stretch credulity. When the obvious faulty explanations have been ruled out, the problem becomes that of choosing between possible explainers. In a commonsense approach, Beardsley[11] recommends asking three questions:

1. *How common is the explainer?* Some explainers could be rejected because they are so rare. Pain in a tooth may be referred pain from other sources, but this happens so rarely that one is unlikely to encounter it. Dental decay, on the other hand, is common. The most common explainer may not locate the truth, but it is a good place to start looking.
2. *How simple is the explanation?* Perhaps the tooth pain could be explained by the possibility of an electrochemical interaction between the amalgam fillings and other restorations in the mouth. Such an explanation might require specific concentrations of materials in the restorations, particular properties of the saliva, and a particular kind of diet. The logical principle to follow is to reject the more complicated explanation if a simpler one can do the job.
3. *Does the explanation check out?* If the explanation is correct, it has consequences that can be tested. In the example, gingival recession can lead to pain in a tooth, but such pain is caused by exposed dentin and has different characteristics from the pain associated with decay.

Evaluation of scientific hypotheses

Aspects of this commonsense approach to evaluating explanations are found in the evaluation of scientific hypotheses. A useful hypothesis must have the following characteristics[1]:

1. *Internally consistent.* The hypothesis should not contradict itself on any specific question. Consider the problems of long-distance romances as analyzed by folk wisdom. On the one hand, it is said that "absence doth the heart make fonder," but, on the other hand, it is said that "out of sight is out of mind." Folk wisdom is not internally consistent; a scientific hypothesis, however, must not contradict itself.
2. *Comprehensive.* The hypothesis should explain all known relevant facts. A hypothesis is supported more strongly if a variety of tests or data agree with the predictions. A proven hypothesis's support is strengthened by the variety of tests, because the more diverse the possibilities covered, the greater the chance of the hypothesis having been falsified.
3. *Testable.* The experiments or observations that test the hypothesis must be feasible. I attended a lecture in 1972 where an economist, after careful consideration of rates of oil use and available supply, predicted the world would run out of oil in 1980. The economist, of course, was wrong, but his hypothesis was good in the sense that it could be tested. Either there would be oil and gas available in 1980 or there would not. For science to progress, a useful hypothesis must do more than simply restate the data. It must extend our understanding by predicting results under conditions that have not yet been observed. If the conditions cannot be realized, then the hypothesis is useless.

   The logician Popper,[13] who is credited with developing our modern conception of scientific method, has argued, "Simple statements, if knowledge is our object, are to be prized more than less simple ones because their empirical content is greater and because they are testable." Indeed, Popper's comparison of the works of Freud and Einstein led him to his important concept that falsifiability of a hypothesis was the key element in scientific method. Freud's theories were sufficiently flexible that they could be adjusted to explain everything; there was no way of testing them. But Einstein's theory of relativity made some startling and precise predictions that could have been (but were not) disproved.[14]
4. *Simple.* Attempts to explain the logical basis for this criterion have not been entirely successful, but it

Box 7-1 Common objections to hypotheses[17]

General principle: Most objections extend the reasoner's current model of the situation under consideration.

1. Challenge to definitions and terms

Hypothesis	If A then B.
Objection	No, that depends on what you mean by A (or B).
Example	Debates and differing criteria on what constituted periodontal disease—1, 2, or 3 mm of loss of attachment or gain in pocket depth?

2. Different conclusion

Hypothesis	If A then B.
Objection	No, if A then not B but C instead.
Example	Hypothesis: Johnny hates girls: he puts their pigtails in the ink well.
Objection:	No, Johnny likes girls: that's his way of getting their attention.

3. Different antecedent or cause

Hypothesis	A causes B.
Objection	No (not necessarily), C or D causes (or could cause) B.
Example	Hypothesis: Periodontal disease is caused by Treponema denticola.
Objection:	No, periodontal disease is caused by a variety of gram-negative microbes.

(continued on page 78)

would be difficult to argue that a complex hypothesis is necessarily better than a simple one. The most widespread use of this criterion occurs in statistical evaluation of data, when a significance level (ie, the probability of the result having arisen entirely by chance) is calculated. If this level is higher than a stated level (usually 5%), then the result likely can be explained in terms of random events, and there is no need to postulate any other reason for differences between groups. The use of this criterion is traced back to the theologian William of Ockham, who decreed that one should not multiply causes without reason—a principle known as *Ockham's razor.* Unfortunately, Ockham's razor is not infallible. Many biologic systems have turned out to be more complex than were originally envisaged. Nevertheless, the intuitive idea that simple explanations are usually better than complicated ones has received quantitative support from Bayesian statistical analysis, which shows, in agreement with Popper, that a hypothesis with fewer adjustable parameters has an enhanced posterior probability, because its predictions are sharp.[15]

5. *Novel.* The point of inductive reasoning is to add to knowledge; if the hypothesis does not do this, it is useless.

6. *Successful predictions.* Because the human mind is so ingenious in coming up with explanations for existing data, successful prediction is usually considered stronger support for a hypothesis than the explanation of a number of observations known when the hypothesis was put forward.

A hypothesis that predicts a mathematical relationship between variables is particularly strong, because the precision of the fit of the observed data to the hypothesis can be calculated. This was evident to Isaac Newton, who, it is said,[16] proposed a universe of precision to replace a universe of "more or less." It remains true today, particularly in hard sciences, such as physics or chemistry, where experiments are designed to test hypotheses framed in complex mathematical relationships.

Criticizing hypotheses

A scientific hypothesis is most effectively criticized by proposing a more plausible alternative. As noted previously, this is an area where expert knowledge can be helpful or even critical. Although scientists have specialized expert knowledge, I think they often use the same strategies in criticizing scientific papers that they use in everyday reasoning. Perkins and coworkers[17,18] found that 80% of objections to arguments in everyday reasoning fall into just eight categories. Box 7-1 presents the nine most common objections to hypotheses.

Box 7-1 Common objections to hypotheses[17] *(continued from page 77)*

General principle: Most objections extend the reasoner's current model of the situation under consideration.

4. Interference

Hypothesis	If A then B.
Objection	Normally perhaps, but because of C, B does not follow from A.
Example	Hypothesis: Plaque causes inflammation.
Objection:	Normally it does, but in these immunosuppressed patients, it does not.

5. Irrelevant reasons

Hypothesis	A implies B.
Objection	No, A has little or no bearing on B.
Example	Hypothesis: Gingival recession is the result of aging.
Objection:	No, gingival recession is not the result of aging per se but rather of the exposure of the tissues to plaque for long periods.

6. Too much/too little

Hypothesis	If A then B.
Objection	No, A is too much (or too little) to bring about B.
Example	Hypothesis: Antifluoridationists believe fluoride in water supplies causes fluorosis.
Objection:	Most dentists believe 1 ppm (common in water supplies) is too little fluoride to cause fluorosis.

7. Factor ignored

Hypothesis	If A then B.
Objection	No, the argument ignores factor C, therefore not B.
Example	Caries studies that ignore the age distribution of the subjects.

8. Counter example

Hypothesis	All As are Bs.
Objection	No, here is an A that is not a B.
Example	Hypothesis: All heavy plaque formers have periodontal disease.
Objection:	Eastern Europeans often have lots of plaque but relatively little attachment or alveolar bone loss (apocryphal data).

9. Saving revision

Hypothesis	A does not imply B.
Objection	No, combined with (or taking into account) C, A does imply B.
Example	Hypothesis: Bleeding on probing does not predict attachment loss.
Obejction:	No, but if bleeding on probing occurs three out of four times in succession, then it does predict loss of attachment.

The general principle is that most objections extend the reasoner's current model of the situation under consideration. This approach is well-suited to the criticism of scientific papers by experts on the topic, because such experts might be aware of some factor or consideration that is unknown to the author. I believe that individuals tend to use only a few common objections; for example, some people focus their critiques almost exclusively on definitions of terms. The list is given here so that readers can expand on the techniques they use to generate alternative hypotheses.

Positivism vs Conventionalism

The approach to scientific method outlined in the previous pages is based on a positivist view of the world. In this view, there are laws of nature that are empirical statements describing the real world. Statements made about this world can be either true or false as a matter of fact. Thus, a positivist would hold that there really are such things as atoms or viruses or complex peptides such as thyrotropin releasing hormone (TRH). It is this view that predominates in biomedical, biologic, and most natural sciences. On occasion, however, this model breaks down. In vacuum-tube electronics, electrons are treated as particles, whereas in good crystalline solids, they must be treated as waves.[19] Positivists might have trouble answering the direct question: Is an electron a wave or a particle? The question can be answered through description of the electron in the terms of quantum mechanics, but this is a description that is a long way from our ordinary conception of reality that includes objects like chairs or doorknobs that can be described in terms of direct sense impressions.

Conventionalists argue that it does not matter whether the laws of nature are true or false but rather under what conditions they provide the most economical, fruitful, and illuminating picture of reality. In this view, a successful experiment shows that a certain way of describing the world is useful. Conventionalism assigns to scientific knowledge no higher status than that of being a useful hypothesis.[20]

When a conventionalist anthropologist visited the laboratory of Nobel laureate Guilleman, who was studying TRH, he portrayed the laboratory's activities as "organization of persuasion through literary inscription." He would describe TRH as a fact that was constructed on the basis of inscriptions provided by various instruments, the interpretive and persuasive powers of the scientists in the laboratory, and the acceptance of those interpretations in the larger community of endocrinologists.[20] By contrast, a positivist biochemist would think of the laboratory's work as isolating and sequencing a particular molecule.

Opportunities for conventionalism in dental research: The case for qualitative studies

The vast majority of biochemists would be positivists, but in the social sciences conventionalists would perhaps form the majority. The social sciences deal with *constructs*, unobservable, constructed variables used to label patterns of observable variables. Examples of constructs include dental aptitude, socioeconomic status, and intelligence. Statistical procedures, such as factor analysis and canonical correlations, have been developed to locate constructs. In an editorial in the *Journal of Dental Research*, Chambers[21] argued that dental research should shed some of its positivist outlook centered on life sciences and embrace the methods of the social sciences. Educational research, for example, has experienced a blossoming in qualitative studies.

Despite the methodologic advances, qualitative field research does not figure as largely as it might in dental research. It seems that various aspects of dentistry could best be investigated by this approach, in particular, providing evidence and theories that enable health professionals to understand their clients better as people.

Summary of the Logic of Criticism of Inductive Arguments

The conclusion of many scientific papers often boils down to either proposing a hypothesis that explains the data or stating that no effect was observed. Some articles contain a conclusion that can be considered a hypothesis. We know from the logic of inductive arguments that the hypothesis can be considered as only more or less credible, depending on the strength of the supporting data. Such hypotheses can be criticized by either: (*a*) assessing the data, including techniques, methods of observation, data analysis, or other components of the study; or (*b*) analyzing the logic by formulating a plausible alternative hypothesis that explains the data better than, or at least as well as, the hypothesis put forward by the author.

Other articles deny the truth of some particular statement. I call these "negative results papers." There are various ways that such denials can be made. A paper might state that some treatment did not have any effect. This means that, as the authors are denying the hypothesis, the logic (modus tollens) is valid. Thus, the most effective strategy for criticizing such papers is to question the data. In particular, we often want to determine if the methods used in the study were sensitive enough to conclude reasonably that some event or effect did not occur.

References

1. Hempel CG. The test of a hypothesis: Its logic and its force. In: Philosophy of Natural Science. Englewood Cliffs, NJ: Prentice Hall; 1966:19–46.
2. Fowler WS. Development of Scientific Method. Oxford: Pergamon, 1962:62.
3. Hume DA. Treatise on Human Nature (1739–1740), ed 2, vol 1, section 15. Revised with notes by Nidditch PH. Oxford: Clarendon Press, 1978:173–175.
4. Stone GK. Evidence in Science. Bristol: Wright, 1966:83–86.
5. Spilker B. Guide to the Clinical Interpretation of Data. New York: Raven Press, 1986:19–26.
6. Kolata G. A new approach to cystic fibrosis. Science 1985;228:167.
7. Kornman KS, Robertson PB. Fundamental principles affecting the outcomes of therapy for osseous lesions. Periodontol 2000;22:22–43.
8. Stebbing LS. A Modern Introduction to Logic. London: Methuen, 1942:339.
9. Skrabanek P, McCormick J. Follies and Fallacies in Medicine. Buffalo, NY: Prometheus, 1990:30–31.
10. Sackett DL. Evaluation: Requirements of clinical application. In: Warren KS (ed). Coping with the Biomedical Literature. New York: Praeger, 1981: 123–140.
11. Venning GR. Identification of adverse reactions of new drugs. III. Alerting processes and early warning systems. BMJ 1983;286:458.
12. Beardsley MC. Writing with Reason. Englewood Cliffs, NJ: Prentice Hall, 1976:122–151.
13. Popper KR. The Logic of Scientific Discovery. London: Hutchinson, 1959:142.
14. Magee B. Philosophy and the Real World: An Introduction to Karl Popper. LaSalle, IL: Open Court, 1985:41–42.
15. Jefferys WH, Berger JO. Ockham's razor and bayesian analysis. Am Sci 1992;80:64.
16. Westfall RS. Newton and the fudge factor. Science 1973;179:751.
17. Perkins DN, Allen R, Hafner J. Difficulties in everyday reasoning. In: Maxwell W (ed). Thinking. Philadelphia: Franklin Institute Press, 1983:177.
18. Nickerson RS, Perkins DN, Smith EE. The Teaching of Thinking. Hillsdale, NJ: Erlbaum, 1985:136–140.
19. Ziman J. An Introduction to Science Studies: The Philosophical and Social Aspects of Science and Technology. Cambridge: Cambridge Univ Press, 1984:53.
20. Latour B, Woolgar S. Laboratory Life: The Construction of Scientific Facts. Princeton: Princeton Univ Press, 1986: 43–90.
21. Chambers D. The need for more tools. J Dent Res 1991; 70:1098.

8 | Quacks, Cranks, and Abuses of Logic

We do not think it necessary to prove that a quack medicine is poison; Let the vendor prove it to be sanative.

—Thomas Balrington Macaulay[1]

Three Approaches to Medical Treatment

Three approaches contribute to our understanding of medical treatment: *anecdotal evidence*, the *numerical method*, and the *pathophysiologic approach*. To some extent, these approaches have been in conflict.[2] The first two approaches are empirically driven, while the third is theory driven.

Personal experience related by *anecdote* is reliable when effects are clear, large, and occur quickly. For example, experienced dentists often teach as part-time instructors in dental school clinics, because, among other reasons, they can provide practical know-how that is not easily delivered in lectures. Students can try the techniques recommended by these clinicians and can readily determine whether they work, at least in the short run. However, anecdotal evidence does not work well for many chronic conditions, where the effects are not clear-cut or are expected to occur over the long run.

Another empirical method, the *numerical approach,* developed by Pierre Charles Alexandre Louis in the 1830s, relied on careful observation and the collection of statistics. Louis found, for example, that patients who were bled early in their treatment for typhoid fever fared worse than those who were not—a finding counter to the theories of the day. Opponents of the numerical approach objected to the lack of consideration given to the unique nature of disease in individual patients. The positivist philosopher Auguste Comte suggested that reliance on a "theory of chances" would reduce practitioners to a servile status, whereby they would have to accept ideas imposed upon them by professors who had collected large numbers of observations.[3]

Evidence-based medicine is the heir to the Louis tradition, and, to some extent, it has attracted the same kind of criticisms that Louis endured. For example, Louis' opponents worried about ignoring the uniqueness of each patient and questioned whether data collected on the Paris poor could be applied to private practices treating the affluent. Moreover, at that time, Louis lacked the statistical expertise that informs present-day evidence-based medicine. Nevertheless, concerns persist about the validity of a doctrinaire rules-based approach, based on assessment by panels of experts far removed from the actual patient-physician encounter, which typically involves thoughtful analysis of the underlying mechanisms of disease.[4]

Developed by Claude Bernard, the *pathophysiologic approach* is experiment-driven, deterministic, and reductionist. In this approach, the control of disease depends on an understanding of physiologic and pathologic mechanisms. Today, the pathophysiologic approach dominates the search for drugs and other treatments and underpins the vast biomedical research enterprise. A mechanism-based approach to developing a new analgesic drug comprises eight steps,[5] the first four of which follow true to the mechanistic/reductionist spirit:

1. *Establishment of a biologic hypothesis of the pathophysiology of pain (such as prostaglandin E_2 release from inflamed tissue).*
2. *Identification of a potential molecular target (such as inhibition of the enzyme COX-2).*
3. *Establishment of a screen to look for small molecules that bind to the target.*
4. *Chemical optimization of any promising molecule found from the screen.*
5. *Test in animals.* Claude Bernard would not be hesitant to undertake the fifth test as well. But at this point, the possibilities of complex interactions become more probable. The drug may have unforeseen effects if it interacts with molecules other than the target. The complexity becomes even more worrisome when the drug is applied to human populations in the final three steps. The demonstrated need for animal and subsequent human testing reflects the lack of predictability of treatments based solely on physiologic mechanisms. Modern cell biology has revealed a massive complexity in cell signaling and processing of stimuli, and Swales[2] goes so far as to suggest that this complexity makes claims to predictive value impossible. Thus, in the last analysis, human testing and principles of evidence-based medicine will eventually be applied.
6. *Test for pharmacokinetic properties and safety in humans.* The US Food and Drug Administration (FDA) nomenclature for this step is Phase I. Such studies are closely monitored and are usually (but not always) conducted in healthy volunteer subjects. The objective is to determine the metabolic and pharmacologic actions of the drug in humans and the side effects associated with increasing doses and, possibly, to gain early evidence on effectiveness.
7. *Test for efficacy in small numbers of patients (around 100 to 300).* The FDA nomenclature for this step is Phase II, and, commonly, new drugs fail because of poor efficacy or toxic effects at this stage.

8. *Test in large-scale (probably greater than 1,000) multicenter clinical trials.* Typically, these Phase III studies are double-blind, randomized controlled trials.

Sometimes complications are seen after the drug is released onto the market; therefore postlaunch safety surveillance must be involved in Phase IV. This was the case when drug maker Merck recalled Vioxx (a COX-2 inhibitor used in treating arthritis) because it was linked to heart problems.

Two questions about any treatment

There are two basic questions that must be asked about any treatment:

1. *Does the treatment work?* This is the primary question asked in evidence-based medicine or dentistry. Other chapters discuss concepts, such as asking appropriate questions, searching for the evidence, evaluating the standard of evidence within a hierarchy, research design, and meta-analysis, that will help the reader uncover this information and assess it.
2. *How does a treatment work?* This question relates to the pathophysiologic model of Claude Bernard and his successors, such as physiologists, biochemists, and molecular biologists. Established medicine and dentistry form a coherent approach to understanding and treating health problems. To return to our pain example: there is evidence that inflamed tissues release prostaglandins; the chemical structures of the prostaglandins are known; and many enzymes that participate in their metabolism have been identified. Moreover, the effectiveness of inhibitors of these enzymes in reducing pain is known. In many instances, histologic studies have characterized the possible negative effects of high concentrations of these inhibitors on tissues. So, when we take an aspirin or ibuprofen to interfere with prostaglandin metabolism, we can be confident of relief of at least some types of pain. Failures—and discomfort—still occur, but, as the processes involved are further understood, research can lead to better inhibitors and reduced side effects.

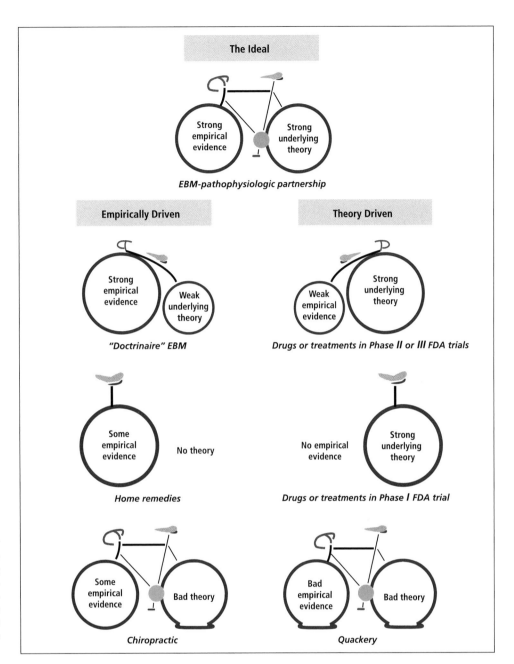

Fig 8-1 Bicycle metaphor for common theory-evidence relationships. A treatment is most reliable when both the empirical evidence for its effectiveness and the underlying theory or mechanism explaining why it works are strong. EBM = evidence-based medicine.

Relationships between theory and empirical evidence

Figure 8-1 illustrates some common theory-evidence relationships using a bicycle metaphor. The ideal occurs when there is strong empirical evidence for a treatment's effectiveness and a strong underlying theory or mechanism explaining why the treatment works. An example would be treating minor head-aches with aspirin. Both empirical evidence and plausible mechanisms of action are present, and we can be confident that the treatment is safe and reliable, just like a regular bicycle.

However, it can happen that only one component is strong, and the other is weak—leading to a relationship that can be compared with a penny farthing bicycle. The penny farthing bicycle had a tendency to crash when it hit unpredictable situations, such as potholes, and the rider came a cropper, falling head-first over the handlebars. At times, there is strong empirical evidence that a treatment works, but the reason the treatment works is obscure. An example of this is afforded by Emdogain (Straumann). There is evidence for the effectiveness of this preparation at the highest level of the hierarchy of evidence[6] (ie, systematic review), but some have questioned whether the result is primarily attained because of the physical nature (gel) of the preparation or because of the presence of the supposed active ingredient. Until this question is resolved, a clinician might be unsure of applying the preparation in situations where the barrier effect provided by the gel might be compromised. Simply put, if either theory or evidence is weak, we cannot predict as reliably as would be desired.

In some cases, there may be either no credible theory or no empirical evidence (exemplified by riding a notoriously unstable unicycle); falls are inevitable in such situations. Almost daily, there are news reports of breakthroughs in the treatment of disease based on experiments in rodents or in vitro studies. The understanding of mechanism in such instances may be very strong, but the predictability of successful application in the absence of evidence from human studies is very low. An FDA official estimated that a drug starting human trials in the year 2000 was no more likely to reach the market than one entering trials in 1985 (roughly an 8% chance), and the product failure rate for drugs in Phase III trials has increased to nearly 50%.[7] The condition can also occur when there is some empirical evidence to support the use of a treatment that, unfortunately, is based on a faulty theory; chiropractic comes to mind as an example. In a review of chiropractic published in a book generally favorable to alternative medicine, a practitioner, Redwood,[8] states, "however, positive health changes have never been convincingly correlated with vertebral alignment. . . . [A]lternative hypotheses are necessary to replace the outmoded bone-out-of-place concept." Thus, the theory underlying chiropractic is viewed as outmoded and incorrect. Chiropractic treatment cannot be expected to be progressively improved, because the current theory cannot fruitfully guide its future development.

Finally, sometimes evidence for the effectiveness of a proposed treatment is either not available or of poor quality, and the theory underlying the treatment is obviously erroneous. This situation is the natural domain of quackery and scientific cranks. Homeopathy, as it is typically applied today, involves dilutions of such magnitude that not a single molecule of the initial solution remains. The theory that the original solution somehow leaves its trace in the water in subsequent solutions—the ad hoc theory used to explain how homeopathic preparations work—is generally regarded as implausible. Believers in homeopathy face an awkward dilemma—either the established laws of chemistry and physiology are wrong, or the purported mechanisms of homeopathy are wrong; the two cannot exist together.[9] Thus, homeopathy is a quintessential example of a bad theory, although it appeared to have some validity from an evidence-based perspective when a 1997 meta-analysis of homeopathy generated the surprising finding of an overall benefit.[10] The study received abundant criticism, however, as mechanistically inclined investigators were incredulous and examined the study more closely. Subsequent analysis of homeopathic effects indicated that, as a general rule, studies showing a benefit were of lower quality and that, when study quality was more rigidly controlled, the findings were compatible with the notion that the clinical effects of homeopathy are placebo effects[11]—a finding that prompted a *Lancet* editorial entitled "The end of homeopathy."[12] The *Lancet* editors are probably guilty of wishful thinking; commercial forces with an interest in promoting homeopathy doubtless will keep the question active for some time.

In summary, the credibility of any theory or study depends on its consistency with diverse sources, particularly sources supported by a large body of evidence. Perhaps building on Kuhn's[13] description of science as puzzle solving, the philosopher Susan Haack[14] likened interpretation of data to solving a crossword puzzle; the clues are analogous to the observational or experimental evidence, and the entries are the analogue of currently accepted background information. The two sources have to blend with and reinforce each other.

Scientific Cranks

Some investigators work in such isolation that they are unaware of what is happening—or has happened—elsewhere. The work of these investigators can be seriously flawed, for inductive logic requires that a researcher consider all available evidence. Often, scientists working in isolation publish in obscure journals or write books that are published by nonacademic presses. A fascinating subset of the isolated scientist is the *crank* who may publish internally consistent work without reference to what others have found. Gardner[15,16] has written entertaining books in which he documents the characteristics of scientific cranks; his criteria for identifying cranks are given below:

1. Consider themselves geniuses but regard colleagues as ignorant blockheads
2. Consider themselves unjustly persecuted
3. Attack the greatest scientists and best established theories
4. Tend to write in complex jargon, often of their own invention
5. Contribute to journals that they edit
6. Publish books privately or with nonacademic publishers

Cranks most likely to disturb dentists are some of the antifluoridationists. The argument for fluoridation is convincing not only to dentists and to dental researchers but also to eminent scientists of other disciplines, who are in a position to consider the issue in its widest context. Sir Peter Medawar, acting as director for the National Institute of Medical Research (UK), said of the fluoridation issue, "Every time an American municipality determined against fluoridation there was a little clamor of rejoicing in the corner of Mount Olympus presided over by Gaptooth, the God of Dental Decay." Medawar[17] states that:

The more difficult part of the fluoridation enterprise is not scientific in nature. I mean that of convincing disaffected minorities that the purpose of the proposal is not to poison the populace in the interests of a foreign power or to promote the interests of a local chemical manufacturing company.

Although fluoridation is a complex issue, there certainly has been a tendency for both sides to argue simplistically. Thus, in considering arguments in support of or against fluoridation, remember that the most obvious flaw is that they most likely will not consider all the evidence.

Lifesavers Guide to Fluoridation by Yiamouyiannis,[18] an active opponent of fluoridation, cites 250 references in support of its claims. When the citations were examined critically by experts, many were found to be irrelevant to community water fluoridation, while others represented unreplicated or refuted research. Some references that supported fluoridation were selectively quoted and misrepresented. Moreover, only 48% of the English-language articles cited came from refereed journals, and a large percentage of the articles were published in outdated or obscure journals.[19] Cranks do not lack perseverance. The editor of the *British Dental Journal*, Grace,[20] wrote several editorials on the benefits of fluoridation; and, as they contained judgments of arguments made by specific people,

these were checked very carefully by lawyers for the *British Dental Journal*. Thus, the editorials were very carefully worded. Nevertheless, the *British Dental Journal* was sued by Yiamouyiannis in ongoing procedures that ended only when the plaintiff died.

Crank science can have tragic effects. Adele Davis is generally regarded by nutrition scientists as a major source of nutrition misinformation. Some reports suggest that newborn infants died as a result of their parents' following of Davis' principles of nutrition.[21-23]

However, honest mistakes also occur. The extant literature is so large and scattered that it is not difficult for an author to be unaware of an article's existence and fail to cite it. Nevertheless, the goal of a good investigator is to consider all the available evidence.

Quacks

The term *quack* has come to mean any dishonest, ignorant, or incompetent practitioner, regardless of formal training. Dentists who practice "holistic" dentistry that includes unproven or refuted methods are considered quacks.

The term *quackery* is derived from the word *quacksalvers*, who were wandering peddlers selling mercury ointments as treatment for syphilis during the Renaissance era. The term was defined for a report on the US House Select Committee on Aging's Subcommittee on Health and Long-Term Care by Congressman C. Pepper as "anyone who promotes medical schemes or remedies known to be false or which are unproven, for a profit."[24] Pepper's definition of *quackery* poses a problem: If stringent criteria for proof were adopted, some accepted medical or dental treatments might well be found lacking, even though they are considered the best current treatments. In the view of Skrabenek and McCormick,[25] quackery can be distinguished from rational therapy in that it does not derive from any coherent or established body of evidence, and it is not subjected to rigorous assessment to establish its value.

Bad science in complementary and alternative medicine

Complementary and alternative medicine (CAM), as defined by the National Center for Complementary and Alternative Medicine (NCCAM) of the US National Institutes of Health (NIH) is a group of diverse medical and health care systems, practices, and products that are not considered part of conventional medicine.[26] Complementary medicine is used together with conventional medicine, such as when aromatherapy is used to lessen discomfort after oral surgery. Alternative medicine is used in place of conventional medicine.

Practitioners of unconventional medicine constitute an economically important group, for the cost of unconventional medicine was estimated to be at least $13.7 billion in 1990. About one in three respondents to a large survey reported using unconventional medicine, mainly for chronic conditions.[27] More recent data indicate an increasing use of CAM; a survey funded by NCCAM found that 75% of respondents turned to CAM at some point in their lifetimes, including 62% who had used it the previous year.[28]

Relatively recently, the NIH established a NCCAM center dedicated to exploring complementary and alternative healing practices in the context of rigorous science, training CAM researchers, and disseminating authoritative information to the public and to professionals.[26] NCCAM classifies alternative medicine into five categories: (1) alternative medical systems, such as homeopathic medicine and naturopathic medicine; (2) mind-body interventions, such as therapies that use creative outlets, such as art, music, or dance; (3) biologically based therapies, such as dietary supplements; (4) manipulative and body-based methods, such as chiropractic; and (5) energy therapies, such as therapeutic touch. The evidence for effectiveness and, indeed, plausibility of these methods varies widely. Clearly, NCCAM is attempting to approach some of these therapies on a rational, evidence-based basis, by funding studies that test their effects. In the document providing justification for its 2006 fiscal year activities,[29] NCCAM highlights some results of NCCAM-funded studies:

1. "Story of Discovery: Ancient Acupuncture Provides Modern Pain Relief for Arthritis" (report on a Phase III trial). However, the article notes that all patients also received standard anti-inflammatory medications.
2. "Science Advance: Popular Echinacea Product Not Effective in Treating Pediatric URIs."
3. NCCAM also supports the largest randomized Phase III clinical trial to date of the potential of gingko biloba to prevent dementia in the elderly. Regardless of its outcome, this trial has set the standard for such studies.

My overall assessment is that there appears to be scant therapeutic return on the NIH NCCAM investment, but at least some attention is being paid to discovering whether there is compelling evidence to support therapies that have considerable public acceptance.

Despite the possibility that NCCAM's entry into the arena may help matters, a problem with many alternative medical approaches remains their development outside the normal peer-reviewed structure of science, where publications are evaluated by skeptical experts and where experiments are repeated and, through repetition and refinement, come to be accepted. An acceptable scientific hypothesis, according to the philosopher Hempel,[30] is internally consistent, comprehensive, testable, simple, novel, and predictive. Some of these criteria, such as simplicity and novelty, are easily met by alternative therapies. For example, the bone-out-of-place chiropractic theory, while anatomically erroneous,[31] is simple and was novel in its time. However, other criteria often pose formidable problems for alternative medical approaches, leaving them open to quackery.

Comprehensiveness

An essential criterion for the acceptability of inductive arguments is the consideration of all available evidence before reaching a conclusion. However, quack and some alternative practitioners seem to live in worlds of their own creation, using concepts unique to their approach. Acupuncture, for example, posits the existence of meridians along which flows Qi (pronounced "chi"), but the meridians do not correspond to any known physiologic or anatomic pathways. Researchers are investigating neurochemical mechanisms that might integrate acupuncture into medical science, but questions about the meridians remain. Skrabanek[32] concluded that acupuncture is effective in some patients with functional and psychosomatic disorders, but that the effects of acupuncture are unpredictable, unreliable, and possibly related to hypothesis and suggestion.

Testability

Some theories of alternative medicine cannot feasibly be tested, and, indeed, their proponents seem to accept having them remain untested. Two modern apologists for homeopathy note, "This study illustrates the difficulty in doing research in homeopathy. Homeopathic medicines are individualized by definition based on a totality of symptoms. Most conventional clinical research involves administering the same medicine to all patients."[33]

Open Publication

A norm of science is that scientific knowledge is public knowledge.[34] Materials and methods, data, and interpretations are published in accessible journals, so organized skepticism and acceptance by consensus occur. Quack science tends to keep secrets. For example, a widely publicized report from India—involving a large number of people undergoing a treatment protocol that includes swallowing live sardines—notes that the exact treatment is a family secret known only by five brothers.[35]

Lack of objectivity

Traditionally, objectivity has been one of the hallmarks of good science. In theory, this means that any qualified scientist could repeat the observations, obtain similar data (within the limits of experimental error), and reach the same conclusions as those published by another scientist. Conclusions are generally conservative, in that they do not extend much beyond the data; extravagant speculations are discouraged in scientific publications. In quack science, claims for treatments are anything but conservative. An advertisement for an instrument known as the *Zapper* claims that it is "the cure for all diseases." Some psychics claim that results bordering on the miraculous can only be obtained by themselves. Thus, their results can never be repeated, and, even if they did occur, the psychic approach could not be considered scientific. In the absence of scientifically repeatable data, quackery often relies on testimonials based on personal experience.

Why and when personal experience can be unreliable

Quackery relies on personal testimony and anecdotal evidence in place of rigorous scientific assessment. Personal testimonies are not used in scientific medicine to prove or disprove a treatment's effectiveness, because the observations are not made objectively under controlled conditions, making the rigorous assessment of the treatment impossible. Yet, personal testimonies of being cured are a powerful means of influencing opinion because of the common belief in

personal experience as the best way of determining whether something works.

Personal experience is reliable when the treatment under consideration has a large effect, occurs quickly, and has a clear outcome. Anyone who has hit a thumb with a hammer while driving nails knows from personal experience not to do it again. But the reliability of personal experience declines markedly in instances where the symptoms are variable, the time course is long, the effects of the treatment are complex, and the outcome measures are ill-defined. Oil from croton seeds exemplifies a complex treatment; the oil has cathartic properties but also contains potent tumor-promoting phorbol esters. An individual taking croton oil might deem the preparation effective and swear to its efficacy, not realizing what the long-term effects might be.

Why ineffective treatments may appear to be successful

Quacks thrive on treating conditions with variable and ill-defined symptoms, for several factors can make treatment of these conditions appear successful.

Placebo effect

Evidence suggests that expectations of a practitioner and patient can markedly affect the outcome of treatment, and this effect is optimum when both practitioner and patient believe strongly that a treatment is efficacious.[36] One study[37] examined the role of these nonspecific effects by analyzing the results of uncontrolled studies of medical and surgical treatments in which both patients and therapists had expectations of a successful outcome. The particular treatments selected for study were later found to be ineffective when examined in controlled trials. Thus, any effects reported in the uncontrolled trials did not occur as a result of the treatment, but were nonspecific and included factors such as expectancy and belief. These nonspecific effects accounted for good-to-excellent improvement in almost 70% of patients treated.[37] More recent studies have provided substantial evidence that expectation of analgesia is an important factor in the engagement of objective, neurochemical antinociceptive responses to a placebo. The responses appear to be mediated by endogenous opioid neurotransmission in the dorsolateral prefrontal cortex.[38] In other words, belief that a treatment will relieve pain causes the brain to respond by releasing its own natural painkillers. Often, quacks' and patients' confidence in a treatment produces the placebo effect and causes the treatment to look effective.

The placebo effect also benefits practitioners of conventional medicine and dentistry. Beck[39] has reviewed the topic for dentistry and advises dentists on how to use the placebo effect. However, it should be noted that different placebos have different effects. In a comparison of two placebos (a sham acupuncture device and an inert pill) the authors conclude that placebo effects are malleable and depend on behaviors embedded in medical rituals.[40]

Variability

Some conditions have high rates of spontaneous remission or long asymptomatic periods (such as herpes simplex virus infection) or are influenced by psychosocial variables. Other conditions are self-limiting, as the body's natural defenses and reparative mechanisms come into play. If a quack treatment is given before natural recovery, a quack or patient might conclude that the treatment is effective. This exemplifies the *post-hoc fallacy*, which occurs when an investigator relies on just one (temporality) of Hume's three criteria for causation.[41]

Regression

Typically, patients seek treatment when their symptoms are bothersome. In a condition with variable symptoms, the intensity of the symptoms likely will regress from the bothersome extreme that sent the patient to a practitioner to the mean value, thereby making the practitioner's treatment look effective. Thus, a person with low back pain will go to a chiropractor when the pain becomes intolerable and will consider the treatment effective when the problem returns to its normal levels—as it probably would have done without treatment.

Reporting bias

People are more likely to report a positive outcome than a negative one for fear of appearing foolish. Who wants to say, "I still feel lousy after spending megabucks on coenzyme Q treatment"? The reporting bias aids quacks, because believers report a quack's success, whereas the wiser (but sadder and poorer) individuals who recognize the treatment's failure keep their knowledge to themselves. Reporting bias can

also be problematic for conventional treatments. Guided tissue regeneration was once widely recognized as an effective means of achieving regeneration (as opposed to mere repair) of the tooth-supporting structures. However, a systematic review found that about 11 patients needed to be treated to produce one extra site gaining 2 mm or more attachment.[42]

Complex treatment

Often, people who consult quacks also elect to undertake conventional therapy. Indeed, Eisenberg et al[27] found that, among those who used unconventional treatment for a serious condition, 83% also sought treatment from a medical doctor. Thus, a successful outcome may be the result of the conventional treatment, rather than the quack treatment.

A more general problem is that treatments can be complex and can be thought of as not only administering a specific agent but also as an associated ritual. As noted earlier, placebo effects seem to be influenced by particular rituals.

Quack strategy and tactics

A tactic used by quacks to promote their services is the principle of providing incomplete information. Those effects that warp the judgment of individuals on the effectiveness of treatments occur so commonly and predictably that a strategy for being a successful crank can be codified (see list below). In general, quacks flourish when conventional medicine can offer no cure.

Freirich's[43] rules for becoming a successful quack:

1. Choose a disease that has a natural history of variability. (For those wishing to become dental quacks, temporomandibular joint disorder is a good candidate.)
2. Wait until a period when the patient's condition is getting progressively worse.
3. Apply the treatment.
4. If the patient's condition improves or stabilizes, take credit for the improvement, then stop the treatment or decrease the dosage.
5. If the patient's condition worsens, report that the dosage must be increased, that the treatment was stopped too soon and must be restarted, or that the patient did not receive treatment long enough.
6. If the patient dies, report that the treatment was applied too late—a good quack takes credit for any im-

provement but blames deterioration in the patient's condition on something else.

Quacks have been quick to promote cures for AIDS, and a wide range of unproven treatments have been offered, only serving to defraud desperate patients.[24] Lacking scientific evidence to support their claims, quacks have developed effective persuasive techniques, some of which are listed below. Some of the tactics employ half-truths. For example, tactic 6 advocates claiming that a treatment is recognized in other parts of the world, but not in North America. Indeed, some successful treatment modalities, such as the Brånemark implant, do get developed outside North America. In Sweden, Brånemark obtained very good evidence that the implant system was successful, and some 15 years passed before it was introduced into North America. However, other remedies developed outside North America are fraudulent; it would be highly irrational to go to the Philippines for so-called psychic surgery. The main issue is not where a treatment was developed, but the evidence supporting its use.

A partial list of quack tactics[44]:

1. Promise quick, dramatic, painless, or drugless cures.
2. Use anecdotes, case histories, or testimonials to support claims.
3. Use pseudoscientific disclaimers, eg, instead of promising to cure a specific illness, claim that the treatment will "detoxify the body," "strengthen the immune system," or "bring the body into harmony with nature."
4. Use dubious credentials, eg, unaccredited schools.
5. Claim product or service provides treatment or cure for multiple illnesses or conditions.
6. Claim secret cure has been discovered or recognized in another part of the world but is not yet accepted in North America.
7. Claim to be persecuted by orthodox medicine, eg, claim that doctors are suppressing the cure so they will not have competition.
8. Claim medical doctors do more harm than good.
9. Report that most disease is caused by a faulty diet and can be treated by nutritional changes; advocate the need for vitamins and "health foods" for most people.
10. Use scare tactics to encourage use of product.
11. Support "freedom of choice," both of individuals to market unproven and unorthodox methods and of consumers to purchase them.

Quackery and dubious dental care

It is unlikely that you think your gluteus maximus influences your mandibular first premolar; however, a *Journal of the American Dental Association* article on dental quackery[45] makes note of a quack dentist inferring such a ludicrous relationship. Dental quackery is performed not only by outright quacks but also by dentists who stray from accepted procedures and attempt fringe treatments.

In a report prepared for the American Council on Science and Health, Dodes and Barrett[46] state that experts on dental health fraud suspect that over $1 billion a year is spent on dubious dentistry. A brief summary of their report follows:

1. Dubious credentials: To be recognized as a specialist, dentists must undergo at least 2 years of advanced training at an institute accredited by organizations such as the ADA Council on Dental Education. Recognized dental specialties include endodontics, oral and maxillofacial surgery, oral pathology, orthodontics, pediatric dentistry, oral pathology, periodontics, prosthodontics, and public health dentistry. Yet, some dentists claim specialty status based on nutrition degrees from correspondence schools, certificates from organizations with no scientific standing, continuing education courses, or alleged expertise in unrecognized fields—such as "holistic dentistry" or "amalgam detoxification."
2. Controversial care: *Controversial care* refers to treatment modalities that have either been tried and found wanting—such as Sargenti root canal therapy—or to treatments that have not been tested sufficiently to ascertain their usefulness. Temporomandibular disorders (TMDs) have been described as dentistry's hottest area of unorthodoxy and complete quackery. Mohl et al[47] have reviewed some of the devices used for the diagnosis and treatment of TMDs and have concluded that there is no evidence to support the use of surface electromyography or silent-period duration for the diagnosis of TMDs and that sonography and Doppler ultrasound have no particular advantage over conventional stethoscopes or direct auscultation.
3. Other problem areas: Implants, bonding, and tooth bleaching can be useful treatments, but they are occasionally performed by inappropriately trained personnel. For example, in my view, an implant placed by a dentist with only one short training course (possibly as little as 1 day) has a worse prog-

nosis than one placed by an oral surgeon or periodontist.

4. Blatant quackery: Dodes and Barrett give examples of practices that have no scientific basis whatsoever but that, nevertheless, are employed by quacks to treat dental problems:

- Reflexology: Involves pressing on hands or feet to relieve pain and to remove underlying cause of disease in other parts of the body.

- Cranial osteopathy: Based on the view that "manipulation" of the skull's bones can cause "the energy of life" to flow to cure or prevent a wide variety of health problems, including pain—especially pain associated with TMDs. Quite apart from the pseudoscientific theoretical basis, cranial osteopathy is practically flawed because the bones of the skull are sutured together, and the manipulations performed by cranial osteopaths do not produce movements sufficiently large to be detected with sensitive instruments.

- Silver amalgam replacement: Has been advocated to avoid mercury toxicity; however, billions of amalgam fillings have been used successfully, and fewer than 50 cases of allergy have been reported in the scientific literature since 1905.[45] The ADA reported that no credible evidence exists to show that mercury in dental amalgam, when used in nonallergenic patients, constitutes a general health hazard or is related to any specific disease.

- Nutrition quackery and holistic dentistry: Occur under the guise of nutritional counseling and unnecessary dietary supplements, including herbal remedies, which are advocated and sold. Greene[48] believes that many of these treatments are not directed at dental disease, but rather at the overall condition of patients. When applied by dentists, such treatments push dentistry into unorthodox medical care, which, as exemplified by herbal medicine, can endanger patients.[49]

- Applied kinesiology: Practiced mostly by chiropractors, it is a technique used to assess nutritional status on the basis of muscles' response to mechanical stress. Operationally, the approach typically involves the practitioner pushing down on a patient's outstretched arms before and after vitamins or other substances are placed under the patient's tongue. Treatment can consist of expensive vitamin supple-

ments or a special diet. A controlled test found that applied kinesiology was no more useful than random guessing in evaluating nutrient status.[50]

- Auriculotherapy: Acupuncture of the ear, based on the notion that stimulating various points on or just beneath the skin can balance the "life force" and enable the body to recover from disease. Some proponents claim that it is effective against dental pain.

Abuses of Logic

Some traditional fallacies of informal logic

Several traditional fallacies of informal logic may be considered arguments that are valid in that the conclusion is logically related to the premises but that are unsound in the sense that at least one of the premises is wrong.[51] It is important to note that the premises and the conclusions of these fallacies are not necessarily wrong. Other common fallacies occur because we do not focus directly on the points of issue but rather on circumstances that are more or less irrelevant.

Some examples of traditional fallacies follow; more can be found in texts (eg, Fearnside and Holther[52]) that specialize on the topic.

Ad hominem and the fallacy of origin

The fallacy of origin occurs when we reject an argument because it comes from an unreliable source. This fallacy can be considered in some ways the opposite of the argument from authority, which is based largely on the reliability of the source. The force of an argument, however, should not lie in its source, but rather on its premises and logic. For example, we may be tempted to dismiss studies funded by manufacturers, but to do so indiscriminately would be erroneous, because some manufacturer studies are sound and introduce valuable innovations into, for example, oral care. In such instances, the key is to examine the studies carefully and to identify their strengths and weaknesses.

A variant on the fallacy of origin is *ad hominem*, or personal attack, whereby the person making the argument, rather than the argument itself, is criticized.

Special pleading

The fallacy of special pleading occurs when we refuse to apply to ourselves principles that we apply to others. For example, a scientist acting as a reviewer for a journal might refuse to allow a statement in a paper because the data underlying the statement were not statistically significant. In his own paper, the scientist may not adopt the same stringent criteria and publish statements that are based on nonstatistically significant trends in the data. Any reason offered for this disparity of standards, such as difficulty in performing experiments or shortage of patients, would be part of the special pleading.

Tu quoque (you also)

When under attack for lacking evidence to support their claims, quacks use the tu quoque argument—agreeing that there may not be evidence to support their claims but noting that much of established medicine or dentistry also lacks evidence. As with the cliché "two wrongs don't make a right," the lack of evidence for some established medical treatments in no way supports the use of quack therapies. Rather, it is an argument for more research. Typically, quacks cite out-of-date studies to support the tu quoque argument; the estimate that only 10% to 20% of medical treatments have an established base has been dismissed as no more than a modern medical myth.[53]

Fallacy of composition

The fallacy of composition occurs when we believe that what is true of all of the parts is true of the whole. This is sometimes untrue. For example, it is said (at least in a logic text) that while an individual baboon is cowardly, a group of baboons is extremely aggressive.[51] On the other hand, it is often true that the whole shares the characteristics of its parts. For example, individual cells are poisoned by cyanide, and an individual, composed of many cells, also is poisoned by cyanide. In fact, much of modern biology is based on the principle of *reductionism*—studying simpler aspects of an organism to get information about the whole. However, there is the danger of missing something because of interrelationships of the parts. An example can be found in the study of chemical carcinogenesis. It appears that some compounds must be metabolized before they become carcinogenic. A once-accepted theory that correlated chemical structure of organic compounds with their carcinogenicity ignored this possibility and has since been discredited.

Ad populum

Occasionally, statements are justified by stating that "there is widespread agreement," a justification based on the suppressed premise that most people are right. The legitimate use of this reasoning process occurs in inductive reasoning, where the people concerned are "reliable authorities."

Genetic fallacy

A genetic fallacy occurs when it is assumed that one of several necessary conditions is the sole and exclusive cause of an effect. This fallacy has occurred in cancer research. As each new area of biochemistry develops, tumor cells are examined closely, and alterations (as compared with "normal" cells) are found. Then it is proposed that the alteration is the cause of the tumor. In most cases, a tumor cell without the alteration is eventually found; such an observation destroys the credibility of that particular alteration as a necessary condition for cancer. Thus, 50 years ago, changes in oxidative enzymes were implicated; in the 1970s, there was extensive interest in altered membrane glycoproteins and/or glycolipids; in the early 1980s, researchers focused on the cytoskeleton; and in the late 1980s, scientists suspected oncogenes. Hopefully, one of these bandwagons will prove useful in cancer treatment.

Post hoc

Post hoc is taken from the Latin expression *post hoc ergo propter hoc*, which, literally translated, means "after this, therefore because of this." In chapter 7, Hume's[41] three criteria for cause and effect are given, but this fallacy would state that only one of them (temporal priority) is necessary. The post hoc fallacy has been of prime benefit to quacks and producers of patent medicines. Someone becomes ill, takes a medicine, and gets better; the individual attributes his or her well-being to the medicine, rather than to a healing process initiated by his or her own body. As someone said of vitamin C, "with it you can cure your cold in 7 days, whereas without it, it will take you a whole week to get better." But the post hoc fallacy is not restricted to the laity; many clinical trials of drugs performed by clinicians are similarly affected. In some instances, an overt statement of the reasoning used is not made but only implied.

Apples and oranges

Often, people try to compare results obtained in one system with results obtained in a different system. If the aspects in which the two systems differ are relevant conditions, then the person is said to be comparing apples and oranges. This criticism usually precipitates an argument about which conditions are relevant. The fallacy occurs frequently in the extrapolation of results from experimental animals to humans. The use of saccharin was banned in the United States, partially on the basis of observations of Canadian scientists, who found that massive doses of saccharin produce tumors in rats. Rather than banning saccharin, a US senator is said to have suggested that a statement be placed on the package: "Warning: Canadians have determined that saccharin is detrimental to your rat's health." In the field of clinical pharmacology, for example, it is difficult to prove that a given chemical will have the same toxicity or efficacy in humans as in experimental animals, but there is much evidence to suggest that, in many instances, this hypothesis is reasonable.

Circular reasoning

Circular reasoning occurs when an alleged proof of a statement eventually involves the assumption of the statement being proved. Circular reasoning can remain undetected for long periods. For example, one of the most often quoted "proofs" of Maxwell's laws of the distribution of molecular velocities assumes one of the features of the final law that it attempts to prove.[54] If circular reasoning is suspected, the best place to look for it is in the definitions, particularly if the definition in question is odd. Circular reasoning is also called *begging the question*, since it begs (assumes) the very thing it tries to prove.

UFO fallacy

Unidentified flying objects are just that: *unidentified*. The question becomes whether they represent some form of visitation by extraterrestrial beings. Users of this fallacy generally argue their case by pointing out what individual sightings were not (it was not a weather balloon; none was released in that area). Chapter 5 defined the disjunctive syllogism as a valid form of deductive argument in which, given only two alternatives, when one is known to be false, the other must be true. Clearly, this technique, which could be called *proof by elimination,* can be effective whenever there is a finite number of possibilities. The problem with the UFO theory is that there is a potentially large number of causes for the phenomena, which may be grouped under the heading "unknown natural occurrences." Faced with such an unlimited list, the disjunctive syllogism becomes ineffective. The UFO fallacy occurs where proof by elimination is attempted without adequate consideration of all the possible alternatives.[55]

In proof by exclusion, clinical diagnosis can proceed by means of the disjunctive syllogism. For example, if, on routine dental examination, a middle-aged woman were found to have a radiolucent area near the apex of a mandibular anterior tooth, two possibilities might come to mind: *(1)* dental infection, ie, a nonvital tooth; or *(2)* periapical cemental dysplasia. The dentist would probably test the teeth for vitality. If the teeth were vital, the dentist could exclude the first possibility—dental infection—and conclude that the most probable diagnosis was periapical dysplasia. However, to do so would run the risk of committing the UFO fallacy, for there are other possibilities—such as a midline cyst of the mandible or a central mucoepidermoid carcinoma—that also fit the facts of the case. According to Murphy,[56] it is largely a myth that you can exclude some diseases as impossibilities and that, by default, the diagnosis must be something else. One difficulty is that there may be a problem with the sensitivity of the test; vitality testing, for example, does give false-positive results. But a far greater problem with proofs by exclusion is that, in practice, they rarely exclude, because it is difficult to prove that the list of possibilities is exhaustive.

Fallacies of clinical dentistry

Greene[57] has noted several fallacies in the evaluation of clinical treatment procedures. Several of these arise from the nature of inductive logic, in particular, from failure to consider alternative explanations. Greene classifies these potential problems into the fallacies of success and failure.

Fallacies of success

The following factors have to be considered before reaching any conclusion about a treatment's effectiveness:

1. *Spontaneous remission.* Because some conditions are self-limiting, spontaneous remission is an alternative explanation of the supposed success of a clinical procedure. Individuals usually enter treatments when their symptoms are at their worst, and some symptoms naturally become less severe, regardless of whether therapy is instituted.

2. *Placebo response.* When dealing with pathologic pain, about 35% (or perhaps a higher percentage) of the population responds favorably to a placebo, regardless of whether their problem is real or imagined, and this rate increases when a strong positive suggestion is added. The placebo effect is a plausible alternative hypothesis for many successes, and the rate of clinical success for any treatment must be compared with the placebo response for that particular problem.

3. *Multiple variables of treatment.* Often, dentists devise treatments composed of several parts applied either together or in sequence. However, from Mill's canons of induction, we know that you can only assess the effectiveness of each component by varying one factor at a time. Thus, in a complex procedure, it is difficult to determine whether all parts of the treatment are essential or if some are meaningless. Irrelevant variables may be credited for the success, while the critical variable is overlooked. Greene[57] cites the example of pontics in fixed partial dentures, where research attention focused on the compatibility of various materials (eg, gold, porcelain, and acrylic) with the edentulous ridge tissues. After many studies, researchers concluded that it was not the material, but the design of the pontic and its cleansability, that determined tissue response.

4. *Treatment of nonexistent problems.* According to Greene,[57] the most common treatment error is *overtreatment*. If there is no problem at the onset of treatment, and if the treatment does no harm (Hippocrates' first rule of medicine), there will be no problem after treatment, and the procedure will be classified as a success. Greene believes that some extensive reconstruction procedures or certain prophylactic measures—such as preventive equilibration—are applied to patients who could be helped with a more conservative approach or who need no treatment at all.

5. *Short-term successes but long-term failures.* Some procedures that seem successful at the time of treatment may fail later. For example, a successful pulpotomy done with calcium hydroxide in a permanent tooth may fail years later and result in dys-trophic changes in the canals, which preclude root canal therapy. Some treatments may also produce side effects. This principle is recognized in pharmacology, where both efficacy and safety of drugs are evaluated prior to introduction of a drug to the market, but—as shown by the problems with intrauterine devices—the same kinds of rigorous standards are not always applied to nonpharmacologic treatment procedures or devices.

Fallacies of failure

The fallacies of failure are related to the problem of negative results. There are always a host of possible reasons why success was not seen, including:

1. *Wrong diagnosis.* An incorrect diagnosis can lead to the use of an unsuitable treatment.

2. *Incorrect cause-effect correlations.* If the cause of the clinical problem is unknown or is incorrectly identified, a clinician might expect the treatment to fail. Greene[57] states that this type of error usually is made by clinicians who have a theoretical bias about certain problems, which leads them to analyze all patients with those problems in a narrow frame of reference. The clinician who attributes myofacial pain dysfunction problems solely to occlusal disharmony may fail to help myofacial pain dysfunction patients with stress problems, and perhaps may make their situation worse.

3. *Multifactorial problems.* Problems can be caused by more than one factor. For example, if a patient has a necrotic pulp in a tooth that also has a periodontal problem, conventional periodontal therapy may fail without concomitant root canal therapy. Such a failure would not result from the periodontal therapy being an ineffective treatment, but rather from the complex nature of the problem.

4. *Methodologic problems.* Normally effective treatments might fail because of defective methods, such as improper execution of the treatment, lack of patient cooperation, premature evaluation, and even the patient's psychological state. The latter phenomenon is exemplified in severely depressed patients, who simply do not respond well to conventional treatment of their physical problems.

5. *Insufficient statistical power.* Treatments can fail to show a statistically significant effect because there are too few subjects in the experiment to either establish or conclusively rule out the existence of effects of clinically meaningful magnitude.

References

1. Macaulay TB. Westminster reviewer's reference of Mill. In: Macaulay TB. The Miscellaneous Writings of Lord Macaulay, vol 2. London: Longman, Green, Longman, and Roberts, 1860. Available at: http://www.infomotions.com/etext/gutenberg/dirs/etext00/2mwsm10.htm.

2. Swales J. The troublesome search for evidence: Three cultures in need of integration. J R Soc Med 2000;93:553.

3. Rangachari PK. Evidence-based medicine: Old French wine with a new Canadian label? J R Soc Med 1997;90:280–284.

4. Kassirer JP. The quality of care and the quality of measuring it. N Engl J Med 1993;329:1263–1265.

5. Woolf CJ, Max MB. Mechanism-based pain diagnosis: Issues for analgesic drug development. Anesthesiology 2001;95:241–249.

6. Esposito M, Coulthard P, Thomsen P, Worthington HV. Enamel matrix derivative for periodontal tissue regeneration in treatment of intrabony defects: A Cochrane systematic review. J Dent Educ 2004;68:834–844.

7. Gottlieb S. Modernizing development science to unlock new treatments. Available at: http://www.fda.gov/oc/speeches/2006/modernizing0206.html. Accessed June 26, 2007.

8. Redwood D. Chiropractic. In: Micozzi MS (ed). Fundamentals of Complementary and Alternative Medicine. New York: Churchill Livingstone, 1996:91–110.

9. Brunette DM. Alternative therapies: Abuses of scientific method and challenges to dental research. J Prosthet Dent 1998;80:605–614.

10. Linde K, Clausius N, Ramirez G, et al. Are the clinical effects of homoeopathy placebo effects? A meta-analysis of placebo-controlled trials. Lancet 1997;350:834–843.

11. Shang AJ, Huwiler-Muntener K, Nartey L, et al. Are the clinical effects of homoeopathy placebo effects? Comparative study of placebo-controlled trials of homoeopathy and allopathy. Lancet 2005;366:726–732.

12. The end of homeopathy [editorial]. Lancet 2005;366:690.

13. Kuhn TS. Normal science as puzzle-solving. In: The Structure of Scientific Revolutions, ed 2. Chicago: Univ Chicago Press, 1970:35–42.

14. Haack S. Manifesto of a passionate moderate. Chicago: Univ of Chicago Press, 1998.

15. Gardner M. Fads and Fallacies in the Name of Science. New York: Dover, 1957:3–27.

16. Gardner M. Science: Good, Bad, and Bogus. Buffalo, NY: Prometheus, 1981.

17. Medawar PB. The Limits of Science. Oxford: Oxford Univ Press, 1984:18.

18. Yiamouyiannis J. Lifesaver's Guide to Fluoridation. Delaware, OH: Safe Water Foundation, 1983.

19. Wulf CA, Hughes KF, Smith KG, Easley NW. Abuse of the Scientific Literature in an Antifluoridation Pamphlet, ed 2. Columbus, OH: American Oral Health Institute, 1988.

20. Grace M. Facts on fluoridation. Br Dent J 2000;189:405.

21. Jarvis W. Dangerous fleece. The Scientist. February 4 1989:Letters.

22. Wetli CV, Davis JH. Fatal hyperkalemia from accidental overdose of potassium chloride. JAMA 1978;240:1339.

23. Oseas RS, Phelps DL, Kaplan SA. Near fatal hyperkalemia from a dangerous treatment for colic. Pediatrics 1982; 69:117.

24. Zwicky JF, Hafner AW, Barret S, et al. In: Hafner AW (ed). American Medical Association: Readers Guide to Alternative Methods. Milwaukee: American Medical Association, 1993:5.

25. Skrabanek P, McCormick J. Follies and Fallacies in Medicine. Buffalo, NY: Prometheus, 1990:30–31.

26. National Center for Complementary and Alternative Medicine. NCCAM Facts-at-a-Glance and Mission. Available at: http://nccam.nih.gov/about/ataglance/. Accessed June 27, 2007.

27. Eisenberg DM, Kessler RC, Foster C, Norlock FE, Calkins DR, Delbanco TL. Unconventional medicine in the United States: Prevalence, costs, and patterns of use. N Engl J Med 1993;328:246.

28. National Center for Complementary and Alternative Medicine (NCCAM). A new portrait of CAM use in the United States. NCCAM Newsletter 2004;11(343).

29. National Center for Complementary and Alternative Medicine. 2006 Congressional Justification [PDF]. Available at: http://nccam.nih.gov/about/congressional/index.htm. Accessed June 27, 2007.

30. Hempel CG. The test of a hypothesis: Its logic and its force. In: Hempel CG. Philosophy of Natural Science. Englewood Heights, NJ: Prentice Hall, 1966:19–46.

31. Crelin ES. A scientific test of chiropractic theory. Am Sci 1973;61:574–580.

32. Skrabanek P. Acupuncture: Past, present, and future. In: Stalker D, Glymour C (eds). Examining Holistic Medicine. Amherst, NY: Prometheus, 1984:181–196.

33. Jacobs J, Moskowitz T. Homeopathy. In: Micozzi MS (ed). Fundamentals of Complementary and Alternative Medicine. New York: Churchill Livingstone, 1996:67–78.

34. Ziman J. Reliable Knowledge: An Exploration of the Grounds for Belief in Science. Cambridge: Cambridge Univ Press, 1978.

35. Live sardine "cures" asthma. Vancouver Province. June 9, 1997: World.

36. Beecher HK. Pain, placebos and physicians. Practitioner 1962;189:141.

37. Roberts AH, Kewman DG, Mercier L, Hovell M. The power of nonspecific effects in healing: Implications for psychosocial and biological treatments. Clin Psychol Rev 1993;13:375.

38. Benedetti F, Mayber HS, Wager TD, Stohler CS, Zubieta JK. Neurobiological mechanisms of the placebo effect. J Neurosci 2005;25:10390–10402.

39. Beck FM. Placebos in dentistry: Their profound potential effects. J Am Dent Assoc 1977;95:1122.

40. Kaptchuk TJ, Stason WB, Davis RB, et al. Sham device v inert pill: Randomised controlled trial of two placebo treatments. BMJ 2006;332:391–397.

41. Hume DA. Treatise on Human Nature (1739–1740), ed 2, vol 1. Oxford: Clarendon Press, 1978:173–175.

42. Needleman I, Tucker R, Giedrys-Leeper E, Worthington H. Guided tissue regeneration for periodontal intrabony defects—A Cochrane Systematic Review. Periodontol 2000 2005;37:106–123.

43. Freirich EJ. Unproven remedies: Lessons for improving techniques of evaluating therapeutic efficacy. In: Cancer Chemotherapy: Fundamental Concepts and Recent Advances. Chicago: Year Book Medical, 1975:385–401.

44. Cornacchia HJ, Barrett S. Consumer Health: A Guide to Intelligent Decisions. Toronto: Mosby, 1989:44–45.

45. Berry JH. Questionable care: What can be done about dental quackery? J Am Dent Assoc 1987;115:681.

46. Dodes JE, Barrett S. Dubious Dental Care. New York: American Council on Science and Health, 1991.

47. Mohl ND, Lund JP, Widmer CG, McCall WD Jr. Devices for the diagnosis and treatment of temporomandibular disorders. Part II: Electromyography and sonography. J Prosthet Dent 1990;63:334.

48. Greene CS. Holistic dentistry: Where does the holistic end and the quackery begin? J Am Dent Assoc 1981;102:25.

49. Tyler VE. Hazards of herbal medicine. In: Stalker D, Glymour C (eds). Examining Holistic Medicine. Buffalo, NY: Prometheus, 1982:323.

50. Kenney JJ, Clemens R, Forsythe KD. Applied kinesiology unreliable for assessing nutrient status. J Am Diet Assoc 1988;88:698.

51. Capaldi N. The Art of Deception. New York: Brown, 1971: 102–103.

52. Fearnside WW, Holther WB. Fallacy: The Counterfeit of Argument. Englewood Cliffs, NJ: Prentice Hall, 1959.

53. National Council Against Health Fraud (NCAHF). The making of a modern medical myth: "Only 10–20% of medical procedures are proved." NCAHF Newsletter. November 1995.

54. Wilson EB. An Introduction to Scientific Research. New York: McGraw Hill, 1952:34.

55. Giere RN. Understanding Scientific Reasoning. New York: Holt, Rinehart and Winston, 1979:149–155.

56. Murphy EA. A Companion to Medical Statistics. Baltimore: Johns Hopkins Univ Press, 1985:25.

57. Greene CS. The fallacies of clinical success in dentistry. J Oral Med 1976;31:52.

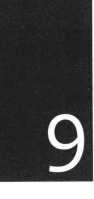

Elements of Probability and Statistics, Part 1: Discrete Variables

Probability does pervade the universe—and in this sense the old chestnut about baseball imitating life really has validity. The statistics of streaks and slumps, properly understood, do teach an important lesson about epistemology and life in general. The history of a species, or any natural phenomenon that requires unbroken continuity in a world of trouble, works like a batting streak. All are games of a gambler playing with a limited stake against a house with infinite resources. The gambler must eventually go bust.

—Stephen Jay Gould[1]

Probability and Distributions

Statistics is the scientific methodology used to make probability statements; it is generally divided into two types: *(1) descriptive* statistics involves gathering, displaying, and summarizing data, and *(2) inferential* statistics is the science of drawing conclusions from specific data. These conclusions can be helpful in making decisions such as how to bet in card games or on elections. Statisticians first determine how the data are distributed—that is, *what* and *how many* data points have particular outcomes or scores—and then use that information to make statements about probability of specified occurrences. For example, in interpreting the results of a clinical trial for any treatment, the question is whether the treatment had any effect or whether differences between treated and control groups happened by chance. Certain distributions of data, such as the normal distribution and the binomial distribution, feature prominently in scientific research and can be described mathematically. Knowing that data follow such distributions enables statisticians to make statements about particular situations, such as the probable value of the average of a large population based on a single sample. Statistical statements have an element of quantified uncertainly. For example, most readers are familiar with election opinion polls, of which a typical result might state that a

candidate is favored by 51% of the voters with a margin of error of 4%. Statistics is grounded in probability theory; this chapter starts with the laws of probability, shows how these yield particular distributions of data, and examines how statisticians make inferences from data and distributions. Typically, the inferences of scientific interest include how well the results conform to a theory, whether there are significant differences between groups (such as a treated group and a control), and estimation of values and differences.

Probability theory was conceived to satisfy gamblers' desire to calculate odds of outcomes of various events, such as rolling dice or being dealt certain cards. The 17th-century mathematicians Blaise Pascal and Pierre de Fermat are widely regarded as the founders of a general theory of probability. Pascal's curiosity about probability was prompted by a gambling friend, the Chevalier de Mere, who had discovered through personal experience that a seemingly well-established gambling rule led to unsatisfactory results and sought Pascal's help. Pascal ultimately carried his interest in probability into the realm of the "Four Last Things"—death, judgment, heaven, and hell—and concluded that to live one's life as a devoted Christian was a good wager (henceforth referred to as *Pascal's Wager*), reasoning that the small bet entailed in the costs of living a Christian life paled in comparison to the infinite rewards of heaven.[2] My approach here, however, will be limited to more mundane issues.

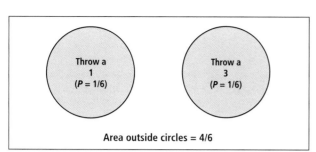

Fig 9-1 Diagram illustrating the probability of throwing a 1 or a 3 (ie, two mutually exclusive events).

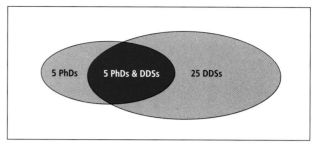

Fig 9-2 Example of nondisjoint outcomes. Probability of PhD or DDS degrees must be adjusted by subtracting those faculty who have both.

Probability[3] is a term that has different meanings depending on the context in which it is used. Three approaches follow:

1. *Classical probability*, or *a priori* approach, was developed for making intelligent wagers, and it applies the fundamental assumption (rather than empirical evidence) that the game is fair (for example, that a fair die is equally likely to show 1, 2, 3, 4, 5, or 6).
2. *Frequentist probability*—the prevailing approach used in science—was formally defined by the mathematician John Venn (of the diagrams), who stated in 1872 that the probability of a given event is the proportion of times the event occurs over the long run.
3. *Subjective* or *personal probability* judgments (as in "I think it's 50:50 that the Cardinals will win the World Series this year") are often the only tools available for complex predictions about the future, since obtaining the type of data needed for a frequentist approach is impossible and a strong theoretical base for making any prediction is lacking. Improbably perhaps, this approach forms the first step in Bayesian statistics, which have found wide application in dentistry and medicine (see chapter 10).

Probability calculations

To make probability calculations, several rules must be observed:

1. Probabilities always take a value between 0 (an impossible event) and 1 (an inevitable or totally certain event). An *event* is defined as a set of elementary outcomes. In turn, *elementary outcomes* are the possible results of a *random experiment*, which, for prob-

ability purposes, is defined as the process of observing the outcome of a chance event. The *sampling space* is the set of all elementary outcomes. In probability problems, one often tries to determine the probability of combined events, such as: event A occurs and event B occurs; either event A or event B occurs; or neither event A nor event B occurs. In tackling probability problems, one normally divides the number of outcomes of interest with the total number of outcomes, ie, the sampling space.

For example, in the roll of two fair dice, the sample space comprises 36 elementary outcomes (each of the six faces of one die can be combined with each face of the second die), of which all are equally likely. The event that the total of the two dice equals 2 can occur in only one way—when both dice show 1—so its probability is 1/36. In contrast, the event that the two dice total 4 can occur in three ways:

Die 1	Die 2
1 +	3
3 +	1
2 +	2

Therefore, its probability is 3/36.

2. The addition rule for mutually exclusive events. If events are mutually exclusive, they cannot occur together. The probability of one or the other occurring is the sum of their individual probabilities. Thus, the probability of throwing either a 3 or a 1 on the single roll of a die is:

$$P(1 \text{ or } 3) = P(1) + P(3) = 1/6 + 1/6 = 1/3$$

This outcome can be illustrated in a Venn diagram (Fig 9-1), where probability is indicated by area. The probability of the total sample space area is 1 (ie, it is certain that one face of the die will turn up—the die will not balance on an edge). The area for each outcome represented by circles is 1/6, and the sum

Table 9-1 Probability distribution for the random variable X = sum (no. of dots on first die) + (no. of dots on second die)*											
	Value of x										
	2	**3**	**4**	**5**	**6**	**7**	**8**	**9**	**10**	**11**	**12**
Probability that X = x	1/36	2/36	3/36	4/36	5/36	6/36	5/36	4/36	3/36	2/36	1/36

*x = particular values of X, which can vary from 2 to 12.

of the areas within the circles is 1/3 (1/6 + 1/6). Thus, the addition rule is applied to determine the likelihood that any one of several mutually exclusive events will happen.

3. The general addition rule for nondisjoint outcomes. *Nondisjoint outcomes* are outcomes that have elements in common. Suppose a dental school employs 200 faculty. Of these, 30 hold dental degrees (P[DDS] = 30/200 = .15) and 10 hold PhD degrees (P[PhD] = 10/200 = .05). Upon closer examination it is found that 5 people hold both a dental degree and a PhD degree. To estimate the probability that a randomly selected employee has a PhD or a dental degree, therefore, it would be necessary to avoid counting twice those individuals who hold both degrees (Fig 9-2). That is, it would be inaccurate to count the total number of PhD degrees (10) and the total number of dental degrees (30) and arrive at a value of 40/200, yielding P = .2, because the 5 individuals holding both degrees would be counted twice. The general addition rule for nondisjoint outcomes adjusts the probability by subtracting those who have both degrees, as follows:

$$P(\text{PhD or DDS}) = P(\text{PhD}) + P(\text{DDS}) - P(\text{DDS and PhD}) = (10/200) + (30/200) - (5/200) = 35/200 = .175$$

4. The multiplication rule for a series of independent events. *Independent events* are events where the occurrence (or not) of one is completely separate from the occurrence (or not) of the other. Using a fair die, the probability of each face turning up on a second roll is not influenced by the number that turned up on the first roll.

The multiplication rule states that the probability that two independent events will occur is the product of their individual probabilities. Thus, the probability of throwing a 1 on the first roll of the die and a 3 on the second roll of the die is:

$$P(1) \times P(3) = 1/6 \times 1/6 = 1/36$$

5. Conditional probability. *Conditional probability* refers to the probability that one event will occur if some other event has already occurred; it is generally expressed as P(X|Y) (the probability of event X given that event Y has already occurred). If two dice are thrown sequentially and the result of the first throw is a 1, then the probability that a 1 and a 3 will be thrown equals the probability that a 3 will be thrown on the roll of the second die. The sample space would be 36 if we did not know that a 1 had already been thrown. However, only 6 outcomes are now possible, representing the sample space, and therefore the probability is 1/6 (P[3|1] = 1/6). Conditional probabilities are particularly important in the interpretation of diagnostic tests, which are discussed in chapter 14.

Distributions of outcomes

A *random variable* is defined as the numeric outcome of a random experiment. Consider the random variable X = sum of the dots on two dice. As noted earlier, there are 36 possible outcomes, but since some values of X can be obtained in more than one way, the total number of values is only 11. The value 4, for example, can be obtained by a 3 on the first die and a 1 on the second; by a 1 on the first die and a 3 on the second; and by both dice showing a 2. Similar calculations could be done for all of the possible outcomes, yielding a probability distribution for X. To distinguish the random variable X from the particular values of the total on the dice, we will label the particular values *x*. Thus, a table can be constructed (Table 9-1).

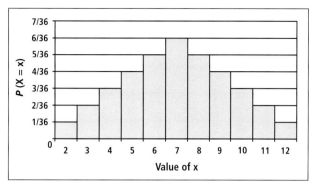

Fig 9-3 The probability of the value of the sum of the dots of two dice. The most probable is seven.

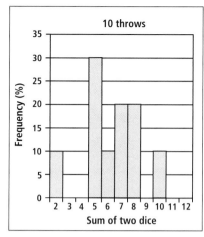

Fig 9-4a Observed frequency distribution of the total number of dots on two dice when thrown 10 times.

Two aspects of this table should be noted. First, the total sum of all probabilities equals 1. This makes sense because when two dice are thrown, only the values of x shown in the table can be obtained, and x must have some value since no die will land and balance on its edge. Second, X may be called a *discrete* variable in that it is made up of a finite number of values. Note that one cannot get a sum of the dice equal to 3.44; only integers can be obtained by summing the number of dots.

This probability distribution can be drawn as a relative frequency histogram (Fig 9-3), with the ordinate given by the probability and—by convention—with the bars of the relative frequency centered on the outcome values. Also by convention, the total area of the histogram is assigned a value of 1. By following these conventions, we can compare the relative probabilities for specified outcomes simply by comparing the areas of the bars representing those outcomes. For example, we can see that the chance of two throws totaling 6 equals the chance of two throws totaling 8. The chance of the two dice yielding a value of 2 equals the chance of them totaling 12, and so on.

money bet that the total number of dots on two dice would total 7 more times than they would total 6. If the dice followed the classic probabilities, we could expect that in 36 throws of the dice, the total 6 would show up five times whereas the total 7 would show up six times. Over several throws of the dice, the person betting on 7 would win more times than the person betting on 6.

The preceding example is based on classical probability, but frequency distributions also can be generated by actual events or experiments. To demonstrate, we could throw pairs of dice again and again, each time recording the sum of the dots. Intuitively, one would expect the empirical distribution to more closely match the classical (*a priori*) distribution as the number of throws increased. Figures 9-4a to 9-4d show the results of a computer simulation in which two dice were thrown 10, 100, 500, and 5,000 times, respectively. By recording the results in the form of a frequency histogram—that is, the number of times each of the possible totals occurred—we can see that the experiment representing 5,000 throws yielded results closer to the classical (a priori) distribution than did the lower number of throws.

Statistical Inference

Frequency distributions can help us make decisions. In light of the frequency distribution in Fig 9-3, for example, it would be reasonable to accept an even

An example of statistical inference: Hypothesis testing

In the preceding sections on logic, we assumed that test predictions of the hypothesis could readily be

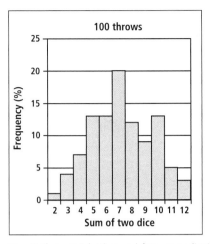
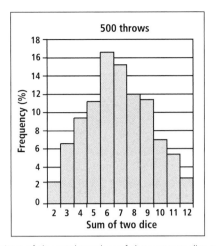
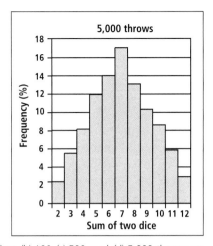

Figs 9-4b to 9-4d *Observed frequency distributions of the total number of dots on two dice when (b) 100 (c) 500, and (d) 5,000 throws are made. As more throws are made, the observed distribution resembles to a greater extent the unexpected (a priori) distribution.*

found true or false. In fact, this often is not the case; rather, statistical testing of a hypothesis requires a standard ritual as outlined by Larkin[3]:

1. Propose a research question.
2. State an alternative hypothesis H_1 based on the research hypothesis.
3. State a null hypothesis H_0.
4. Choose a level of significance.
5. Sample.
6. Choose a probability distribution appropriate to the problem.
7. Find the distribution of possible values if H_0 is true.
8. Find the probability of getting the sample value or a value more extreme.
9. Decide whether to accept or reject H_0.

Let us consider a mock example. Suppose there are four University of British Columbia (UBC) dental graduates—A, B, C, and D—who plan to hold a reunion after each has completed 20 endodontic cases. At this reunion, they will determine how their patients have fared as compared with patients treated by other dentists in general practice.

Step 1: Research question

Their research question is: Does a recent UBC graduate differ from other practicing dentists in the proportion of successes in endodontic therapy?

Although reports in the dental literature claim a 95% success rate for endodontic therapy, a more realistic figure for dentists in general practice would be around 80% (Dow P, personal communication, 1982).

Step 2: Alternative hypothesis

The alternative hypothesis is $P_{UBC} \neq P_{Others}$ where P_{UBC} is the proportion of endodontic successes for each recent UBC graduate. P_{Others} is the proportion of successes for other dentists, which is estimated as .80.

Step 3: Null hypothesis

Testing the null hypothesis is analogous to the mathematics strategy of proof by contradiction: We begin testing the null hypothesis by assuming it is true. In this example, then, the UBC graduates and other dentists are both random samples from the same target population.

The null hypothesis is $P_{UBC} = P_{Others}$ or, as expressed differently for a constant-sized sample, number of successes of UBC graduates = number of successes of other dentists. The question to ask is: Are the results obtained by a UBC graduate better or worse, or different in any way, from those obtained by others? To answer it, we will calculate the consequences of the null hypothesis—that is, the probability of the observed results if the null hypothesis were true. If this probability is low, we will reject the null hypothesis because it contradicts the observed evidence.

Step 4: Significance level

The dental students agree to accept a difference as being real if the possibility that their results could be explained by chance is less than 5%. This is an arbitrary decision, but it conforms to the commonly used value of 5%. By this standard we reject the null hypothesis if the observed result occurs by chance less than 5% of the time (ie, 1 time out of 20). But there are really no formal rules for setting this standard, which is called the *level of significance* and designated α. The commonly used level of significance of 5% was described by Fisher[4] as:

> Usual and convenient for experimenters . . . in the sense that they are prepared to ignore all results, which fail to reach this standard, and, by this means, to eliminate from further discussion the greater part of the fluctuations which chance causes have introduced into their experimental results.

Fisher pointed out that there is always a risk of error and asserted that 5 mistakes in 100 repetitions constitutes a reasonable rate of risk.

It is important to note that, relative to the decisions made in everyday life, a 5% risk of error is conservative. Brides and grooms promise to stay together "'til death do us part," but many more than 5% of marriages end in divorce, not death. Racetracks, lotteries, and stock markets would go out of business if everyone insisted on a 95% chance of their investments increasing in value. The standard of a ⅟₂₀ risk of accepting error is intended to prevent any branch of science from collapsing like a house of cards built on poorly supported observations. (However, such a conservative standard probably results in some interesting and useful studies languishing in file drawers.)

Step 5: Sample

The four dentists each treat a sample of 20 patients. At the reunion, the dentists report their data (Table 9-2).

The question is, can these data be explained by chance? To find the answer, we must compare the observed set of facts with some expected values. The various techniques to do so constitute a subject in themselves and are taught in probability and statistics courses. In this section we are primarily concerned with the logic behind statistical tests rather than the computational details.

In all subsequent calculations, we will assume that the sample is obtained randomly and is therefore rep-

Table 9-2 Successes and failures of four dentists		
Dentist	Successes	Failures
A	20	0
B	16	4
C	13	7
D	11	9

resentative of the population. This assumption is common to all statistical inference, though in many instances random sampling is not possible.

Steps 6 and 7: A probability distribution

One possibility is that the observed data result from chance. The goal is to determine, from probability considerations alone, the frequency of success in samples of 20 when the predicted rate of success is 80%.

Step 6: Generating a distribution

The particular distribution of interest for this example is called the *binomial distribution*, which results when there are only two choices—in this case, success or failure, with fixed probabilities of .80 and .20, respectively.

One approach that could be used to calculate the frequencies of success and failure would be to rent a machine that mixes balls and selects them randomly, like those used in a bingo hall. Using white balls to represent success and black balls to represent failure, we would add them to the machine in a ratio of 80:20. This ratio is chosen because the proportion of 80% represents the success rate generally found for endodontic therapy—ie, P_{Others} = .80. To collect the data, we would let the machine select a sample population of 20 balls representing the number of patients treated by each of the four dentists. The number of black and white balls would be tabulated, then thrown back into the machine and another sample of 20 balls would be randomly selected, tabulated, and so on. These collected data are the *reference distribution*.

When 1,000 random samples had been collected in this manner, a table of the results could be prepared (Table 9-3). Using this table, we could plot the reference distribution as a frequency distribution, known as a *relative frequency histogram* (Fig 9-5).

Table 9-3 Results of random selection of a population containing 80% white ping-pong balls and 20% black ping-pong balls (sample of 20; white = success)

No. of white balls (successes)	Frequency (%)
0	0
1	0
2	0
3	0
4	0
5	0
6	0
7	0
8	0
9	0
10	0.2
11	0.7
12	2.2
13	5.5
14	10.9
15	17.6
16	21.8
17	20.6
18	13.6
19	5.9
20	1.0

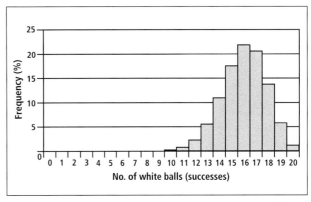

Fig 9-5 Relative frequency histogram of average number of black balls in samples of 20 from a population containing 80% white balls and 20% black balls.

$$P(S) = \text{binomial coefficient } p^S(1-P)^{n-S}$$

The binomial coefficient is derived by the formula

$$\binom{n}{s} = \frac{n!}{s!\,(n-s)!}$$

Some readers might remember that the formula for the binomial coefficient is the same one used in determining the number of combinations of n objects taken S at a time. Other readers might recall that another way of finding the binomial coefficient is to use Pascal's triangle, in which each entry is the sum of the two numbers just above it:

```
            1
         1     1
      1     2     1
   1     3     3     1
1     4     6     4     1
```

No matter how it was generated, the graph displays two points to consider:

1. The peak of the frequency distribution—16 successes, or 4 failures out of 20—is exactly the result expected because the parent population contained 80% white balls. This peak, called the *mode*, is considered the most representative value. However,

Step 7: Frequency distributions

In the preceding example, we generated the frequency distribution using a bingo hall apparatus to mix and select black and white balls randomly. In generating this distribution, we adopted the *frequentist* approach to probability, in which the probability of a given event is the proportion of times the event occurs over the long run (here 1,000 random samples).

We did not need to resort to a mechanical model; a mathematical formula could have been used to calculate the frequencies (and, in fact, was used to generate the data above). In brief, the probability of success is the same for every trial. The probability of obtaining S successes in n trials is derived by the formula

only 21.8% of the samples had this modal (ie, most commonly occurring) value that is characteristic of the parent population. Thus, a sample value is more likely to differ from the true population value than to represent it exactly, and this rule is true of most, but not all, sampling distributions.

2. None of the samples drawn had 0 to 5 successes. This is not surprising; any dentist would intuitively know that if he or she had only 5 successes out of 20 attempts, the results could not be explained by chance. The logic behind this intuition will now be explored.

Steps 8 and 9: Calculation and judgment

Typically, investigators will report the results of statistical testing as a value of P, which is the probability of the result occurring by chance. If the investigator adopts the 5% level of significance, the statement "$P < .05$" means that the results are statistically significant—that is, they are unlikely to be explained by chance.

We know from the experiment with the bingo balls that, because of fluctuations of random sampling, it is unlikely that the difference between the value actually observed minus the value expected from the frequency distribution will exactly equal zero. Thus, we assume that any variation from the expected value is due to chance until demonstrated to be otherwise. This assumption is reasonable. Since we know that random fluctuations always occur, there is no need to postulate any other effect if random fluctuations alone can explain the difference between the observed and the expected values. This conclusion demonstrates the philosophical principle called *Ockham's razor*: One should not multiply causes without reason.

As noted previously, the proposition that (observed minus expected) = 0 is called the *null hypothesis* (often symbolized as H_0). Expressed another way, it could be said that the null is H_0:$P = .80$, where P is the probability of success in the population from which we are sampling. The observed fraction of successes (such as 13 successes out of 20) is tested for its consistency with a true underlying probability of .80. It is always tested for rejection.

If the difference (observed minus expected) is too large to be explained by chance, there must be some other effect operant; the hypothesis that another effect exists is designated as H_1. Thus, the decision of whether the data are consistent with the null hypothesis can be expressed as follows: (observed minus expected) = 0, ie, H_0 true, only random fluctuation operant; (observed minus expected) $\neq$ 0, ie, H_1 true, some other effect operant.

The logic is similar in form to the disjunctive syllogism:

premise 1   *Either H_1 or H_0.*
(where H_1 is the alternative hypothesis, something happened, and results cannot be explained by chance; and H_0 is the null hypothesis, which states that results can be explained by chance)
premise 2   *Not H_0.*
(null hypothesis is rejected)
conclusion   *Therefore H_1.*
(alternative hypothesis is true)

This form of argument is not a deductive syllogism in the strict sense because the statement "not H_0" is not absolute but rather probabilistic. The net result of this argument is that if we can reject the null hypothesis, we can accept the alternative hypothesis. The problem now is, how do we decide that the null hypothesis is false?

For illustration purposes, let us suppose that the results from the four UBC dentists relative to their frequency on the frequency distribution are given in Table 9-4.

Recall that the null hypothesis in this case is that there is no difference in the proportion of successes found in their patients and the proportion of successes for dentists generally. Therefore

Observed	–	Expected	= 0
No. of successes of recent UBC graduate		No. of successes based on experience of all dentists	

We can see that the results of Dentist A, who had 20 successes, are hard to explain by chance because 20 successes in 20 trials would be expected to occur only 1.1% of the time if the sample were drawn from a population with an 80% success ratio.

We should consider that there are two ways in which the UBC graduates could differ from other dentists: They could be better than average or worse than average. In considering performance relative to our reference probability distribution, before collecting data we would consider a result to be different from the reference distribution in two possible ways:

1. More successes than expected. That is, on the basis of the reference distribution, the number of observed successes or a greater number of successes would be predicted to occur 2.5% of the time or less.

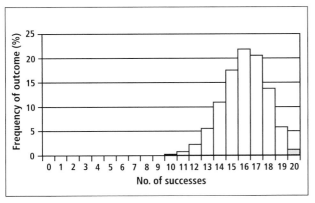

Fig 9-6a Relative frequency histogram for Dentist A.

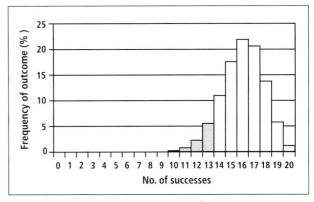

Fig 9-6b Relative frequency histogram for Dentist C.

Table 9-4 Results relative to frequency distribution

Dentist	Success	Failure	Percentage of time this no. of successes expected by chance	Percentage of time this no. of successes or more extreme values expected by chance*
A	20	0	1.1	1.1
B	16	4	20.5	100
C	13	7	5.5	8.6
D	11	9	0.9	1.0

*Successes includes both tails of failures distribution.

2. More failures than expected. That is, on the basis of the reference distribution, the number of observed successes or a smaller number of successes would be predicted to occur 2.5% of the time or less.

In this way, the reference distribution is divided so that the left and right tails are both used and the dividing line is placed 2.5% from each end. In our example, the crude reference distribution does not allow us to place cutoff points at exactly 2.5%, but we can still calculate the expected frequencies.

Therefore, we can conclude that Dentist A's high success rate is unlikely to be due to chance because P = .011, which is less than .025. Such a high success rate would be expected only 1.1% of the time if the null hypothesis were true (Fig 9-6a). Dentist A's result falls outside the 2.5% cutoff line.

On the other hand, we can conclude that there is no evidence to suggest that Dentist B is any different—better or worse—than the average dentist. After all, Dentist B had a success rate of 80%, which matches the most frequently occurring success rate for other dentists. Thus for B, (observed minus expected) = 0. This is not proof that the null hypothesis is true; we

can surmise only that there is insufficient evidence to conclude that it is false. Nevertheless, if the data are such that the null hypothesis cannot be rejected, then it is often said (following Ockham) that one accepts it.

Dentist C is in an awkward position: C's record of 13 successes is below average but not significantly so. We see from Table 9-4 and Fig 9-6b that even if Dentist C's true rate was 80%, observing 7 or more failures occurs more than 2.5% of the time. That is, if C regarded 7 failures as rare, C would also have to classify 8, 9, 10 . . . 20 failures as rare.

If we had chosen a larger sample—say, 300 patients—we might decide that more extreme values are needed. There would be 300 results possible rather than just the 20 results possible in our example. Thus, the number of cases distributed into each result would be spread thin, and the percent frequency for many of these possible results would be low—indeed, less than 5%, even for results not far from the most likely value of 240 successes. Thus, in determining whether a particular result differs from the expected value, the question of interest is not the *frequency* of the particular result (which is determined in part by the number of possible results), but rather the *location* of the result in the distribution. The result can be located by a method similar to that used to find a particular home by its address; rather than searching for the number, however, one uses the cumulative frequency of all results more extreme than the observed result. In the case of Dentist A (20 successes), we are at the end of the street—there is nothing more extreme, and therefore the cumulative frequency equals the number for that particular result—that is, 1.1%. To locate the position of Dentist C's result, we would have to add the frequencies for 7 failures (5.5%) plus 8 failures (2.2%) plus 9 failures (0.7%) plus 10 failures (0.2%) plus 11 to 20 failures (approximately 0%) to get a total of 8.6%. Thus, the probability of getting at least the number of failures obtained by Dentist C is greater than 5%, and Dentist C can accept the null hypothesis.

Dentist D, however, cannot accept the null hypothesis. D can determine that 11 successes in a sample of 20 from a population with an 80% success rate would occur only 0.9% of the time, and the total frequency for 9 or more failures is less than 2.5%. For D, (observed minus expected) $\neq 0$; chance alone cannot explain his low success rate. D must reject H_0 and sadly conclude that his failure rate is higher than expected.

Some issues in statistical inference

One-tailed vs two-tailed tests

In our example, the dentists—prior to treating the patients—agreed to determine whether their results differed from the accepted value of 80% success for endodontic treatment, meaning they would be willing to accept results that were better or worse than average. An extremely modest dentist might decide—once again prior to treating the patients—that it would be impossible (for example, because of the dentist's inexperience) to achieve a better than average success rate. Such a modest dentist would then accept results as being significantly different only if there were more failures than expected. Moreover (assuming the 5% significance level was adopted), the unlikely 5% of the samples would have to be located on the left side of the distribution curve—that is, only one tail (as opposed to both tails) would be examined. Dentist A, for example, would have to accept the null hypothesis. The cutoff line for the lower frequency of success, however, is moved to the right. In our example above, 12 successes would be significantly less (at the 5%

level) than the number of successes expected from a trial of 20 with a probability of success of .80.

Two types of error

Suppose that you are omniscient God and you know that Dentist B is actually worse than average and that B's patients have only a 70% chance of success. Thus, you know that B committed an error upon accepting the null hypothesis. Statisticians say that B has committed a *type II error* and label the chance of erroneously accepting the null hypothesis as β. The power of the test is given by the formula $1 - \beta$. The power quantifies the chances of detecting a real difference of a given size. The calculation of the probability of making a type II error is a complex function of level of significance (ie, α), sample size, and actual magnitude of the difference between the populations (a value often unknown). Moreover, different formulae apply depending on how the data are distributed. Sample size issues, as well as formulae for various applications, are discussed in van Belle.[5]

In the preceding examples, we have considered the dentists' performance relative to a fixed success rate of 80% and a predetermined number of patients (20). However, suppose that two dentists want to compare their success rates relative to one another. We would then want to compare two proportions, each of which can be considered a sample of the outcome for each dentist, for example Dentists B and C:

Null hypothesis H_0 $p_B - p_C = 0$

A common formula for making this comparison follows[4]:

$$Z = \frac{p_B - p_C}{\mathrm{SQR}\left(\dfrac{pq}{n_1} + \dfrac{pq}{n_2}\right)}$$

Z = the z-score for the normal distribution
p_B, p_C are the proportions of successes for Dentists B and C (ie, $p_B = X_B/n_B$, $p_C = X_C/n_C$).
$q = 1 - p$.

$$p = \left(\frac{X_B + X_C}{n_B + n_C}\right)$$

Let X_B, X_C represent the number of successes for Dentists B and C, respectively, when they treated n_B and n_C patients.

This test uses the normal distribution to approximate the binomial distribution and is considered a good approximate test provided that n is large and neither np nor nq is very small. The normal distribution and the reason it is used to approximate other distributions will be discussed in the next chapter.

Suppose one wishes to know how many patients would be required to determine whether patients treated by Dentist B experienced a different success rate from those treated by Dentist C? A simplified formula suggested by van Belle—if one assumes equal sample sizes and a two-tailed test—follows:

$$n = 16 \left(p_{avg} \right) \frac{(1 - p_{avg})}{(p_B - p_C)^2}$$

where $p_B = 0.80$ (Dentist B's success rate was 16/20);

$p_C = 0.65$ (C's success rate was 13/20).

The variance is given by

$$p_{avg} = \frac{(p_B + p_C)}{2} = \frac{(0.80 + 0.65)}{2} = 0.725$$

Substituting the values in the equation,
n = 16 × .725(1 − .725) / (0.15)²
n = 141.8

Thus, each dentist would have to treat about 142 patients to ensure a comparison of reasonable power. This sample size, of course, is much larger than the sample size (20) used to examine the performance of one dentist relative to a fixed success rate, because two samples or sources of variability are present.

Note that type II errors are highly probable. For example, it would be difficult to distinguish between *populations* of 80% and 79% success rates; however, it is probably not a large enough difference to have any practical significance.

The other type of error is called α or *type I error*. This might occur in our example of testing observed vs expected success rates if the dentist's patients actually had an 80% chance of success but, through bad luck, the particular sample that was drawn happened to have 10 failures. The dentist would then reject the null hypothesis even though it was true.

This type of error is at least under the control of the investigator. Setting a higher significance level of, say, 1%, would lower the probability of a type I error. However, for a given sample size, lowering the value of α would increase the chance that an actual difference between groups would fail to be detected. The only way to reduce both α and β simultaneously is to increase the sample size. But a larger sample size may be difficult to obtain because of factors such as cost and subject availability.

Table 9-5 Types of errors

Decision based on data	Actual situation H_0 true	H_0 false
Accept H_0	Correct True negative $1 - \beta$	Type II error False negative β
Reject H_0	Type I error False positive α	Correct True positive $1 - \alpha$

Table 9-5 summarizes the possible outcomes of making a decision based on data and the probability of the outcome in terms of α and β.

Lessons to be learned from these examples

Statistical inference has the following features:

1. It is based on probability (ie, the observed results are compared with samples selected randomly from a specified probability distribution). There is no possibility of attaining absolute certainty in any statistical test of significance.
2. An arbitrary decision must be made on the level of significance. In some instances investigators do select levels of significance other than 5%, on account of considerations such as the consequences in given situations of committing a type I error.
3. The sample size influences the possibility of observing a significant difference.
4. Only two possible hypotheses—which are mutually exclusive and exhaustive—are assumed: the null hypothesis and the alternative hypothesis. In other words, if you reject the null hypothesis, you must accept the alternative hypothesis.

Goodness of Fit

Example of goodness of fit: Mendel's experiment

One class of experiments is specifically designed to determine how well the results fit a theory. Comparison is made not between the results of two or more treatments but between the observed result of a single kind of event and a predicted result based on theory. A classic example of this type of trial is used in genetics, whereby the outcomes of breeding experiments are tested to see if the results can be explained by Mendel's laws. In such experiments, which utilize nominal scale data, the results are normally expressed as counts. With counts, results obtained are whole numbers. This property of discreteness leads to the distinctive methods used in their statistical analysis.

The simplest cases feature only two categories: In Mendel's pea-breeding experiments, color was used as a category. If homozygous yellow seed–producing and green seed–producing pea plants are bred and the yellow color is dominant, all of the progeny in the first generation will be yellow, as shown below:

YY   crossed with   yy
homozygous yellow seed   homozygous green seed
parent   parent
All progeny are Yy

In the first generation, all progeny produce yellow seeds because they all possess the dominant Y. If the first generation is crossed with itself, however,

Yy   crossed with   Yy
YY   +   Yy   +   Yy   +   yy
yellow   yellow   yellow   green
3:1

some green seed producers will be segregated, producing a ratio of 3 yellow:1 green.

From a statistician's point of view, the mechanism is irrelevant. The problem is how to test given sets of data to see how well they fit a hypothesis. Among others (including Fisher[6]), Zar[7] has applied this test to Mendel's data. In 10 experiments (which can be pooled because the samples are homogeneous) involving 478 plants, one would expect 358.5 to be yellow ($\frac{3}{4} \times 478$) and 119.5 to be green ($\frac{1}{4} \times 478$), according to Mendel's law. Mendel actually found 355 yellow peas and 123 green peas. Because of the relatively primitive statistical concepts used at the time, Mendel accepted the findings as close enough to 3:1 to prove the point. Modern statisticians, however, use a chi-squared test where:

χ^2 = Sum of all categories (observed minus expected)^2/expected

$$\chi^2 = \sum_i \frac{(f_i - F_i)^2}{F_i}$$

where f_i = observed frequency in category i and F_i = expected frequency in category i.

Note that if the observed frequency equals the expected frequency, $\chi^2 = 0$, whereas a large discrepancy between expected and observed values produces a high value for χ^2.

Two rules must be observed with the χ^2 test: (1) The actual frequencies must be employed in the calculations (ie, it is not valid to convert the data to percentages and then to compare observed percentages with expected percentages); and (2) the expected value in any comparison should not be less than 1, and less than 20% of the expected values should be less than 5.[6] Given the formula for χ^2, it is obvious that the value would be inflated significantly by having low numbers in the denominator.

From Mendel's data:

$$\chi^2 = \frac{(355 - 358.5)^2}{358.5} + \frac{(123 - 119.5)^2}{119.5} = 0.137$$

But if $\chi^2 > 0$, the question we must ask is, how often could we expect to get results that deviate from the expected values by at least that much, based on random samples of a population that is $\frac{3}{4}$ yellow and $\frac{1}{4}$ green? In theory (for this case), we could generate such a distribution by making a tetrahedral die with three sides marked yellow and one side marked green, then tossing it 478 times and documenting the number of times green faced down and the number of times yellow faced down. We would repeat this die-tossing experiment many times to see how often the deviations of the observed ratio exceeded those of Mendel. To save us the trouble of making tetrahedral dice (not to mention all the tossing), probability theorists have devised a χ^2 distribution to analyze such data. The shape of the χ^2 curve depends on the number of degrees of freedom (df), which in turn is related to the number of categories compared. The mathematics used to derive the χ^2 distribution (and thus the Table of Critical Values [appendix 4]) is complex and need not concern us here. Use of the table, however, is quite simple. If the ratio obtained by Mendel occurred reasonably often, we would not be in a position to reject the hypothesis that the ratio is 3:1. On the other hand, if the results with such a large deviation seldom occurred—say, less than 5% of the time—then we would conclude that it is unlikely the sample came from a population where the color ratio was 3:1.

Of course, the results of Mendel's experiment fit well with his 3:1 hypothesis. Since there are only two groups (yellow or green), the df is calculated as follows:

(No. of groups − 1) = 2 − 1 = 1.

When we consult the Table of Critical Values (see appendix 4), we find that with 1 *df*, the critical value at the .05 level of significance is χ^2_1 = 3.841, which of course is much greater than the 0.137 value calculated from the observations. Therefore, the observed numbers do not differ significantly from those expected from a population with a 3:1 ratio. Note that the same reasoning applied earlier in another statistical test is applied here: There is an arbitrary level of significance (here α = 5%), and the null hypothesis is tested for rejection. Moreover, the test is directional in the sense that it does not prove that the sample came from a population with a color ratio of 3:1 but only that the data are compatible with such a proposal.

Many, including Fisher,[4] have speculated that Mendel's results are "too good to be true"—that finding the data to be in such close agreement with a hypothesis would be extremely rare, raising the possibility that Mendel cooked his data to agree with his hypothesis. More recent research[6] has tended to look at Mendel's results less critically. For example, it is known that Mendel also published data that did not agree with his hypothesis, and it is difficult to understand why he would cook his data in one case and not the other. In the time since Mendel performed his experiments there have been many developments in statistics, of course, including the practice modern scientists adopt of "stopping rules" to determine when an experiment should be curtailed. One explanation that has been proposed is that Mendel simply collected data until it supported his hypothesis and then stopped. In any case, Fisher was reluctant to assign personal blame to Mendel and noted the possibility "that Mendel was deceived by some assistant who knew too well what was expected."

Why use nonparametric statistics?

In statistics, the term *parameter* refers to a quantity used in defining the distribution of a variable (such as age) in a population. The binomial distribution, for example, uses parameters defined by the number of trials and the probability of success in each one. Unlike tests that are based on a normal distribution of values, in the χ^2 test used in the Mendel example, no parameters, such as a mean or a variance, were calculated from the data. The χ^2 test in that example is a nonparametric statistic; it is *distribution-free*, which means that the form of the distri-

bution does not have to be specified and only the expected values are required.

There remains the assumption that the difference between the observed values and the expected values arises from a random sampling. Another requirement is that the expected values, as noted earlier, should not be less than 5 in more than 20% of the cells. It should also be noted that measured values of variables can follow a χ^2 distribution, in which case parameters such as *df* and mean are involved.

The logic of nonparametric inference is based on the principles of finite probability and makes use of the concept that an event's probability can be thought of as the frequency of that event relative to other events over the long term. In addition to χ^2, a number of other nonparametric tests have been developed to analyze other types of comparisons.

The major limitation of nonparametric tests is that they are generally less sensitive compared with a classical test used on parametric data (eg, t test).[8] Nonparametric tests are less likely to detect a significant difference between groups, if such a difference is present, and hence more likely to accept the null hypothesis even when it is false. For some data, one could choose to use a parametric test or a nonparametric test. Willemsen[9] offers three reasons investigators use nonparametric tests:

1. The assumptions prevalent in common parametric tests about distribution and parameters are not met by the measurements used in a study.
2. A general attitude dictates that research conclusions should be based on as small a number of untested assumptions as can possibly be arranged.
3. Investigators determine that a particular nonparametric test is the one most likely to reject the null hypothesis being tested if it is indeed false.

Example of goodness of fit to a probability distribution: Poisson's distribution

The binomial distribution deals with situations in which it can be determined when an event (eg, success or cure) occurred or did not occur (eg, failure) and the total number of possible outcomes (eg, patients treated) is known. Often for natural phenomena, however, the occurrence

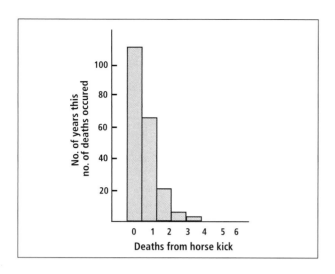

Fig 9-7 Relative frequency histogram.

Table 9-6 Distribution of no. of deaths per year by horse kick for the Prussian cavalry

No. of deaths per year per corps	0	1	2	3	4
Frequency taken from actual data	109	65	22	3	1
Probability	.543	.331	.101	.021	.003
Frequency expected by Poisson (m = 0.61)	109	66.3	20.2	4.1	0.6

of events can be measured (such as flashes of lightning), whereas the frequency of occurrence of nonevents is not evident. Because a flash of lightning can occur in an infinitesimally small amount of time, it would be difficult to calculate in how many of these units of time a flash of lightning did not occur. Often, the probability of a given number of occurrences can be calculated using the *Poisson distribution*, which describes isolated events or occurrences in a continuum, such as space or time. The only condition is that the expected number must be constant from trial to trial. Sometimes called the *law of small numbers*, the Poisson distribution is often used in describing rare events and can be considered an approximation of the binomial distribution, where P (probability of event occurring) is very small and n is relatively large.

A widely used example of this distribution is the data collected on the number of men in the Prussian army who were killed by horse kick over 20 years in 10 army corps (Fig 9-7). A full analysis of the data by Moroney[10] reveals that the condition of constant expectation was met. Had the 10 corps varied greatly in number of men or horses, for example, or had the Prussian cavalry instituted a "Safety with Horses" campaign during the period of the study, then that condition

would not have been met. As we can see, the distribution is highly skewed.

The equation for the Poisson distribution is:

$$P(r) = e^{-m} \times \frac{m^r}{r!}$$

$P(r)$ = probability of event (in this example, death by horse kick) occurring r times

where $r! = r \, (r - 1) \cdot (r - 2) \cdot (r - 3) \ldots 1$
(eg, $5! = 5 \cdot 4 \cdot 3 \cdot 2 \cdot 1 = 120$) and

m = mean number of events per unit of time (in this example, year)

e = base of natural or Napieran logarithms
$= \frac{1}{0!} + \frac{1}{1!} + \frac{1}{2!} + \ldots = 2.7183$

The Poisson distribution is defined by just one parameter—the mean or variance (since, for the Poisson distribution, the variance equals the mean). Because it is often used to look at rates or number of events with time, the Poisson distribution sometimes expresses the mean as mean = r t, where r is the rate per unit time and t is the length of time under consideration.

The data from the Prussian cavalry deaths by horse kick yield an estimate of 122/200 deaths per year per corps (ie, m = 0.61). Using the formula, we can calcu-

Table 9-7 Observed frequencies of caries in Saudi naval men*

Carrier type	Caries present	Caries absent	Row total
e carriers [+]	52	4	$56 = R_1$
Non-e carriers [–]	110	30	$140 = R_2$
Column total	162	34	196 total N

*Data from Keene et al.[12]

late the probability for 0, 1, 2, 3, and 4 deaths per year as expected by the Poisson distribution (Table 9-6)

Inspection of these numbers reveals that the Poisson distribution demonstrates a very good fit with the actual observed data. One could do a χ^2 analysis as follows:

$$\chi^2 = \frac{(109-109)^2}{109} + \frac{(65-66.3)^2}{66.3} + \frac{(25-24.9)^2}{24.9}$$

(The last three cells have been combined so that the expected value for any cell is not < 1 and so that less than 20% of the expected values are < 5^3.)

$$\chi^2 = 0 + 0.02549 + 0.0004 = 0.02589$$

For $df = 2$ and $\alpha = 0.05$, the $\chi^2_{2crit} = 5.99$

Thus, because the χ^2 value for the fit to the null hypothesis is much less than the critical value, we must accept the null hypothesis and conclude that the observed fluctuations from those predicted by the Poisson distribution could be explained by chance.

Note that the Poisson distribution does not produce the normal bell-shaped distribution—also called the *Gaussian distribution*—that is used most widely in statistics (see chapter 10).

Knowing the distribution of values that occurs in a sample is important because it allows estimates to be made about the parent population. Kac[11] recounts the story of the mathematician Steinhous, who was forced to live under an assumed name in Poland during the Second World War and to hide in the forest most days and nights. The only information he had of the war was from a German-controlled newspaper, which functioned for propaganda purposes and emphasized the great victories of the German armies. Steinhous wondered about the true losses of the German army. He noted that the authorities allowed a fixed number of obituaries of the form "Hans the son of Klaus and Hildegard Schmidt fell for the Fatherland." However, some of the obituaries read "Dieter the second son of Klaus and Hildegard Schmidt to fall for the Fatherland. . . ." Knowing that the number of male offspring in a family follows a Poisson distribution and knowing the average number of male offspring, Steinhous could determine the proportion of soldiers killed. From this he could estimate the true losses of the German army, and these vast numbers gave him hope that Germany would eventually lose the war. The estimate proved to be quite accurate, which is a tribute not only to Steinhous but also to the power of understanding probability distributions.

The Poisson distribution has many applications: It describes situations such as the distribution of Simplified Oral Health Index (OHI-S) scores; the number of blood cells found in one square of a hemocytometer; radioactive decay; cohort studies of diseases with rare events; and even the number of goals in a soccer match.

Contingency Tables: An Especially Useful Tool in Evaluating Clinical Reports

Contingency tables, also known as *bivariate frequency distribution tables*, allow investigators to identify an association between two variables. These tables can be particularly useful in evaluating clinical dental research articles because the results are often presented in a form that can be considered as nominal scale data. Patients will be either male or female, their problem will fall into some category, and the treatment will be a success or failure. The relationship among these variables can be elucidated through contingency-table analysis. For example, consider the data of Keene et al[12] on Saudi naval men (Table 9-7). As presented, this is a contingency table. It has four cells and shows

Table 9-8 Expected frequencies of caries in Saudi naval men*

Carrier type	Caries +	Caries –
e carriers [+]	46.3	9.7
Non-e carriers [–]	115.7	24.3

*Data from Keene et al.[12]

Table 9-9 χ^2 values for Table 9-7

	Observed – expected	After continuity correction	(Observed – expected)^2	$\dfrac{\text{(Observed – expected)}^2}{\text{Expected}}$
Row 1 column 1	52 – 46.3 = 5.7	5.2	27	0.58
Row 1 column 2	4 – 9.72 = –5.7	–5.2	27	2.78
Row 2 column 1	110 – 115.7 = –5.7	–5.2	27	0.23
Row 2 column 2	30 – 24.3 = 5.7	5.2	27	1.11
Total χ^2				4.70

the totals for the rows and columns. The frequency f_{rc} refers to the value found in row r and column c. Thus, in this example, $f_{11} = 52$. The *df* for this test is:

$$df = (\text{no. of rows} - 1) \times (\text{no. of columns} - 1)$$
$$= (2 - 1) \times (2 - 1) = 1 \times 1 = 1$$

The total frequency for the row (R_i) is the sum of all frequencies in the row, where i = the row number and j = the column number.

In our example,

$$R_1 = \sum_{C=1}^{2} f_{1c} = 52 + 4 = 56$$

Similarly, for column 1,

$$C_1 = \sum_{r=1}^{2} f_{r1} = 52 + 110 = 162$$

Next, we can calculate the expected frequencies if there was no association between the variables according to the formula:

$$F_{rc} = \frac{R_r \times C_c}{n}$$

where n = total in the sample. In our example,

$$F_{11} = \frac{56 \times 162}{196} = 46.3$$

The values of the expected frequencies are calculated in Table 9-8. Now the χ^2 value can be calculated for each cell (Table 9-9).

The calculated χ^2 is 4.70 with *df* = 1. The critical value of χ^2 is (α = .05, *df* = 1) = 3.84. Because 4.70 > 3.84, we must reject the null hypothesis and conclude that for these Saudi naval men, the presence of caries is significantly associated with the possession of e-type *Streptococcus mutans*. Despite this statistically significant association, however, an analysis to be presented later shows the strength of the association to be quite weak. Thus, this example demonstrates that statistical significance and size of effect are separate facets of data interpretation.

An assumption of some commonly used statistical tests is that the samples are drawn from a parent population with a Gaussian (normal) distribution. However, measurement of some characteristics might show frequency distributions that are decidedly non-normal.

Often when we measure any sample of objects, we are trying to infer something about the parent population. Suppose we had only a small number of sample values, and consequently we did not get a frequency distribution curve. We could first calculate the mean, m, from our (small) sample. If we assumed that the parent population was Poisson distributed, we would make our inferences on the basis of a skewed curve, whereas if we assumed the parent population was normally distributed we would use a curve that was symmetrically centered around m. Thus, our assumptions would have influenced our conclusions—clearly undesirable. As noted earlier, some scientists prefer to keep the number of assumptions to a minimum and to use distribution-free tests. Others appear to assume that the normal distribution applies to every measurement. This is a dubious assumption. Apparently, in many instances in which large bodies of data on observational variation have been tested against the normal distribution, they have shown disagreement. The essential point here is that the assumption of a particular distribution can influence the conclusion.

References

1. Gould SJ. The New York Times Review of Books 18 August 1988:35.
2. Gleason RW. The Essential Pascal. Toronto: Mentor-Omega, 1966:89–97.
3. Larkin PA. Notes for Biology 300 (Biometrics). A Handbook of Elementary Statistical Tests. Vancouver, BC: Univ of British Columbia, 1978:15–22.
4. Fisher RA. The Design of Experiments, ed 8. New York: Hafner, 1966:13.
5. van Belle G. CH^2 Sample Size. Statistical Rules of Thumb. New York: J Wiley, 2002:29–51.
6. Piegorsch WW. Fisher's contribution to genetics and heredity, with special emphasis on the Gregor Mendel controversy. Biometrics 1990;46;4:915–924.
7. Zar JH. Biostatistical Analysis, ed 2. Englewood Cliffs, NJ: Prentice Hall, 1984:70.
8. Porkess R. Collins Web-linked Dictionary of Statistics, ed 2. Glasgow: HarperCollins, 2005.
9. Willemsen EW. Understanding Statistical Reasoning. San Francisco: Freeman, 1974:170.
10. Moroney MJ. Facts from Figures. Harmondsworth, England: Penguin, 1965:96–107.
11. Kac M. Marginalia: Statistical odds and ends. Am Sci 1983;71:186.
12. Keene HJ, Shklair IL, Anderson DM, Mickel GJ. Relationship of *Streptococcus mutans* biotypes to dental caries prevalence in Saudi Arabian naval men. J Dent Res 1977;56:356.

Resources for Statistics

A number of reference texts are available that present statistical concepts and calculations in greater detail than occurs here:

Norman GR, Streiner DL. Biostatistics: The Bare Essentials, 2nd ed. Hamilton, Ontario: Decker, 2000.

Staff of Research and Education Association. The Statistics Problem Solver. New York: Research and Education Association, 1982.

Zar JH. Biostatistical Analysis, ed 2. Englewood Cliffs, NJ: Prentice Hall, 1984

A number of websites perform calculations and enable you to see the effects of manipulations (for example, seeing the effects of sample size on the distribution of means):

http://www.stat.tamu.edu/~west/applets/
http://departments.vassar.edu/~lowry/tabs.html
http://www.quintpub.com/CriticalThinking

10 | Elements of Probability and Statistics, Part 2: Continuous Variables

> *Probability theory is nothing but common sense reduced to calculation.*
> —Pierre Simon Laplace[1]

The previous chapter largely concerned *discrete variables* (mainly counts), but most measurements deal with *continuous variables,* which, at least in theory, can take on an infinite range of values. An example of a discrete variable is the value found on the throw of a die. The mean value for a single throw of a die is (1 + 2 + 3 + 4 + 5 + 6)/6 = 3.5; however, we do not actually observe the value 3.5, because only the discrete integers 1, 2, 3, 4, 5, and 6 are possible. A continuous variable, conversely, is a variable for which there is virtually an infinite number of possible values (given a scale of sufficient magnitude). Recent work on the weight of an electron, for example, has described it to 17 decimal places. When describing the frequency distribution of measurements of continuous variables, it is not possible to put every measurement into its own frequency cell or bin, as we could in the frequency histogram in the example for the binomial distribution (which had 20 bins for the 20 possible values) (see Fig 9-5). Indeed, most of the infinite number of bins representing the infinite measured values of a continuous variable would not contain any measurement if the measurements were taken from a finite population.

To calculate the distribution of values for a given range of a continuous variable, statisticians apply the concept of *probability density.* A simple application of this concept is demonstrated in the uniform distribution (Fig 10-1), which has a constant probability density that is equal to 1 throughout the range of the variable from x = 0 to x = 1. Because the ordinate is 1

throughout this range and because the highest possible x value is 1, the total area of the uniform distribution is 1 (ie, 1 [the width] × 1 [the height] = 1). The uniform distribution of a variable is useful for comparing the relative probability of mutually exclusive events. For example, to calculate the probability that a value selected at random is ≤ 0.4, we would measure the area under the uniform distribution curve from x = 0 to x = 0.40 and find that this area is equal to 0.4. In other words, the probability (P) = .4. The probability that a value selected at random is greater than 0.4 is mutually exclusive of the event that P ≤ .4, so its probability can be calculated as equal to 1, or P = .6. Graphically, this can be illustrated as shown in Fig 10-2.

The uniform distribution is a simple relationship, and calculation of areas, as shown above, is straightforward. For more complex distributions, integral calculus is used to calculate areas under probability density curves. Just as differential calculus concerns rates of change in infinitesimally small steps, integral calculus calculates the cumulative effect of many small changes in a quantity—such as occurs when the values of a continuous variable are spread over a range specified by a probability density function. In other words, integral calculus allows us to calculate the area under the curve of a probability density function for a given range of a continuous variable, and that area corresponds to the probability that values in that range will occur (given the condition that the total area under the probability density curve is 1).

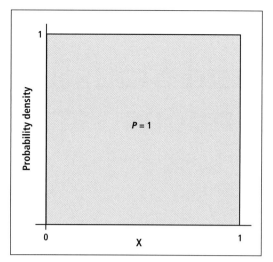

Fig 10-1 The uniform distribution in which the probability density is constant throughout the range of possible values from x = 0 to x = 1, and "0" elsewhere. Total area = 1.

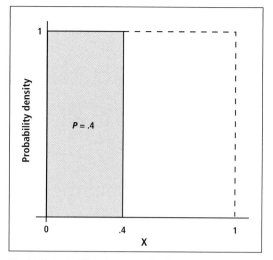

Fig 10-2 Probability that a randomly selected value of x ≤ 0.4.

The Normal Distribution

In the preceding chapter, we looked at sampling from the binomial distribution, as well as possible outcomes from the sum of two dice; both of these examples used discrete variables. We now look at what we expect when we sample a variable with a continuous distribution. Empirically, many types of scores have been found to follow the so-called normal or Gaussian (after the mathematician Carl Gauss, 1777–1855) distribution. The distribution is called *normal* because some early statisticians mistakenly believed that most probability distributions followed the "normal" curve, whose mathematical equation is given by:

$$p(x) = \frac{1}{\sigma\sqrt{2\pi}}\, e^{-\frac{1}{2}\frac{(x-\mu)^2}{\sigma^2}}$$

where p(x) = probability density function
σ^2 = variance
x = the variate
μ = mean value of x for the population—ie, the average

Note that, by convention, one uses the Greek symbols μ for the mean of the population and σ^2 for the variance of the population. When describing samples from the population, one uses $\overline{X}$ for the mean and s^2 for the variance.[2]

For a number of applications, it is useful to consider the so-called *z-score*, defined as:

$$z = \frac{x - \mu}{\sigma}$$

If the mean μ = 0, and the standard deviation (SD) σ = 1, equation 1 reduces to:

$$p(x) = \frac{1}{\sqrt{2\pi}}\, e^{-\frac{1}{2}z^2}$$

This is called the *standard normal distribution*. The constant

$$\frac{1}{\sqrt{2\pi}}$$

is a scale factor to make the total area under the normal curve equal to 1.

The standard normal distribution curve (Fig 10-3) has many uses, but it is perhaps most commonly used to calculate the percentage of values beneath some portion of the curve or the likelihood of any particular value. For example, if you scored 90 on a test in which the mean grade was 70 and the SD was 10, you could infer—if the grades were normally distributed—that you performed better than about 97.5% of the class, since your grade was 2 SDs above the mean. Similarly, the teacher would expect the percentage of students whose grades fell between 70 and 80 to be 34%. Interestingly, the normal curve never touches zero—it extends out to infinity in both directions, so the existence of some particular high or low value is rare but never theoretically impossible as an illustration of this principle. The tallest man in recorded medical history was said to be Robert Wadlow, who was measured at 8 feet, 11 inches (2.72 m), almost 6 SDs above the mean height of American males.

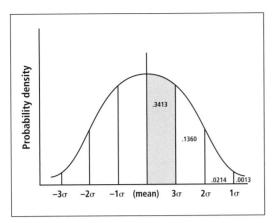

Fig 10-3 Standard normal distribution curve. (Areas not to scale.)

Confidence Intervals

Sample from a population of known dispersion

Suppose we want to estimate the amount of foul-smelling CH_3SH in air expelled from the human mouth under a certain condition. Moreover, suppose that the only material we can get is provided in one sample that is representative of the population of measurements that may be taken under that condition. We want to use the information from that sample to estimate the true value of CH_3SH level for the population.

We take the sample to be run on a gas chromatograph under the direction of the father of malodor analysis, Dr J. Tonzetich. After the analysis, Tonzetich reports that there are 147 ppm of CH_3SH in that sample. However, we do not know the accuracy of that determined value and want some estimate of how random fluctuations affect the value. Because Tonzetich has been running the gas chromatograph machine for 30 years, we decide to ask him, and he replies that his experience, based on 10,000 measurements on a calibrated reference standard, is that the SD is 5 ppm. We are now in a position to calculate the range within which the true value for the population may be found.

First, we must decide on a level of certainty, and, like many biologists, we will be satisfied with 95% certainty. If we know (for example from plotting

Tonzetich's population of 10,000 samples) or assume that the values are normally distributed, then we can infer that 95% of the values fall within 1.96σ (where σ is the population SD) of the true value. Therefore, if we take the determined value and go 1.96σ in either direction, there is a 95% chance that the range so defined—called *confidence limits* (CL)—will include the true value.

Hence, we calculate as follows:

Confidence interval (CI) = range in which true value will be found 95% of the time = determined value ± 1.96σ SD = 147 ± 9.8 ppm.

Technically, a 95% CI (ie, mean ± 1.96σ) means that if we performed the sampling experiment repeatedly, we would get a value within the CI 95% of the time.

Sample from a normal distribution

Suppose that, instead of one sample, we had four samples. Clearly, this puts us in a better position, since the chance that all four samples were drawn from some extreme of the population distribution is smaller than the chance of that occurring with one sample. When calculating the mean of the four samples, we would expect a better estimate of the mean of the population than if we simply took a single sample. But exactly how much better? If we are sampling from a population with a normal distribution, the distribution of the means for any given sample size is also normal, with an SD given by $\sigma/\sqrt{n}$. This new statistic, which describes the sample-to-sample variation in the mean from samples of size n, is called the *standard error* (SE):

$$SE = \frac{\sigma}{\sqrt{n}}$$

We can illustrate graphically how the distribution of means changes with the sample size. Figure 10-4b shows the expected distribution of means when a sample size of 2 is used to construct the means, 10-4c for a sample size of 4, 10-4d for a sample size of 8, and 10-4e for a sample size of 12.

The CL for these distributions can be shown mathematically:

$$CI = \bar{X} \pm z\frac{\sigma}{\sqrt{n}}$$

where z (based on the normal distribution) = 1.96 for 95% CI and 2.58 for 99% CI, etc.

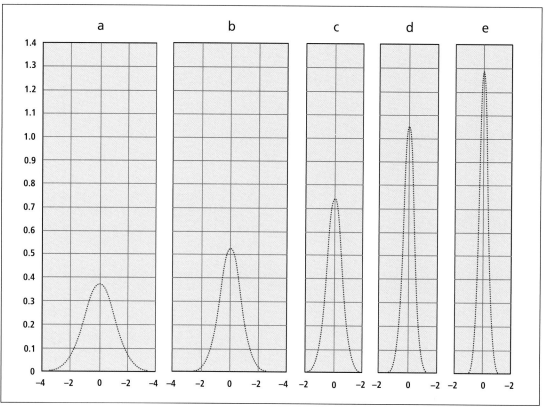

Fig 10-4 Effect of sample size on the expected distribution of means: *(a)* original distribution, *(b)* distribution of means of sample size of 2, *(c)* 4, *(d)* 8, *(e)* 12.

Assuming for the sake of illustration that the four samples have a mean of 147, the CI becomes:

$$CI = 147 \pm 1.96 \frac{5}{\sqrt{4}} \text{ ppm} = 147 \pm 4.9$$

Note that the CI has been halved by using a sample of 4.

Sample from a population whose dispersion is not known "a priori"

Once again, suppose we want to measure sulfur levels in air expelled from the mouth, but we have offended Tonzetich because we refused to drink his homemade wine, Chateau Tonzetich. Therefore, we consult another biochemist; however, lacking Tonzetich's experience, this biochemist does not have data to provide us with the SD of the measurement. But, because we (again) have four samples and hence four values, we can calculate an SD for our combined samples. The problem becomes how to use the SD calculated from the sample to arrive at the population's SD. Fortu-

nately, this mathematical problem has been solved by Gosset, who published under the pseudonym *Student* so competitors would not know the sophisticated statistical control measures being used by his employer, Guinness Brewery. Gosset found that values could be calculated that could convert the samples' SD s to the population's SD σ. In brief, he derived these numbers, called the *Student distribution,* or *t distribution,* by sampling from a normal population. This exercise in probability theory yielded a distribution curve, the shape of which was found to depend on the size of the sample, or the number of *degrees of freedom (df)* of the sample. As the number in the sample increases, his curve approaches the normal curve. Based on Gosset's work, CLs can be calculated as follows:

$$CI = \bar{X} \pm t \frac{s}{\sqrt{n}}$$

where $\bar{X}$ = mean of sample (in this example, $\bar{X}$ = 147)
s = SD of sample
n = number of observations
t = a constant for a given number of *df* (n – 1) and certainty

The actual value of t can be located in statistical tables (see appendix 3).

Thus, if the mean of the four samples was 147 and the SD was 10, the 95% CIs would be:

$$CI = 147 \pm t \times \frac{10}{\sqrt{4}} \text{ ppm}$$

From the table, t ($df = 3$, $\sigma = .05$) = 3.182
$$CI = 147 \pm 15.9$$

Estimation

Calculation of CIs is an example of *estimation*, the process whereby one calculates the value of an unknown quantity—here the level of sulfhydryl components—on the basis of a particular sample of data. There will always be some uncertainty associated with an estimate; that uncertainty is indicated by the CI—typically 95%. If, for example, one measured sulfhydryl levels in a subject's mouth air with another four times (ie, four new samples) one would probably get a slightly different mean and a slightly different 95% CI. However, if the sampling process were repeated many times, we would find that the CIs calculated from our samples would cover the true population mean about 95% of the time.

From the perspective of dental clinicians, an important use of CIs arises during meta-analysis of the literature, in which the effects of a treatment found in different studies are compared. For example, Worthington[3] compared the change in attachment level in four studies of guided tissue regeneration. Figure 10-5 demonstrates that only one of the studies (Study C) included the value indicating no effect, and three of the studies had CIs that fell in the region favoring the control—ie, the untreated group. In meta-analysis, studies are often combined and weighted by such variables as number of subjects in the study to produce a combined CI.

An advantage of using CIs, as opposed to simple null hypothesis testing, is that one sees immediately the relative variation and range of possible effect sizes, rather than basing one's decision on a single test. Moreover, as shown in the meta-analysis example, one can compare different studies directly or with regard to other methods of treatment. Another common use of CIs is to calculate the CI of the difference between two means, typically the difference between control and treated populations. If the CI includes

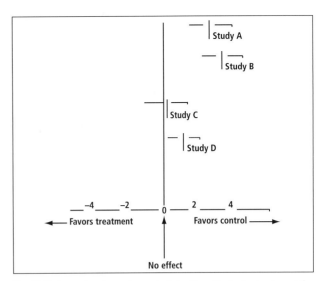

Fig 10-5 Example of a meta-analysis for the effect of a treatment for continuous outcome variable. Three studies (A, B, D) found the treatment to be less effective than the control. Study C found no effect.

zero, then the treatment has not been demonstrated to have a significant effect.

One might wish to use CIs to predict the results of hypothesis testing in comparing means directly. Intuitively, it would seem that if the 95% CIs for the estimated mean of two populations overlapped, then the means for the two populations (say, treated and control groups) would not differ significantly at the 5% level. However, CIs for two statistics can overlap by as much as 29% and yet the statistics can be significantly different.[2]

Relationships Between the Normal, Poisson, and Binomial Distributions

The binomial distribution discussed earlier (and illustrated in Fig 9-5) lacks the familiar symmetrical bell-shaped appearance of a normal curve. However, if p (proportion of successes) or q = (1 – p) = 0.5, then the binomial distribution is symmetrical. Moreover, as n, the number of trials, increases to become at least greater than 20, and for any given probability P such that .2 < P < .8, it turns out that the binomial distribution can be approximated by the normal curve with:

the mean μ = np, and

the SD $\sigma = \sqrt{np\,(1-p)}$

The value of n required to get a reasonable approximation is smallest when $P = .05$ and increases as the value of p or q increases, because the underlying binomial distribution is less symmetrical.

An advantage of using the normal distribution to approximate the binomial is computational; tables giving the probability represented by various areas on standard normal curves are common, and scientists are accustomed to working with them. An example is the use of z-scores of the standard normal distribution to calculate probabilities of events. For example, one might wonder how rare it is to flip a coin 100 times and get 55 or fewer heads. Assuming a fair coin (that is, the expected number of heads is 50), one could calculate:

$$Z = \frac{x - \mu}{\sigma}$$

where
x = number of heads
μ = mean
σ = SD

Thus,

$$\mu = np = 100 \times 0.5 = 50$$
$$\sigma = \sqrt{npq} = \sqrt{100 \times 0.5 \times 0.5} = 5$$
$$P\,(\chi \le 55) = P\left(Z \le \frac{55-50}{5}\right) = P\,(Z \le 1)$$

Looking up a table of Z, one finds that the area of the standard normal curve between 0 and 1 is 0.341. Another 0.5 of the standard normal curve area is found for values less than z-scores of 0. So the total probability of getting 55 heads or fewer in 100 flips of a coin is .841, or 84.1% of the time.

One can also use the normal approximation to calculate CLs for the expected number of events using the formula:

$$SE = \frac{SD}{\sqrt{n}}$$

Thus, as with the earlier discussion of parametric data having means, the 95% CI for the expected number of events will be:

$$95\%\,CI = np \pm 1.96\sqrt{np\,(1-p)}$$

Finally, the binomial distribution can also be approximated by the Poisson distribution, when either p or q is fairly small; the closer p or q is to zero, the better the approximation.

Concluding Remarks

This and the preceding chapter provide an elementary introduction to the statistical concepts most widely used in science. More information, such as simple calculations for estimating sample sizes for parametric data and effect sizes, are given later. However, statistics is a complex field, and the information presented in this book would be sufficient for some types of statistically simple laboratory and clinical research but insufficient for others. For those readers planning an investigation, it is worthwhile to consult a statistician prior to embarking on a study, so that common statistical pitfalls can be avoided. It should also be noted that the field of statistics is continually developing, and, as in dentistry, specialists—for example, experts in cluster sampling—have emerged. Thus, just as in dentistry, where you may or may not want a specialist endodontist to do your root canal, in designing your investigation, you may or may not want a specialist statistician providing advice.

References

1. Laplace PS. Théorie analytique des probabilités, 1812. Cited in CIM Bulletin no. 11, December 2001, Gallerie: Diogo Pacheco d'Amorim.
2. van Belle G. Statistical Rules of Thumb. New York: Wiley, 2002:39.
3. Worthington H. Understanding the statistical pooling of data. In: Clarkson J, Harrison J, Ismail A, Needleman I, Worthington H (eds). Evidence-Based Dentistry for Effective Practice. London: Martin Dunitz, 2003:75–87.

For a list of statistics resources, please see under References in chapter 9.

11 | The Importance of Measurement in Dentistry

At a meeting of the Evolution Committee of the Royal Society, Weldon had read a paper on the sizes of the carapaces of a certain population of crabs. Bateson, who considered the results of no biological importance, when asked by the Chairman of the Committee to comment did so in a single devastating sentence: Though all science might be measurement, all measurement was not necessarily science.
— Vernon Herbert Blackman[1]

A Canadian *Reader's Digest* article published in 1998, entitled "How Honest Are Dentists?," described the experiences of an investigative reporter who was examined by and received treatment recommendations from 45 dentists randomly chosen from across Canada.[2] The results, which to a certain extent impugned dentists' honesty, revealed that the cost of the recommended treatments ranged from $18 to more than $18,000. While some of the difference in cost estimates could doubtless be ascribed to treatment philosophy, much of it resulted from dentists' inability to agree on which teeth have caries. Categorization is the simplest method of measurement, and yet the 10 dentists who examined the reporter in British Columbia and Alberta, for example, differed significantly. Three of the 10 pronounced the reporter caries free, while others identified caries in 9 different teeth. The diagnosis of caries, surely one of the most important activities in clinical dentistry, thus appears to be less than exact in practice, and, indeed, developing new methods of caries detection constitutes an active area of dental research.[3] As new technologies are applied to dentistry, new measurement techniques are often required to assess their effectiveness. For example, the widespread use of dental implants combined with the growing consumer interest in esthetics led to the need for an index to evaluate the soft tissue around single-tooth implant crowns, and new indices have been developed.[4,5] Measurement is an important compo-

nent of dental research; this chapter reviews the basic concepts.

Operational Definitions

By performing certain operations, we can obtain numbers that describe an object; such description involving the use of numbers is *measurement*. For a measurement to be well-specified, the conditions and procedures that define it must be stated in such explicit detail that anyone could perform the same operations and obtain the same number. The physicist Bridgman[6] argued that every scientific term must be specifiable by a definite testing procedure that provides criteria for its application. These criteria are called *operational definitions*. One operational definition for the presence of plaque is to stain it by having the subject rinse with a solution of dye; if plaque is present, a specific result is obtained, namely the presence of visible stained material on the tooth. The testing procedure could be performed in various ways, such as with or without rinsing, thus introducing the possibility that loosely held stained material would be eliminated. Thus, the nature of the testing procedure determines what is being measured. Although many techniques claim to measure the same property or characteristic, they actually differ markedly in what they measure. For example, the following substrates have been proposed to measure the clearance of food debris ingested for experimental purposes.[7]

- Gingerbread biscuits containing copper or iron
- Standard biscuits with ferric oxide as a marker
- Peanut butter with radio-iodinated serum albumin as a marker
- Soda cracker debris stained with iodine

Since soda crackers and peanut butter vary considerably in stickiness, the measurement of retention or clearance of ingested food debris clearly depends very much on the manner in which the test is performed.

Different definitions can give rise to markedly different estimates of the prevalence of disease: Two radiographic studies of the prevalence of chronic periodontitis in 13- to 15-year-old adolescents in England and Denmark gave estimates of 0.06%[8] and 51.5%,[9] respectively. The radical difference appears to be the result of varying diagnostic radiographic criteria used in the two studies.

Wilson[10] proposed that a full-fledged operational definition of a scientific quality has four stages:

1. An intuitive feeling for the quality
2. A method of comparison that allows the determination that A has more of the quality than B
3. A set of standards against which the quality can be compared and by which categories can be devised
4. The interrelation of standards as may be required if there are different ways of measuring the same property

Resolution

Resolution expresses how finely detailed a measurement can be. At first it might seem that resolution is a straightforward concept. For example, it would seem self-evident that a ruler marked in centimeters could provide measurements to the nearest centimeter and no smaller. If we were using the ruler to compare the lengths of two lines and both lines fell between the 7- and 8-cm marks, we would have to conclude that they were the same length. However, if one of the lines was 7.1 cm and the other 7.9 cm, it would be obvious to even a casual observer that the lines differ in length. Typically, scientific observers in-

terpolate between the markings. Indeed, there is a fairly general belief that a trained observer can carry the measurement to one significant figure beyond what is strictly justified by the absolute resolving power of the system. Nevertheless, my own experience contradicts this belief. When I studied analytical chemistry, students were expected to make readings to the nearest 0.01 mL on a burette marked in quantities of 0.1 mL. Neither I nor any student I knew was able to do this with any degree of accuracy, but this inability did not change our instructors' expectations.

While resolution is subject to certain fundamental limitations, some proposed limitations are illusory. Introductory textbooks on cell biology usually report that a light microscope cannot distinguish two points that are separated by a space of less than 0.2 to 0.5 µm. This limit is said to be controlled by the properties of visible light and the mechanism by which images are formed in a microscope. A 35-mm slide of a microscopic image projected at high magnification does not yield any additional information; such magnification is said to be "empty." Before accepting this limitation, however, we need to define what we mean by the term *distinguish*. In light microscopy, resolution can be discussed in terms of Abbe's specification for the limit of a diffraction-limited microscope; or according to Lord Rayleigh's criterion concerning the spatial relationship of the diffraction patterns; or in relation to the Sparrow limit, which refers to the spatial frequency in which the modulation transfer function becomes zero. Moreover, modern techniques such as video-enhanced microscopy allow objects to be "seen" that theoretically could not be resolved by applying Rayleigh's criterion.[11]

Taking the changing values in microscopic resolution as a cautionary caveat, let us consider two examples of instrument resolution in dentistry: oral radiology and periodontal probing. Dental radiographic films have an estimated resolution between 14 and 20 line pairs (lp) per mm, which is equivalent to a pixel size of 25 to 36 µm; images from a charged-coupled device (CCD) with a pixel size of 40 µm have an estimated resolution of 12.51 lp/mm,[12] but some high-resolution systems claim 26 lp/mm.[13] Conventional periodontal probing has a resolution of 1 mm (or 0.5 mm if interpolation is used); electronic probes can resolve to around 0.1 mm. However, it is possible that other contributors to measurement variability (such as angulation of the probe and probing force for periodontal probes) may make a greater contribution to error than that imposed by the resolution of the instrument.

Precision

Precision refers to the distance that lies between repeated measurements of the same quantity. Murphy[14] notes that the concept of precision is usually applied only to those measurements in which random variation is at least comparable in size with the limit of uncertainty of measurement. For such a measurement the precision is not indicated by the number of significant figures in the result, but rather by multiple determinations of what purports to be the same quantity. The standard deviation (SD) often serves as the criterion for the precision of a result; less frequently it is indicated by, among others, the variance, the mean deviation, the range, the standard error (SE), and confidence intervals. A measurement is said to be precise if there is only a small spread of numbers around the average value. Yet the definition of precision cited above implies that repeated application of a given measuring technique to a given system will yield results that apply to a single statistical population. Mandel[15] argues that such an assumption is not supported by a detailed examination of actual measuring processes in which populations are nested within populations. This complication is typically ignored. One reason investigators seek to make their measurements as precise as possible is to increase the possibility of detecting effects. The *true score* theory of measurement states that every measurement—ie, every observed value—can be considered to consist of two components: *(1)* the true value, and *(2)* an error.

> Observed value = true value + error.

The various types of error—random, systematic, the result of observation, etc—are discussed in chapter 12. For now, it should be noted that in the absence of error, the observed value would equal the true value and therefore would be perfectly reliable. Alternatively, if the measurement did not actually measure anything present in the sample, then the observed value would merely reflect the error and therefore be perfectly unreliable.

A relationship between the variances (to be discussed later) of these three elements can be described as follows:

> Variance (observed value) =
> variance (true value) + variance (error).

For values obtained from groups of individuals, the variance of the true value may be understood as being derived from the real differences between individual members of the group.

As a general rule, a clinical measurement of an individual contains two major sources of error: *biologic variation* that results from variation over time and *analytic variation* of the measurement technique. When these components are independent of one another, we do not need to consider the covariance between them, and the total variability of the observed values expressed as the SD_{total} can thus be described as:

$$SD_{total} = \sqrt{SD_{biologic}^2 + SD_{analytic}^2}$$

For example, the pH of saliva in an individual involves the measurement of many factors that vary over time, and each measurement of pH involves the use of a pH meter, a technique that could be affected by analytic error. The section on analysis of errors using analysis of variance (ANOVA) (see chapter 12) presents one approach to sorting out the relative importance of different factors.

In designing an investigation, it is important to recognize the futility of worrying about analytic variability if biologic variability is great. Klee[16] demonstrates that the reduction in total variability is minimal even when the analytic variability is reduced below 50% of the biologic variability.

Measurements are often reported to have greater precision than the resolving power of the technique. Many students of periodontics are confused to see measurements of probing depth reported in papers to the 0.01 mm since they know that periodontal probes are marked only to the nearest 1 mm. In such instances, the authors are combining individual measurements to make a statement about a group of measurements. The mean of a series of pocket measurements is a corporate property; it refers to an aggregate, not an individual measurement.

Accuracy

A measurement is *accurate* if its performance on average is close to the true value to be determined. The criterion for accuracy is the absence of bias. Among other possibilities, bias can be contributed by the observer, the subject, the instrument, and the environment. Part of the skill of being a competent investigator involves determining how such biases can be detected and removed. When assessing the accuracy of a measurement it is often the case that the true value cannot be determined. Some measurements can be related indirectly to a reference value; for example, measurements of length made with a yardstick could be expressed in terms of the international standard (eg, the wavelength of the orange-red line of krypton-86). Some reference values can have assigned values arrived at by common agreement of a group of experts.[15] In biology and medicine, the problem of obtaining reference values is particularly acute because the measuring technique often significantly affects the value. A good example is the technique used to take blood pressure: Because an apprehensive subject can give an inaccurate value, there is said to be an art to taking blood pressure measurements so that the subject relaxes.

In the physical sciences, several approaches have been taken for estimating accuracy. In one, investigators calculate the contribution of all systematic errors that could affect the measuring process to estimate the amount of error in their measurements. This approach, based on scientific judgment, requires experience of the behavior and properties of the materials and the instruments as well as access to previous measurement data, calibration data, and so forth. Another technique is to compare the results with those obtained by different and independent measuring processes in the plausible belief that our confidence in the value is increased if several measuring methods unrelated to each other yield the same value.[11] For well-established techniques, uncertainty estimates would be based on standard statistical techniques such as estimating parameters of a curve, ANOVA, and SDs.

Validity

Validity expresses the relationship between what a test is intended to measure and what it actually measures. Validity can also be thought of as the extent to which a measure predicts something important about the object measured. For example, there are a number of methods for estimating the amount of plaque on teeth, some of which involve staining the plaque with a dye. However, because the dyes most commonly used (such as basic fuchsin) also stain the overlying pellicle, the measurements of stained areas correlate poorly with the weight of plaque present. Thus, the validity of the staining procedures as an estimate of the amount of plaque present is dubious. In this instance, the disparity between intended and actual measures is related to the physical-chemical aspects of the

measurement. But the validity of some techniques of plaque measurement could also be questioned on clinical grounds. From the standpoint of the initiation of periodontal disease, the area of greatest concern is the deposition of plaque close to the gingival margins, and yet the various methods of scoring plaque do not always emphasize this fact. For this reason, Schick and Ash modified the plaque-measuring portion of the Ramfjord Periodontal Disease Index (PDI) to restrict the scoring to the gingival half of the tooth surfaces.[17] Another example from periodontics is the validity of attachment-level measurement, the question being how reliably the coronal level of the connective tissue attachment can be determined by clinical probing.

In the discussion of accuracy, it was noted that comparing the same property using different techniques is sometimes of value. *Predictive validity* refers to the estimated value of a new measuring technique relative to that of an existing instrument or technique that is already validated or highly accepted—ie, a gold standard. For continuous data, a correlation coefficient for the standard and the new measurement can be calculated. For example, the McGill Pain Questionnaire (MPQ) is a standard reference for the measure of pain. However, some investigators prefer to use a less cumbersome and more convenient method, such as a visual analogue scale. If an an experiment on pain is performed and a visual analogue scale is used as the method of measuring pain, the results would be accepted more readily if a high correlation could be shown between the scores recorded by the new test and those from the MPQ.

The section on specificity and sensitivity in chapter 14 shows the calculations used to evaluate the diagnostic performance of new tests relative to a gold standard (ie, the best available test to determine if disease present or absent). This can be thought of as an example of concurrent validity a measures ability to distinguish between groups that it should theoretically be able to distinguish between.[18]

Research in education has necessarily had to consider the validity of tests measuring student performance. Frey[19] has outlined several measures of test validity:

- *Face validity.* At first glance the test must appear to measure what it is intended to measure. This is simply a matter of human judgment and yields no numerical data. A test on oral histology, for example, might be expected to include questions on odontoblasts, ameloblasts, fibroblasts, osteoblasts, and mucosal epithelium, among others.

- *Content-based validity.* This measure concerns how well the test questions cover a certain well-defined domain of knowledge. Validity at this level generally involves some organized method of selecting and forming questions. In a test of knowledge of oral biology, professors are normally required to include various components, such as the histology, biochemistry, microbiology and neurophysiology of the oral cavity.

- *Construct-based validity.* This measures how well the score on the test represents the characteristic that it is designed to measure? Trochim[18] defines it as the degree to which inferences made from the operationalization in the measurement to the theoretical constructs on which the operationalizations were based. In measuring intelligence quotient (IQ), for example, the operationalization might be a question like the following: What number follows next in the series 1, 2, 3, 5, 8, 13 . . .? In this example, the theoretical construct would be that one aspect of intelligence is the recognition of numerical patterns.

- *Consequences-based validity.* This measure focuses on the effects on the subjects of taking the test and whether the test is biased against certain groups. For example, there are data reporting that the distribution of IQ scores are such that American blacks score significantly lower than American whites (Fig 11-1). In other words, the mean IQ score for blacks is lower than the mean IQ score for whites. In the controversial book, *The Bell Curve*, Hernstein and Murray[20] used this data as well as other assumptions or data—including the relationship between economic success and IQ—and antisocial behavior and IQ, to recommend a broad range of social policies.

The publication of Hernstein and Murray's book has resulted in an abundance of critical reviews, many of which criticize of the quality of the data as well as interpretations of the bell curve (see, for example, Jacoby et al[21]). Several critiques are based on the validity of the IQ test; ie, does it really measure intelligence? For example, one explanation of the difference is that black people typically had a lower socio economic status (SES) than whites, and it is possible that IQ tests were measuring social background rather than intelligence. This could be tested by plotting SES of parents versus the IQ of the children to see if nurture rather than nature had some role in IQ scores. In fact, IQ scores go up with SES . . . but for both blacks and whites. So although it does not explain the IQ difference between blacks and whites, the finding does indicate that IQ measurement may include some component of home envi-

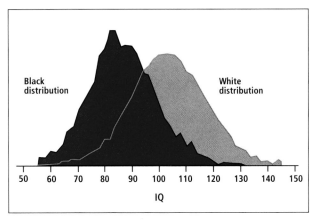

Fig 11-1 Frequency distributions of IQ for equal-sized populations of blacks and whites. Adapted with permission from Hernstein and Murray.[20]

ronment. Contrarily, it could also be argued by proponents of the IQ test that the higher SES parents were in fact smarter than the lower SES parents and that their native intelligence was passed on to their children. Another approach to criticizing IQ test validity has been to look closely at the construction of the tests. Richardson,[22] suggests that IQ testing is primarily a reformatting exercise in which ranks in one format (teacher's ratings) are converted into ranks in another format (IQ scores). This reformatting is accomplished by selection from the pool of items used in the construction of the test. Moreover the test items are also selected so that the distribution of results mimics the characteristics of physical characteristics, such as height or strength, that is they are distributed normally, forming a bell curve.

In any case, if researchers adopted the consequences-based criteria for validity, IQ scores would not be considered valid, because it appears to discriminate between racial groups.

Types of Scales

Scales are required for making comparisons between measurements. The hierarchy of measurement levels ranges from nominal scales that categorize observations through ordinal and interval scales to ratio scales that have an absolute zero and a fixed interval of measurement. The information content is relatively low for nominal scale data in comparison with ratio scale data, and different statistical approaches are required to make comparisons. Typically the statistical approaches for nominal scale data are less sensitive than those used for ratio scale data. Because each level of scale adds some new information and statistical sensitivity, it is generally preferable to use the highest level of measurement possible and not to convert data on a higher level scale to a lower one. For example, there would be a loss of sensitivity if we were to convert ratio scale data to rank values and then compare groups using a nonparametric test.

Nominal (or qualitative) scale

A nominal scale is used primarily for systematic classification (eg, gender, race, hair color). While a number may be assigned to each class to simplify record-keeping, it would be chosen arbitrarily and would carry no value. A nominal scale can be used to sort objects or individuals into groups according to gender or hair color (red, brunette, blonde), for example. The key to sorting by nominal scales is to construct well-defined categories. In most instances, sorting people by gender is fairly clear-cut; a person is either male or female. Sorting by hair color is more difficult. Would you place a person with auburn hair in the brown- or red-haired group? Should peroxide blondes be classified with natural blondes, and what of people who have their hair streaked? A good nominal scale has a sufficient number of well-defined categories to prevent objects from being put into inappropriate groups. Ideally, independent observers will sort the objects into the same groups; however, this ideal is difficult to achieve. For some conditions such as premalignancies, the groups are not well-defined, leading to widespread disagreement among oral pathologists when diagnosing this condition.

Nominal scale data are analyzed using *nonparametric tests*. In contrast with *parametric tests* (eg, t test), which usually assume the data are sampled from populations that follow a normal (Gaussian) distribution, nonparametric tests are used to analyze nominal scale data (and occasionally interval or ratio scale data) that depart from the expected distributions. (Distributions of data are discussed in more detail in chapters 9 and 10.) For present purposes, it should be noted that some nonparametric tests rely on binomial

or other non-Gaussian distributions; perhaps shockingly, when the number in a sample reaches a certain threshold (eg, > 30), a normal approximation to a binomial distribution might be used. The tests used most often for nominal scale data and the criteria that favor their use are presented in Table 11-1.

Ordinal scale

An ordinal scale is used to analyze data when increasing amounts of the measured characteristic are associated with higher values (Table 11-2). Hence, an ordinal scale both sorts and orders subjects or objects. In theory, ordinal scale data should not be averaged. For example, some components of the various indices used to assess periodontal disease rely on ordinal scale data. However, because of how it is defined, a plaque score of 3 on the Ramfjord PDI cannot be added to a plaque score of 1 to obtain an average of 2: a score of 1 means plaque is present on some but not all scale surfaces; a score of 3 means plaque extends overall and covers more than half of the surfaces. A score of 3 does not indicate three times as much plaque as a score of 1. Therefore, in theory at least, certain common statistical tests that calculate means and variances (ie, parametric tests) should not be used to analyze such data. In theory at least, statistical comparisons of groups rated by ordinal scales should be performed with nonparametric techniques, and sophisticated techniques for analyzing data from periodontal examinations have been proposed.[23]

Nevertheless, despite considerable doubt about equal intervals between the categories, it is common practice to summarize subjective ordinal scale data, calculate means, and apply the usual parametric tests. Fleiss et al[24] have investigated the degree to which the distribution of values of several periodontal indices in a sample of patients approximates a normal distribution, as well as the capacity of these indices to detect treatment differences. They concluded that the distribution of whole-mouth means was too skewed to warrant the application of parametric statistical analysis. However, they found that the square root of the whole-mouth means appeared to have a near-normal distribution and the power to detect treatment effects. They recommend using the square root of the whole-mouth mean as the preferred transformation in clinical trials of antigingivitis agents. Similarly, Labovitz[25] has shown that in appropriate circumstances certain ordinal statistics can be exchanged with interval statistics. To

Table 11-1 Nonparametric tests commonly used with nominal scale data

Name of test	No. of groups	Matched/ Unmatched	No. of cells	Comment
χ^2	2	Unmatched	Total should not be < 20; expected (or theoretical) value in all cells should not be < 5	Assigns approximate P value; makes calculation easy Values in cells should be counts (not %) Cells must be mutually exclusive and exhaustive Can be used with observed data and calculated expected values, or theoretical model as a "goodness of fit" test
Fisher exact	2	Unmatched	Used when expected value in any cell is < 5	Used when there are only two responses (eg, success or failure). Assigns exact P value; calculations messy, tables tricky to use, values in cells should be counts (not %)
χ^2 with Yates' correction	2	Unmatched	Large	Whether Yates' correction should be used remains controversial
McNemar χ^2	2	Matched	Large	Used for two response categories (eg, alive and dead) in paired, matched, or pre/post designs
Sign test	2	Matched	Large	Two response categories (+ and –); based on binomial distribution

Table 11-2 Statistical tests commonly used with ordinal scale data

Name of test	No. of samples/ groups	Matched/ unmatched	Comment
Mann-Whitney U (Wilcoxon Rank Sum Test)	2	Unmatched	Tests the null hypothesis that there is no difference in the distribution of two populations by examining the relative ranks of values from two independent samples (cf, t test for parametric data)
Kruskall-Wallis	> 2	Unmatched	Compares means of more than two samples when (a) only ordinal data are available, or (b) when a one-way ANOVA would be used for parametric data but the underlying distributions are far from normal
Freidman two-way ANOVA	> 2	Matched	Analogous to two-way ANOVA for parametric data. Independent variables (treatments) are the columns; rows are matched groups or repeated measures on individuals

achieve this end, he recommends assigning as limited a scoring system as possible based on available evidence and to use all available categories rather than collapsing them into just two or three.

In using ordinal scales, the investigator assumes that the measured objects can be placed in some type of order, although this is not always possible. The so-called Bo Derek scale of rating attractiveness (10 is a

Table 11-3 Some statistical tests commonly used with interval and ratio scale data

Name of test	No. of samples	Matched/ unmatched	Comment
z-score	1	Unmatched	Examines differences between a sample and a population
t test	2	Unmatched	Compares two means Assumes both samples randomly derived from normal populations with equal variances, but considered robust enough to withstand considerable departures from these assumptions
Paired t test	2	Matched	Assumes that differences in paired values follow a normal distribution; if paired values correlate, a paired test will be more powerful than two in dependent sample tests
One-way ANOVA	> 2	Unmatched	Determines whether significant differences exist between means of the samples; subsequent tests are needed to find differences between given pairs of means Assumes normal distribution and equal variances for the samples but is fairly robust to departures
Two-factor ANOVA Randomized Block	> 2	Unmatched	Similar to pairing, it enables assessment of interaction between factors as well as primary effect of factors Assumes the effect of block is a fixed factor

perfect score) assumes that beauty can be ranked. However, Somerset Maugham tells us that beauty is in the eye of the beholder. If Maugham is right, the Bo Derek scores would be uninterpretable.

A second major consideration in using ordinal scales is the number of categories to construct. If the number of categories is small, the scale will be crude and unable to detect subtle differences. Conversely, if the number of categories is large but each one is not well defined, there will be poor agreement between observers.

Interval scale

An *interval scale* sorts and orders objects in the same manner as an ordinal scale, but in addition it uses a fixed unit of measurement that corresponds to some fixed quantity of a particular characteristic (eg, °C or °F) (Table 11-3). The problem associated with interval scales is linearity. It might be said that happiness is re-

lated to income; the more you earn, the happier you are. However, *Fortune* magazine reported that the relationship is not linear; rather, happiness increases as the cubic root of income. Thus, if you double your income you will be only 26% happier. Therefore, you would need to earn eight times your present income to be twice as happy as you are now.[26] (This explains why some dentists work only 4 days a week. The 25% increase in work between a 4-day and a 5-day week would yield only an 8% increase in happiness.) Consequently, though it has a fixed unit of measurement, income is not a valid quality for measuring happiness on an interval scale.

Ratio scale

A *ratio scale* is an interval scale with a known point of origin (zero point) (see Table 11-3). As the name implies, a ratio scale allows us to compare values directly. For example, Kelvin (K) is a ratio scale because it is zeroed at absolute zero, the temperature at which there is no molecular motion. Thus, 200°K is twice as hot as 100°K, and °K is used in the gas law equations. In contrast, Celsius (C) is an interval scale and could not be used directly in the gas law equations; 20°C is not twice as hot as 10°C. Periodontal probing indices are a ratio scale because some pockets measure 0 mm.

A problem associated with ratio scales is that some qualities have a value of zero when some amount of the quality is present. Suppose that a 10-question quiz on the timing of tooth development was given to a graduating dental class. Because 3 years would have elapsed since the class studied oral histology, it is possible, indeed likely, that some individuals would score zero. Yet it is highly unlikely that those individuals know nothing about oral histology. If some other questions were asked, the individuals who scored zero might answer at least one or two questions correctly. Moreover, we could not be sure that individuals who scored 10 on the test knew twice as much as those who scored 5. Thus, although examination results look like ratio scale data, in reality they are not.

It should be evident that when ordinal measurements are made, the results can be expressed only in terms of *greater than* or *less than*. More precise statements can be made on an interval scale, and effects can be compared via differences. For example, the difference between a bathwater temperature of 50°C and one of 30°C is twice as great as the difference that exists between two baths that measure 20°C and 10°C, respectively. Ratio scale measurements can be compared directly.

Units

The *units* of measurement—that is, the size of the scale intervals—are arbitrary. Historically, the arbitrary determination of units caused major problems in trade because of the variability of measures used in different towns and countries. One proposed solution to this problem was to devise universal measures based on the perfection of nature. The length of a meter was intended to equal one ten-millionth the distance from the North Pole to the equator as measured along a segment of a meridian (in France), so established as to exclude all that is arbitrary[27] (at least in the eyes of its French proponents). Nevertheless, convenience dictates that the size of some units (and hence the scale intervals)

should remain arbitrary. For example, the temperature interval of 1°C differs from that of 1°F. Units can be defined only if the set of standards used is additive (as with a 1-m ruler, which comprises 100 cm).

How unit size affects the conclusion

Obviously, a unit that is too coarse may not be capable of detecting differences. A ruler graduated only in 1-m lengths would not be a practical tool for measuring the height of individuals. Pearce[28] has recommended that for the proper use of ANOVA techniques, the unit of measurement should not exceed one tenth of the total range encountered in the experiment. Wilson[29] states that it can be shown mathematically that substantial gains in efficiency can be made by reducing the scale interval to a fraction, perhaps a third or a fifth, of the SD of the population being measured. Practical considerations may also apply. In periodontics, Glavind and Loe[30] measured all surfaces of 1,530 teeth and showed that the method error for periodontal probing was less than 0.5 mm. Because this amount of error was not considered clinically significant, the markings of 1 mm on the probe were considered to be appropriate.

Strange as it might seem, it is possible to obtain data that are more precise than the units of the scale originally used in the measurements. It is not unusual to see reports in the periodontics literature of probing depths or level of attachment expressed to the nearest 0.1 mm. Because the marks on a periodontal probe are only by millimeter, this might seem impossible. However, you can demonstrate this effect yourself by making two sharp pencil marks 7.5 cm apart. Now measure the distance to the nearest centimeter. By placing a ruler, marked in centimeters, with no finer markings (ie, no numbers between the centimeter markings), randomly between the points (ie, do not always start the measurement on zero or any other predefined point), sometimes you will obtain values of 8 cm and other times 7 cm. By averaging many values, you could not only obtain a value closer to the true value of 7.5 but also have an SE of less than 0.1 cm—which would be less than one tenth of the markings on the ruler! The actual limit to this approach is set by the systematic error in the markings of the ruler; that is, by measuring the distance millions of times, you could still not gain accuracy in the range of micrometers.[29]

Wrong units

Difficulties also can arise from use of the wrong scale of measurement. In studying the effects of nutrients on growth, for instance, it has been found that the logarithm of weight produces a better variate than the weight itself; this is because a change in nutrition does not immediately make an animal larger or smaller but may well lead to a change in its growth rate. Hence, some difficulties can be met simply by converting the data into a more useful form. This topic is discussed in greater detail by Pearce[28] and Zar.[31]

Ratios

It is common for some values to be reported as the ratio between two measurements. Income is expressed as dollars/y, ATPase activity as moles Pi/h/mg protein, collagen production as moles/h per 10 cells, and so forth.

In considering complex values, several factors must be taken into account:

1. *In dental journals it is not unusual for authors to report the percentage of successes.* However, this can lead to pseudo-precision. If the denominator is small, the precision of the percentage is small. For example, a paper on reinjection of local anesthetic into the periodontal ligament concluded that the injection should be done so that a strong back pressure is noted.[32] Among the data offered to support this view was the finding that if strong back pressure is not observed, anesthesia is achieved in only 7 of 22 cases, or 32% of the time. Using the table in appendix 2 taken from Mainland,[33] we can see that if there are 7 successes out of 22 attempts, the 95% confidence limit for this percentage is between 14% and 55%. Thus, it is possible that the majority of patients would experience anesthesia even when a strong back pressure was not obtained.

   Because percentages with low denominators lack precision, some clinical medical journals publish percentages only for fractions with denominators greater than 50. As far as I can determine, however, most dental journals have not adopted this practice.
2. *The accuracy (and/or precision) of the ratio is influenced by both the numerator and the denominator.* This means that the ratio will be less accurate than either of the measurements used to construct it.
3. *The use of ratios often carries the assumption that a linear relationship exists among the components in the calculation.* If this is not so, the comparison may be meaningless. For example, the amount of enzyme in a solution is often measured by incubating the solution with a known amount of substrate for a known time, and measuring the amount of product. However, the amount of product is linear only with respect to the amount of enzyme for a limited range of enzyme concentrations. If sufficient enzyme to react with all of the substrate is already present, the addition of more enzyme will not yield more product. Thus, to compare the relative amount of enzyme present in two solutions, both solutions would have to be assayed in the linear portion of the activity vs enzyme-concentration curve.
4. *In appropriate circumstances, the distribution of the ratio of two Gaussian-distributed variables* (discussed in chapter 12) *can be bimodal.* This may lead an investigator to conclude that a population is heterogeneous when it is not.[34]

References

1. Blackman VH. Botanical retrospect. J Exp Botany 1956;7:ix.
2. MacDonald J. How honest are dentists? Readers Digest Canada. September 1998. Available at http://www.readersdigest.ca/mag/1998/09/think_01.html. Accessed August 20, 2007.
3. Huysmans MC, Longbottom C. The challenges of validating diagnostic methods and selecting appropriate gold standards. J Dent Res 2004;83(spec no.):C48–C52.
4. Meijer HJ, Stellingsma K, Meijndert L, Raghoebar GM. A new index for rating aesthetics of implant-supported single crowns and adjacent soft tissues—The Implant Crown Aesthetic Index. Clin Oral Implants Res 2005;16:645-649.
5. Furhauser R, Florescu D, Benesch T, Haas R, Mailath G, Watzek G. Evaluation of soft tissue around single-tooth implant crowns: The pink esthetic score. Clin Oral Implants Res 2005;16:639-644.
6. Bridgman PW. The Logic of Modern Physics. New York: Macmillan, 1927.
7. Mandel ID. Indices for measurement of soft accumulations in clinical studies of oral hygiene and periodontal disease. J Periodontal Res 1974;9(suppl 14):7.
8. Hull PS, Hillam DG, Beal JF. A radiographic study of the prevalence of chronic periodontitis in 14-year-old English schoolchildren. J Clin Periodontol 1975;2:203–210.
9. Blankenstein R, Murray JJ, Lind OP. Prevalence of chronic periodontitis in 13- to 15-year-old children: A radiographic study. J Clin Periodontol 1978;5:285–292.
10. Wilson EB. An Introduction to Scientific Research. New York: McGraw Hill, 1952:164.

11. Heintzmann R, Ficz G. Breaking the resolution limit in light microscopy. Brief Funct Genomic Proteomic 2006;5: 289–301.

12. Folk RB, Thorpe JR, McClanahan SB, Johnson JD, Strother JM. Comparison of two different direct digital radiography systems for the ability to detect artificially prepared periapical lesions. J Endod 2005;31:304–306.

13. Berkhout WE, Verhiej JG, Syriopoulos K, Li G, Sanderink GC, van der Stelt PF. Detection of proximal caries with high-resolution and standard resolution digital radiographic systems. Dentomaxillofac Radiol 2007;36:204–210.

14. Murphy EA. A Companion to Medical Statistics. Baltimore: Johns Hopkins Univ Press, 1985:192.

15. Mandel J. The Statistical Analysis of Experimental Data. New York: Dover, 1964:103–125.

16. Klee GG. Toward more effective use of laboratory results in differential diagnosis. In: Hamburger HA, Batsakis JG (eds). Clinical Laboratory Annual. New York: Appleton-Century-Crofts, 1982:119.

17. Ramfjord SP. The periodontal disease index (PDI). J Periodontol 1967;38(suppl):602–610.

18. Trochim WMK. The Research Methods Knowledge Base, ed 2. Cincinnati: Atomic Dog, 2001:68.

19. Frey B. Statistics Hacks. Sebastopol, CA: O'Reilly, 2006.

20. Hernstein RJ, Murray C. The Bell Curve. New York: Free Press, 1994.

21. Jacoby R, Glaubeman N (eds). The Bell Curve Debate: History, Documents, Opinions. New York: Random House, 1995.

22. Richardson K. The Making of Intelligence. London: Weidenfeld and Nicolson, 1999:35.

23. Zimmerman S, Johnston DA. Non-parametric tests and RiDiTS. J Periodontal Res 1974;9(suppl 14):193.

24. Fleiss JL, Park MH, Bollmer BW, Lehnhoff RW, Chilton NW. Statistical transformations of indices of gingivitis measured non-invasively. J Clin Periodontol 1985;12:750–755.

25. Labovitz S. The assignment of numbers to rank order categories. Am Sociol Rev 1970;35:515–525.

26. Seligman D. Keeping up. Fortune December 5, 1988;229.

27. Alder K. The Measure of All Things. New York: Free, 2002:89–93.

28. Pearce SC. Biological Statistics: An Introduction. New York: McGraw Hill, 1965:56.

29. Wilson EB. An Introduction to Scientific Research. New York: McGraw Hill, 1952:251–254.

30. Glavind L, Loe H. Errors in the clinical assessment of periodontal destruction. J Periodontal Res 1967;2:180–184.

31. Zar JH. Biostatistical Analysis. Englewood Cliffs, NJ: Prentice Hall, 1974:236–242.

32. Walton RE, Abbot BJ. Periodontal ligament injection: A clinical evaluation. J Am Dent Assoc 1981;103:571–575.

33. Mainland D. Elementary Medical Statistics. Philadelphia: Saunders, 1963:358–363.

34. Murphy EA. A Companion to Medical Statistics. Baltimore: Johns Hopkins Univ Press, 1985:204–209.

12 | Errors of Measurement

Everybody believes in [the law of errors] because mathematicians imagine that it is a fact of observation and observers that it is a theorem of mathematics.

—Gabriel Lippman[1]

In experimental biologic research, *error* can be viewed as the result of any factor that affects the results in a manner that is not precisely known to the experimenter. Even in disciplines as precise as physics or chemistry in which results are the product of physical measurement, the numerical value obtained depends on the accuracy of the experiment that measured it. There is no such thing as the exact value of a physical constant.[2]

Given this uncertainty, results should be presented as a range of values that will fit the experimental data. In physical science, this is accomplished implicitly, by conforming to the rules of significant figures, or explicitly, by calculating the probable sources of error and their contribution to the total error in the experiment. In biologic science, the data may often be expressed as a mean plus an estimate of variability, which is determined by statistical techniques. *Statistics*, as the old joke goes, means never having to say you are certain, and one common means of presenting data is to use a confidence interval (CI). Whatever the means used, the intent is to give the reader an estimate of the probable accuracy and precision of the data. The following sections provide an introduction to assessing errors of measurement.

Precision vs Accuracy

A distinction is made between precision and accuracy. *Precision* refers to the dispersion of values around the measure of central tendency used; a measured value with a small standard deviation (SD) or CI is considered *precise*. In contrast, a measurement is *accurate* if the result, expressed as a range of possible values, includes the "true" value. For example, Winter[3] used a Boley gauge, accurate to 0.1 mm, to examine the markings on various manufacturers' periodontal probes (Fig 12-1). He found that Williams probes manufactured by Hu-Friedy under an old process were both imprecise and inaccurate (see Fig 12-1d). At the 7.0-mm mark of the probes, the true length ranged from 6.8 to 7.9 mm, with most ranging from 7.4 to 7.6 mm. The process used by another manufacturer yielded a product that was inaccurate but precise (see Fig 12-1c): 10 of the 13 probes examined fell in the 7.4 to 7.6 mm group, and the others in the 7.1 to 7.3 mm group. Finally, the process used in the (Hu-Friedy) manufacture of new Williams probes produced accurate and precise probes (Fig 12-1a). Thirty-five of the 42 examined were accurate at the 7.0-mm mark, and the total range was only 6.8 to 7.3 mm.

When there is little random or systematic error, the results are clustered around the true mean (see Fig 12-1a). The presence of random error increases the variability of response around the true mean, thus reducing the precision (see Fig 12-1b). Systematic error displaces the clustered result values away from the mean, rendering them inaccurate (see Fig 12-1c), and when both errors are present, confusion reigns, for the results are neither precise nor accurate (see Fig 12-1d). Error can be classed as *determinate* or *indeterminate*. These categories will be discussed separately, but first the inevitability of some error in every experiment will be examined.

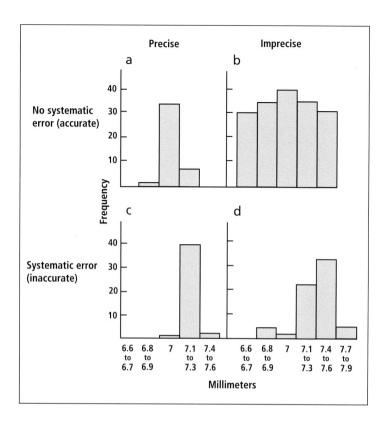

Fig 12-1 Analysis of precision and accuracy of markings on various periodontal probes. *(a)* New Williams probes with little systematic or random error; *(b)* probes with little systematic error and significant random error; *(c)* probes with significant systematic error and little random error; *(d)* old Williams probes with significant systematic and random errors.

Error as the Result of Observation

In any experiment, it is always possible for the method chosen for observing the object to somehow alter it. In extreme cases, when the method of observation grossly alters the object, the result is called an *artifact*.

The *indeterminacy principle* is perhaps the most sophisticated example of error resulting from observation. The principle was first postulated in quantum mechanics by Heisenberg, who noted that it was impossible to know accurately both the position and the momentum of electrons at the same time. To prove this, he showed that any conceivable instrument that could accurately measure the electron's position would affect the electron's momentum and vice versa. The indeterminacy principle has been the center of a methodologic controversy about whether uncertainty is inherent in nature or results from the imperfect state of our knowledge and methods. But we do not have to look to quantum mechanics for examples of observation affecting the quantity being studied. In dentistry, Shaw and Murray,[4] stated:

Some of the differences in diagnosis observed between the first and second examinations may be due to systematic changes introduced by the examination method. The use of a probe to test for the presence or the condition of the gingiva inevitably alters the environment and can affect the scores of a second examination.

Similarly, the use of disclosing dyes to measure the deposition of plaque has been questioned, because the dyes possibly inhibit plaque growth.

Although physicists have debated the indeterminacy principle at length, as a general rule, biologists have not concerned themselves too much with this issue. An exception is Hillman,[5] whose critical analysis of some common techniques used in biochemistry consisted of:

1. Describing all the steps in a procedure;
2. Examining the agents in each step that might influence the final answer;
3. Identifying the assumptions necessarily implied in the use of the procedures;
4. Discussing their validity;

5. Suggesting control experiments to analyze quantitatively how each step affects the conclusions of experiments.

Hillman[6] concluded, "At the moment biochemistry is in a state of uncertainty because elementary control experiments for complex procedures have never been done."

I have never seen Hillman's theoretical analysis of the problems inherent in standard biochemical techniques refuted, but it has made little impression on biochemists. It seems that biochemists adopt a more pragmatic and less theoretical approach of simply using different means or methods of observing the same object and determining whether the different techniques corroborate each other.

Early electron microscopists tried different ways of fixing, dehydrating, and staining biologic material. They argued that if you could see similar structures despite using different procedures, the structures likely existed prior to the treatments. Although each procedure could produce some kind of artifact, the different procedures were unlikely to produce the same artifact. Hence, the ordered structures observed were considered to be real. Similarly, electron microscopy and histochemistry have, on the basis of biochemical study of isolated subcellular fractions, confirmed some of the inferences made by biochemists.

Determinate Error

Determinate error results when one part of the observing system or the design of the experiment is inaccurate or defective. In principle, determinate errors can be removed. I divide determinate error into several classes.

Systematic

Systematic errors are the same for each observation. Measurements made with the Hu-Friedy old Williams periodontal probes described in Winter's[3] study would have a systematic error. Systematic error can result from chemical reagents that contain impurities, or even from choice of method. Some methods consistently overvalue or undervalue the quantity measured.

In clinical studies, systematic error can be introduced by any of the biases that cause the study population to be selected or examined nonrandomly in the target population. For example, partial-mouth scores are often used to estimate the prevalence of periodontal disease, but such estimates systematically underestimate the prevalence of the disease.[7]

Personal

Some errors are attributable to the idiosyncrasies of the person making the measurement. Wilson[8] states that almost everyone displays number prejudices, which markedly influence the frequency with which the different digits occur in the estimation of tenths of a division on a scale. The distribution of numbers chosen for Lotto 6/49 (a Canadian national lottery game in which one tries to choose the 6 numbers drawn out of 49 available numbers) provides evidence for number preferences. The numbers 7 and 25 are popular, while few people select 10, 20, 30, 39, or 40 (Fig 12-2). The magnitude of these personal number preferences is such that statisticians can formulate betting (ie, number selection) strategies that guarantee success over the long run.[9] Personal errors can also enter into techniques where, on the surface at least, there appears to be little chance of idiosyncrasies influencing the results. For example, in counting blood cells with a hemocytometer, it is not unusual for consistent differences to exist between operators.

It is possible for bias, either conscious or subconscious, to influence the results. Bias can be demonstrated in another example from hematology. In red blood cell counts with a hemocytometer, the random standard error (SE) of observation used commonly under normal conditions has been estimated at 8% to 10% of the observed count. In the past, laboratory technicians were told erroneously during their training that the error was much less ($\approx$1.4%), and this value was used to set a standard of agreement that was required to be reached before the worker's results were considered reliable. The result was an impossible standard of precision. Because the standard could not be reached with accurate counting, technicians learned to count very rapidly and to make unconscious adjustments to ensure that all counts agreed with the first count.[10] In this example, it was possible to analyze data to prove the existence of bias, but in subjective measurements, such as are often performed in a clinical setting, the problem of uncon-

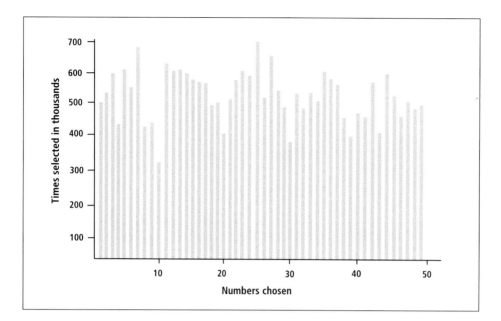

Fig 12-2 Distribution of numbers chosen for Lotto 6/49.

scious bias is even greater. Modern experimental designs, such as the double-blind procedure, have been utilized in an attempt to minimize the contribution of personal bias; in some instances, even elaborate precautions are not successful.

Assignable causes and blunders

An experimenter may overlook relevant variables. If the values of these variables change, the results will be affected. If a researcher were investigating the relationship between pressure and volume using gases at different temperatures, the results might fluctuate wildly. If the researcher learned later that temperature affected the relationship between pressure and volume, the experiment could be repeated at constant temperature. Moreover, if the relationship of temperature to the other variables was known, the researcher could calculate how the temperature affected the original measurements and remove that source of error. Hence, the original error could be assigned to a specific cause.

I suspect that one particularly common—but often difficult to detect—source of error is the blunder. A *blunder* is a failure to follow a protocol or properly ex-

ecute a procedure. Graduate students perform much of the research that forms the basis of publications, but they are often inexperienced in procedures and can make mistakes. When students find unexpected or unusual results, experienced supervisors normally question them closely on the procedures they followed, because it is more likely that the student made an error than that a previously published study or existing lab protocol was erroneous.

Importance of determinate error

In terms of effective criticism of scientific papers, the detection of determinate errors is often more important than statistical issues, because determinate error can result in errors much larger than those arising from random fluctuations.

Several probable instances of systematic error are described in a monograph published by the National Academy of Sciences on the need for critically evaluated physical and chemical data. In one example, two independent measurements of a value of a property of atomic nuclei differed by 25%, 10 times the uncertainty estimated by those making the measurements.[11]

Indeterminate or Random Errors

Even when all known relevant variables are controlled, and the method of measurement is the same, the values obtained for similar samples usually vary. These variations result from a number of uncontrolled variables, each of whose effects is individually small. Such variations, called *random errors,* are dealt with by statistical methods, which provide a means for estimating the variability of results and minimizing the chance of making false conclusions about them. Statistical techniques are generally used only after a reasonable effort to reduce determinate error has been made. Ordinary statistical procedures are not applicable if the errors are not random.[12]

The normal law of error

The usual analysis of data in experimental biology assumes that the indeterminate errors are distributed according to the *normal law of error.* This "law" of error has been the subject of some confusion as to whether it is an empirically derived rule or a theoretical construct. Both views are supported. It has been found experimentally that the normal or Gaussian distribution adequately describes systems in which the measurements under study are affected by a very large number of errors all acting independently. However, according to Wilson,[12] the theoretical argument for the normal law is based on the rapid approach to normality, which can be demonstrated mathematically to occur when the error is caused by the sum of a number of independent causes, each cause being distributed in any arbitrary manner but having a finite SD. It appears safe to use the normal law for observations, in which it is clear that four or five or more sources of error enter with about equal weight. Random error affects measurement of a variable across all the members of a sample and thus increases the variability of the distribution around the average for the sample.[13] In engineering and the physical sciences, random error is sometimes described as the "noise" in the system that interferes to a greater or lesser extent with the meaningful information found in the "signal."

For some measurements, one source of error could be much greater than the others. In such instances, the usual approach would be to attempt to control the major source of error either experimentally (eg, by changing the conditions of measurement) or statistically (ie, by covariance analysis).

The Gaussian distribution does not apply for some data. For example, Pareto's law applies for the distribution of incomes; in graphed representations, there is a long tail on the right-hand side because of the existence of oil sheiks and oral surgeons. In such instances, special statistical procedures might be applied.

Incidentally, even in such nonnormally distributed populations, there is a way of getting a precise estimate of the mean. According to the *central limit theorem* (one of the most important theorems in statistics), if a population has a finite variance σ^2 and mean μ, then the distribution of the sample mean m approaches the normal distribution with variance σ^2/n and mean m as the sample size n increases, regardless of the distribution of the parent population. The normal distribution and establishing confidence limits for means are discussed in chapter 10.

These concepts can be demonstrated by a physical analogue: the Galton board (named after the pioneer statistician Sir Francis Galton), also known as *quincunx* or *bean machine* (Fig 12-3). The board can be created by hammering equally spaced and interleaved rows of nails on a board. Metal balls, such as BB shot, are dropped through a funnel into the array of nails; a series of bins collect the balls as they leave the array. As a ball hits each nail, it has an equal probability of deflecting to either the right or left. The number of balls that accumulates in the bins will resemble a normal distribution graph, where the number of rows of nails corresponds to the number of trials, and P = .5. If there are 15 rows of nails, the location of each ball is the sum of 15 random variables (ie, randomly determined direction of deflection in each row). A consequence of the central limit theorem is that the sum of *n* random variables approximates a normal distribution when *n* is large. With 15 rows of nails, a distribution of balls in the bins resembles a normal distribution. Websites provide animated graphic demonstrations of the Galton board for varying numbers of rows of nails to convince watchers empirically of the truth of the central limit theorem.[14]

Least squares method

Given that measurements are often distributed according to the Gaussian distribution, the question arises

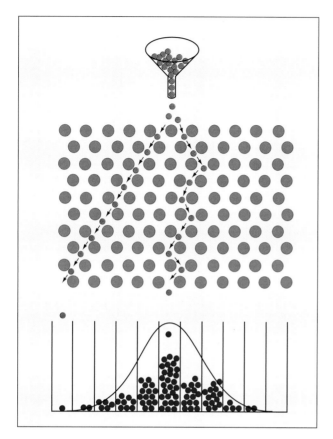

Fig 12-3 Galton board. A series of binomial events (ball deflecting either left or right of each nail, with 50% probability for either direction at each level) will yield a symmetrical curve approximating a Gaussian distribution. The paths of two balls are traced, one of which was deflected to the left at every level, and another that had the more likely outcome of some deflections to the left and some to the right.

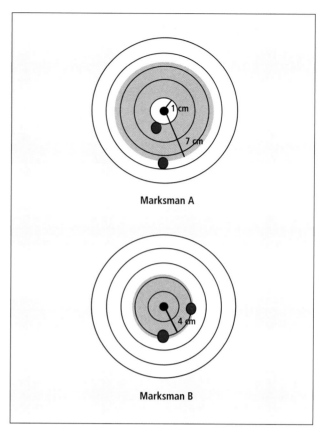

Fig 12-4 Least squares principle. Two marksmen, A and B, have the same average deviation of the distance from where their bullets hit to the center of the target (4 cm). Most people would consider marksman B was the better rifleman, because his shots are scattered over a lesser area of the target. By the laws of geometry, the area of the target is related to the square of the radius from the center.

as to the best method for determining a representative value for a set of observations and the associated error. According to Mellor,[15] the Belgian army once evaluated the ability of its riflemen by adding up the distances, regardless of direction, of each man's shots from the center of the target. The man with the smallest sum won the "le grand prix" of the regiment. However, this rule is clearly faulty; if marksman A scored a 1 and a 7, and marksman B scored two 4s, the Belgian army's rule would rank them equal, though most people would believe that B was the better marksman.

Mellor points out that the second shooter is thought of as more accurate, because his shots fall into a lesser area (see Fig 12-4); that is, marksman B's error is not related to the magnitude of the straight line of where the bullet hits the target, but to the area of the circle described about the center of the target with that line as the radius. Intuitively, it seems that, because the area of the target is proportional to the square of the radius from the center, a valid evaluation should involve the sum of the squares of the distance of each shot from the center. That is, in fact, the case. Legendre's *least squares method* states that "The most probable value for observed quantities is that for which the sum of the squares of the individual errors is a minimum." Gauss reached the same conclusion possibly earlier than Legendre but did not publish his work until 1809.[16] In modern terminology, the sum of squares of deviations is called the *residual sum of squares* or *error sum of squares*.

The least squares method has wide application. It is used in calculating the best estimate for values of physical constants determined by different methods as well as for determining the best fit of experimental data to a straight line (regression), where the best values for the slope and the intercept are calculated.[16] The mathematics can be quite complex; the general objective is to obtain a formula for a parameter that provides the best estimate (ie, produces a minimal least squares difference), which will be called $\hat{P}$. To accomplish this, equations must be produced that specify the difference of observed values to the, as yet, undetermined parameter. The resulting function is then differentiated with respect to each parameter in the equation. The laws of calculus confirm that the value at which $\hat{P}$ is a minimum will be where the derived function is zero. Equating the derived expression to zero enables a formula for $\hat{P}$ to be determined. Application of the least squares method can show that the best value to represent a number of observations of equal weight is their arithmetical mean.[16,17]

Confidence intervals

CIs indicate the precision of the sample that resulted in the estimated value for the population. The wider the CI, the less the precision. Confidence limits are now expected in a number of medical journals, but some of these are not readily available in standard statistical textbooks. This book includes appendix 2, which gives the limits of binomial population expressed as percentages. Appendix 3 contains critical values of the *t* distribution, which can be used to construct CIs as outlined in chapter 10. However, CIs for many other important statistics are not covered in this book, such as regression coefficients, correlation coefficients, relative risks, odds ratios, survival data, and nonparametric analyses (eg, medians). Fortunately, a specialized and accessible text by Gardner and Altman[18] provides the necessary information.

Error of Combined Measurements

A common problem is estimating the error correctly when independent measurements are combined. This consideration becomes particularly important in evaluating derived measurements when the variables are related by other than simple relationships. It can be shown that when the derived quantity u is some function of j independent variables, ie, u = f (v1, v2, . . . vi):

$$s_u^2 = \sum_{i=1}^{j} \left(\frac{\partial f}{\partial v_i} \right)^2 s_{vi}^2$$

where s_u^2 = variance of u, and s_{vi}^2 = variance of variable i.

This relationship is called the *law of propagation of errors*.[15] The law can be reliably used when the errors are reasonably small (10% or less) with respect to the measured values. Mandel[16] states that the law is exact for linear combinations of random variables but only approximate for nonlinear combinations.

A simple case: Sums or differences

Consider an experiment where the quantity of interest is simply the difference between two measurements. This type of calculation occurs in periodontics when comparing probing depths before and after treatment:

$$f\left(v_1, v_2 \right) = v_1 - v_2$$

Propagation of errors theorem gives us:

$$s_u^2 = s_{v_1}^2 + s_{v_2}^2$$

which, in terms of SD of the difference between measurements, becomes:

$$S_u = \sqrt{S_{v_1}^2 + S_{v_2}^2}$$

In this simple case, because the squares of the SD of the measurement of each variable are combined, a large error in one component tends to overshadow small errors in the other component. Note that the SD of the difference (or a sum) is less than the sum of the SDs of the components.

Ratios

Ratios are common in biologic science; for example, enzyme activity is often expressed as a specific activity—eg, units per milligram protein or tooth support as ratio of length of tooth root adjacent to total alveolar bone per root length.

The function of a ratio may be described as:

$$u = \frac{V_1}{V_2}$$

Applying the propagation of errors theorem noting that:

$$\frac{\partial_u}{\partial_{v_1}} = \frac{1}{v_2} \text{ and } \frac{\partial_u}{\partial_{v_2}} = -\frac{v_1}{v_2^2}$$

$$s_u^2 = \frac{1}{v_2^2} s_{v_1}^2 + \frac{v_1^2}{v_2^4} s_{v_2}^2$$

$$\text{dividing by } u^2 = \left(\frac{v_1}{v_2}\right)^2$$

$$\left(\frac{s_u}{u}\right)^2 = \left(\frac{s_{v1}}{v_1}\right)^2 + \left(\frac{s_{v2}}{v_2}\right)^2$$

As the coefficient of variation:

$$(CV) = \frac{s_u}{u}, \text{ for } v_1 = \frac{s_{v1}}{v_1}, \text{ for } v_2 = \frac{s_{v2}}{v_2}$$

The relationship becomes:

$$(cv_u)^2 = (cv_{v1})^2 + (cv_{v2})^2$$

Thus, for ratios, the errors compound in proportion to the sum of the fractional (or percentage) error; or the square of the relative error in the function equals the sum of the squares of the relative errors of the component functions.

Standardization and Errors in Calibration

Studies in clinical research sometimes require assessment of exposure to a chemical and/or determination of biomarkers that may predict or influence disease. The amounts of exposure or concentration of biomarkers may vary widely, and it is necessary to devise an assay that can determine concentrations over a range of values. It is common to calibrate an assay in order to determine the concentration of biochemicals by producing a standard or calibration curve. Known amounts of the biochemical are assessed, typically by reaction with some chemicals or substrate, and then measured by a physical technique, such as fluorimetry or optical densitometry at a specific wavelength. The results are then plotted with optical density, for example, on the ordinate and concentration on the abscissa. Then a straight line that provides the best fit to the points is drawn either by eye or by more rigorous calculation using regression and the least squares method; this line is known as the *standard curve*. Unknowns, such as samples of serum from a human population, are then measured in the same way, and their optical density (or fluorescence or other biomarker) is recorded. The amount of the measured value for the sample is then used as the ordinate and located on the standard curve. The concentration of the unknown is determined by the corresponding value of the abscissa.

Although this straightforward procedure is performed regularly in laboratories, a problem arises when it is necessary to determine the errors (eg, as in legal disputes in which exposure to a chemical might be of paramount consideration). There are really two types of errors involved: those that relate to the measurement of the sample itself and those that result from the regression used to produce the standard curve. Typically, lab workers ignore the error due to regression, but rigorous assessment requires that such error be calculated. For further discussion of this complex matter, which is beyond the scope of this book, consult van Belle[19] and Mandel.[16]

Analysis of Errors by Analysis of Variance

Measurements in clinical research as well as basic research using animals are usually subject to three major sources of variation:

1. Variation between individuals, sometimes called *true biologic variation*, is caused by all the factors that make individuals differ, such as age, race, and genetic factors.
2. Variations with time. Some properties of individuals can vary from hour to hour or from one day to the next, and the field of chronobiology is devoted to understanding such time variations.

Table 12-1 Sample ANOVA table

Source of variation	Degrees of freedom	Sum of squares	Mean square
Between patients	19	190	10
Between examiners	1	7	7
Random error	19	1.9	0.1
Total	39	198.9	

3. Measurement error results from all the factors that tend to produce differences when measuring the same phenomena. Examples include fluctuation in line voltages affecting electrical equipment, different technicians performing the same assay, and stability of reagents. In clinical studies, examiner error is often considered separately from other measurement errors.

Analysis of errors may be described in different ways, but an especially informative reporting strategy is to present an analysis of variance (ANOVA) table. In papers analyzing measurement techniques in clinical dentistry, the sources of variance that are often of interest are patients, examiner effects, and errors of measurement. Suppose there were a study in which two examiners made one measurement each on 20 patients. An ANOVA table might look like Table 12-1, and the components of variance would be estimated as outlined by Fleiss and Kingman.[20]

For patients, the variance:

$$s^2_p = \frac{\text{mean square patients} - \text{mean square error}}{\text{no. of examiners}}$$

$$s^2_p = \frac{10 - 0.1}{2} = 4.95$$

For examiners, the variance:

$$s^2_x = \left(\frac{\text{mean square examiners} - \text{mean square error}}{\text{no. of patients}} \right)$$

$$s^2_x = \frac{7 - 0.1}{40} = 0.17$$

For error, the variance:

$$s^2_E = \text{mean square error} = 0.1.$$

This information on variance can be used to estimate the reliability of the measurements, as well as to plan experiments. A quantity that summarizes the relative magnitudes of the estimated components of variance is the intraclass correlation coefficient R:

$$R = \frac{s^2_x}{s^2_x + s^2_E}$$

Values of the intraclass correlation coefficient close to one indicate excellent reliability (for this to happen, $s^2_x + s^2_E$ must be small relative to s^2_x), and conversely, values close to zero indicate poor reliability, as the variance attributed to examiners or random measurement error is relatively large. The purpose of a reliability study is not to test hypotheses but rather to assess the characteristics of the measurements and the relationships between them. Such studies enable an assessment of the reliability of the data, not a determination of whether differences exist between groups.

In some situations, the value of component variances cannot be assessed directly, but can be deduced through appropriate calculation and experimental design. Variance components analysis is discussed by Box et al.[21]

Moreover, by looking at the various components of variance, an investigator can evaluate and improve experimental design. In the given example, it is clear that the major source of variation is between the patients. Thus, to use this system of measurement to look for effects of a certain treatment, it would not help the investigator much to refine the calibration of the examiners, who are not adding significantly to the error. However, it might be useful to try and select subjects from a more homogeneous group, so the variance attributed to patients could be reduced.

References

1. Lippman G. Cited in Cramer H. Mathematical Methods of Statistics. Princeton, NJ: Princeton Univ Press, 1946:232.
2. Leaver RH, Thomas TR. Analysis and Presentation of Experimental Results. London: Macmillan, 1974:5.
3. Winter AA. Measurement of the millimeter markings of periodontal probes. J Periodontol 197950:483–485.
4. Shaw L, Murray JJ. Diagnostic reproducibility of periodontal indices. J Periodontal Res 1977;12:141–147.
5. Hillman H. Certainty and Uncertainty in Biochemical Techniques. London: Surrey Univ Press, 1972: ix.
6. Hillman H. Certainty and Uncertainty in Biochemical Techniques. London: Surrey Univ Press, 1972:114.
7. Kingman A, Morrison E, Löe H, Smith J. Systematic errors in estimating prevalence and severity of periodontal disease. J Periodontol 1988;59:707–713.
8. Wilson EB. An Introduction to Scientific Research. New York: McGraw Hill, 1952:233.
9. Ziemba W, Baumelle S, Gautier A, Schwarz S. Dr Z's 6/49 Lotto Guidebook. Vancouver, BC: Dr Z's Investments, 1986.
10. Mainland D. Elementary Medical Statistics. Philadelphia: Saunders, 1963:155–156.
11. National Research Council. National Needs for Critically Evaluated Physical and Chemical Data. Washington, DC: National Academy of Sciences, 1978.
12. Wilson EB. An Introduction to Scientific Research. New York: McGraw Hill, 1952:246.
13. Trochim WMK. The Research Methods Knowledge Base, ed 2. Cincinnati: Atomic Dog, 2001:90.
14. Center for Technology and Teacher Education. University of Virginia. Quincunx/Random Walk. Available at http://teacherlink.org/content/math/interactive/flash/quincunx/quincunx.html. Accessed August 21, 2007.
15. Mellor JW. Higher Mathematics for Students of Chemistry and Physics. New York: Dover, 1912:498–566.
16. Mandel J. The Statistical Analysis of Experimental Data. New York: Dover, 1964:131–159
17. Wilson EB. An Introduction to Scientific Research. New York: McGraw Hill, 1952:226-229.
18. Gardner MJ, Altman DG (eds). Statistics with Confidence Intervals and Statistical Guidelines. London: BMJ, 1989.
19. van Belle G. Statistical Rules of Thumb. New York: Wiley, 2002:12–127.
20. Fleiss JL, Kingman A. Statistical management of data in clinical research. Crit Rev Oral Biol Med 1990;1:55–66.
21. Box GEP, Hunter WG, Hunter JS. Statistics for Experimenters. New York: Wiley, 1978:571–582.

13 | Presentation of Results

A colleague of Galileo, Federico Cesi, wrote that Galileo's 38 hand-drawn images of sunspots "delight both by the wonder of the spectacle and the accuracy of expression." That is beautiful evidence.

—Edward Tufte[1]

Ideals and Objectives

As noted previously, a scientific paper is an attempt to persuade the reader of the truth of the author's conclusions. A main component of persuasion is the presentation of evidence. Tufte[1] has argued that the point of displaying evidence is to assist the thinking of the producer as well as the consumer of the information. The common experience of practicing scientists suggests that Tufte's concept is true. Lab meetings or student supervisory committee meetings almost always involve some sort of pictorial display of the evidence or the concepts; sometimes these are outlined on blackboards, whiteboards, or paper, and sometimes they are projected using digital displays and sophisticated computer programs. It seems that scientists cannot engage in discussion without using images and diagrams, which seem inherently central to scientific reasoning. But the effectiveness of scientific images varies considerably. Tufte has suggested that the standard of quality of evidence can be judged on three main criteria: integrity, quality and relevance.[2]

Integrity

The amount of faith that readers of scientific articles place in the integrity of the authors is striking. Few readers will be able to repeat the experiments, and, consequently, most readers are forced to accept as true the raw evidence displayed in a paper. Readers must assume that the fields of view presented in micrographs are representative or typical, and are not special occurrences. They also must assume that the data have been obtained in the manner described in the materials and methods section—and that they have not been selected or excluded so as to conform to the hypotheses of the authors.

The advent of digital photography has brought the issue of integrity to the forefront, as authors now have considerable ability to generate a virtual reality that can mislead readers. The manipulation of photographic images has a long and not always honorable history. In a lecture to the Royal Society in 1865, a pioneer in the photography of mental patients claimed that photography "makes them observable not only now but forever, and it presents also a perfect and faithful record."[3] The limitations of photography in providing perfectly faithful records soon became apparent, for it was discovered that both the visual habits of the photographers and available practical techniques influenced the images.[3] Darwin illustrated his study of the appearance of human emotions with photographs. However, rather than presenting raw data of people experiencing emotions, the photographs were staged with actors, in effect, giving their impressions of the emotions.[4]

Dental records, in particular, have been subject to manipulation. One famous case concerned a University of British Columbia (UBC) professor on sabbatical

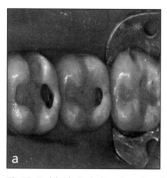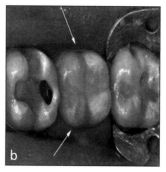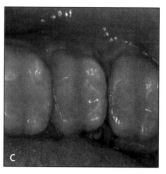

Fig 13-1 *(a)* Clinical situation showing three teeth with caries. *(b)* "Photoshop restoration," in which a lesion has been restored using digital Photoshop manipulations. *(c)* Definitive restoration with three Photoshop-restored teeth in situ.

in Switzerland, whose wife went missing. Police located a body that had been cut up, placed in green garbage bags, and thrown into a ravine. In an attempt to identify the body, the police asked the professor for his wife's dental records. When they looked closely at the records he provided, police discovered that they had been crudely altered. The professor explained that he had altered the records, so that he would not have to face the possibility that his wife was actually dead. Unconvinced by his explanation, the police brought the case to trial, where the professor benefited from the Swiss system that—besides the traditional categories of *guilty* and *not guilty*—has an intermediate result: *not guilty by reason of doubt*.[5] The professor walked away a free man, but it is rumored that UBC students were less convinced of his innocence, and referred to the professor as "the man from Glad" (referring to an actor who advertised green garbage bags). Regardless of his guilt or innocence, by altering the image, the professor cast doubt on his integrity and caused himself much trouble.

The black magic marker has proven to be a versatile instrument for those wishing to alter reality, reportedly being used for such diverse purposes as adding bands to images of polyacrylamide gels and to spot-painting mice to mislead observers into thinking that transplants of black mouse skin to white mice had been successful.[6]

Modern digital techniques improve on the traditional magic marker approach and can be employed to modify images in a manner that can be impossible to detect. Figure 13-1 shows a virtual restoration of a decayed tooth that my colleague Dr Babak Chehroudi completed using Photoshop. A fraudulent dentist could use such techniques to fool insurance compa-

nies into paying for procedures that were never done. Similarly, in science, an investigator could generate images to represent phenomena that did not take place, or modify images to provide support for a central argument. Some journals request access to the raw camera-format images to preclude the possibility that the original observations have been altered.

More subtle compromises of integrity can occur using the tools of rhetoric outlined in chapter 3. The selection and manipulation of data can be guided by the rhetorical principle of cognitive response to direct readers to certain conclusions. This direction can be done stealthily by such methods as choosing indices and scales of graphs to magnify effects (Cialdini's contrast principle), or placing arrows or other indicators to highlight some features present in particular micrographs, while obscuring other features.

The choice of measurement used by the investigator can pose another concern for integrity. For example, in the comic movie *Borat*, the provocateur/protagonist tells members of the Veteran Feminists of America that women cannot benefit from education, because their brains are small, like squirrels' brains. The group protests the conclusion, but, in fact, women's brains are smaller than men's. However, this difference disappears when correction is made for body size. That is, large men and large women have large brains, and small women and small men have small brains; the difference between the sexes is accounted for by the generally greater size of men relative to woman. But the measure of brain size as an indicator of intelligence is inherently flawed and unreliable, and relates back to the discredited pseudoscience of phrenology. For example, Einstein's brain was rather ordinary in size. The 19th-century anatomist Paul Broca, who championed the idea of the relationship of brain size to intelligence, probably would have been saddened by the finding—discovered after his death—that his own brain (at 1,424 g) was not particularly large.[7] The problem with the theory that brain size influences intelligence is that the organization of the brain, rather than its size, determines cognitive ability.[8] Thus, any study using brain size as a surrogate for intelligence would lack integrity, because the concept has been shown to be false.

Quality

The quality of data and illustrations presented in scientific papers can be difficult to assess and can involve technical considerations, numerical considerations, and close examination of results.

Technical quality

Assessing data quality can entail considerable technical expertise. Based on his experience, Lawson[9] has identified no less than 32 common faults in photomicrography. For instance, photomicrographs should meet certain technical standards, such as image sharpness, even illumination, adequate resolution, sufficient contrast, brightness, and proper color balance. When an illustration from a scientist's article is selected for the cover of a scientific journal, it is the mastery of technique that is rewarded. Such an event can cause some puffing out of scientific chests, often accompanied by the appearance on lab walls of framed reproductions of the scientific masterpiece.

Numerical quality

Numeric data also incorporate indicators of quality, such as reporting variation (eg, small standard deviations [SDs] or error bars and the like), resolution (eg, the number, spacing and distinctiveness of protein bands on a polyacrylamide gel), and accuracy, which can be demonstrated through incorporation of standards (eg, molecular weight standards for polyacrylamide gels separating molecules on the basis of size).

Consistency

Often, different tables or figures contain values that are generated under identical conditions. For example, the value obtained for an untreated control sample might appear in several graphs that report the results of different treatments. Ideally, the values from repeated observations should be close to each other; contrarily, a lack of repeatability could cause a reader to suspect that some factors in the experimental methods were not well controlled.

Relevance

Relevance concerns the desirability of having information in context. Two major elements are *comparison* and *mapping*.

Comparison

There is nothing so lonely as an isolated statistic. If the only fact about my income that I reveal is that I earn $136,000 (Canadian) per year, the reader would immediately think of different comparisons to put the salary information in context. What is the average salary of someone living in Vancouver? What is the purchasing power of that salary in American dollars? What does an average UBC professor make? What does the average burnt-out professor make? The exact question that the reader might ask would be related to a specific purpose. No matter whether it be to establish that I earned enough to be able to eat or determine my status (as determined by salary) among other professors at UBC, additional information is required to put the salary number into context. The two major types of comparisons made in scientific papers are: (1) comparisons between different sets of observations, and (2) comparisons between a set of observations and expectations. Specific tests are available for assessing such comparisons. Perhaps the most common statistical test for demonstrating the statistical significance of differences between sets of observations is the t test, as might be used when comparing the value of some outcome variable between a treated group and a control group. A goodness of fit test, such as the χ^2 test, would be commonly used to compare observed vs expected frequencies for categorical data (see chapter 9).

In a scientific paper, the author decides which comparisons will be featured, and there is a temptation to choose those that make the study look important. For many clinical studies of treatments, there are at least two positive possibilities: (1) that the treatment improved some outcome variable with time (eg, the effect of flossing over time on the amount of interproximal plaque), and (2) that one treatment was superior to another (eg, dental flossing might lower interproximal plaque values relative to no treatment or treatment with a mouthrinse). In a study's original design, the authors might have hoped that the treatment was better than the currently accepted treatment, but if they failed to demonstrate statistical superiority of the new treatment (ie, if the statistical test resulted in accepting the null hypothesis of no difference between treatments), they might resort to the lesser claim that the treatment at least worked to some degree, based on a comparison of the values before and after treatment.

Mapping

Tufte[10] has stated that scientific images should nearly always be mapped, contextualized, and placed on a universal grid. In *mapped* pictures, representational images are combined with scales, diagrams, overlays, numbers, and words. Such mapped images can facilitate comparisons and enable explanations. In essence, a mapped picture provides the detailed, specific, and perhaps unique information present in an image (eg, a photomicrograph) in combination with the abstract, focusing, and explanatory power of a diagram. A scale bar gives a universal standard of comparison so that readers can appreciate the actual dimensions involved. An advantage of mapping is that the relevant information is presented within one visual field. Some journals insist on scale bars for micrographs, whereas others allow the magnification to be stated in the figure legend. Having the scale bar directly on the micrograph simplifies comparisons for the reader, who otherwise would have to measure features in the micrograph and divide by the magnification to arrive at the size of a given structure.

The Selection and Manipulation of Data

Because neither the exact length nor the form of a scientific paper is specified, an author is free to decide how much and what data to include as well as how the data are to be presented. In making these choices, authors have an opportunity to make their case as convincing as possible. This section examines some of the strategies and standards for reporting and presenting data.

In reporting lengths, an author is usually constrained to employing the international standard: the meter. But in other situations, there may be more than one way of looking at the data; they may be presented as raw data (just the way they were recorded), as averages, as a ratio of some measured value relative to some standard, or as a ratio relative to some point of time or control. Although there may be many legitimate ways of looking at the same set of data, authors will normally choose a way that makes the data look most convincing. In fact, authors can show extraordinary ingenuity in presenting their data in the best light.

To illustrate several of the ways of looking at data, consider the following hypothetical set of data from an experiment investigating the effect of a mouthrinse on oral malodor. The chemical measurement made is the amount of volatile sulfur compounds (VSC) in nanograms per milliliter of mouth air. In this hypothetical experiment, the mouth air is analyzed for two individuals (A and B) prior to treatment, and at 1, 2, and 3 hours afterward. The results are compared with a control treatment, which comprises rinsing with distilled water.

The data could be processed in several ways, including:

1. The absolute values of VSC (Table 13-1). If replicated, the data could then be analyzed by analysis of variance (ANOVA) or other sophisticated statistical tests for significance.
2. The decrease from the baseline reading (Table 13-2).
3. The amount of VSC relative to the baseline for each individual (Table 13-3). Note that the difference between individuals has disappeared in this treatment of the data, because the baseline for each treatment is set at 100%, and the relative response with time is similar.
4. The percent reduction from baseline (Table 13-4).
5. Disregarding the baseline, and expressing the values in the mouthrinse-treated group relative to the water control (Table 13-5).
6. Data could be averaged for all times after treatment for each individual (Table 13-6).
7. The data could be averaged for all times and individuals (Table 13-7).
8. As in point 7, only expressed as a percentage. Thus, all the data could be reduced to a single statement: "The VSC concentrations in the mouthrinse-treated individuals were 37% of those where water was used," or, alternatively, mouthrinse reduced VSC 63%."

Table 13-1 Total VSC concentrations (ng/mL)

Individual	Treatment	Baseline	1h	2h	3h
A	Water	10	8	9	10
A	Mouthrinse	10	2	3	5
B	Water	4	3	4	4
B	Mouthrinse	4	0.8	1.2	2

Table 13-2 Total VSC concentrations (ng/mL) with time

Individual	Treatment	1h	2h	3h
A	Water	-2	-1	0
A	Mouthrinse	-8	-7	-5
B	Water	-1	0	0
B	Mouthrinse	-3.2	-2.8	-2

Table 13-3 Relative levels of VSC with time

Individual	Treatment	Baseline	1h	2h	3h
A	Water	100%	80%	90%	100%
A	Mouthrinse	100%	20%	30%	50%
B	Water	100%	75%	100%	100%
B	Mouthrinse	100%	20%	30%	50%

Table 13-4 Percent reduction of VSC levels with time

Individual	Treatment	Baseline	1h	2h	3h
A	Water	100%	20%	10%	0%
A	Mouthrinse	100%	80%	70%	50%
B	Water	100%	25%	0%	0%
B	Mouthrinse	100%	80%	70%	50%

Table 13-5 Ratio of treated to control VSC concentrations

Individual	1h	2h	3h
A	25%	33.3%	50%
B	26.7%	30%	50%

Table 13-6 Average VSC levels after treatment

Individual	Mouthrinse	Water
A	3.33	9
B	1.33	3.67

Table 13-7 Average VSC levels after treatment

Mouthrinse	Water
2.33	6.34

9. The author could choose just one time point for a comparison and write, "One hour after treatment, the mouthrinse decreased VSC 80%."

10. Another approach would be to define as *objectionable* any person who had a VSC concentration greater than five. Using these data, it could be said that mouthrinse totally eliminated any objectionable odor from 100% of the people tested for at least 3 hours (not a difficult task, as one of the two individuals was not "objectionable" prior to treatment).

11. Suppose that a third individual, C, had been tested, and the mouthrinse did not affect the VSC in C's mouth air. An unscrupulous author might simply ignore the results. A more creative approach would be to designate C a nonresponder, and then bury somewhere in the materials and methods section the statement that only responders were studied.

The beauty of this approach is that, by setting the definition of who is a responder at an appropriate level, you could get the maximal impact from the results.

This list is not exhaustive. Several other ways of treating the data are available. Any of the above methods of treating the data (save the dishonest ones) might be suitable, depending on the arguments an author might want to make and the relative importance of the particular data set to the author's conclusions.

There are two major points on the author's treatment of data. First, an author selects the data to be presented. The data that appear in scientific papers are condensed from the numbers that fill lab notebooks. Many journals specifically ask referees to point out how a paper could be shortened to reduce the cost of publication. Moreover, because it is not reasonable to expect the author to report every piece of data recorded during a study, an author must walk a tightrope, balancing the merits of an economical description with the benefits of complete data reporting without falling into the abyss of intent to deceive. The reader should be aware that possibly not all collected data are presented. Missing data raise the chance that an author is trying to hide a weakness, such as excessive variability or inconsistencies, or to report only the conditions that gave the biggest effect (as could be done in the example if only the 1-hour time point was considered).

Second, an author determines how data are manipulated. My rule is that the reader's suspicion should be directly proportional to the degree to which the data have been processed. A multitude of problems can be hidden through the ingenious use of relative values or corrections for backgrounds or baselines. The closer the presented data are to the actual observations, the better the chance a reader has of interpreting the data independently. Each manipulation involves an assumption about the underlying process. To return to our example, comparing everything to a baseline is only valid if the baseline is stable. Defining what concentration of VSC is "objectionable" is a value-laden process, as is setting the level of responders or nonresponders. Comparing relative values between individuals would be appropriate only if the response were the same, regardless of absolute level. Presenting only processed data forces the reader to make the same assumptions as the author.

More on derived measures

A common way of manipulating data is for an author to devise an index or other derived measurements.

Example 1: Use of ratios to suppress variation

The cardiac glycoside ouabain inhibits Na^+- and K^+-activated ATPase in isolated plasma membranes. However, the amount of the enzyme activity varies from batch to batch in membrane preparations. Because of this large batch-to-batch variation, an investigator might be unable to discern small effects in cells from rodents, which are not very sensitive to the drug. By calculating the ratio below, it is possible to demonstrate statistically significant effects of even very low concentrations of the drug:

$$\% \text{ inhibition} = \frac{\text{activity in sample with ouabain}}{\text{control activity (ie, no ouabain)}} \times 100$$

For an author, the advantage of this procedure is that the data, freed of troublesome variations, become much cleaner and more convincing. For the reader, the problem of such data is that you cannot find out what variation in the original measurements existed, or what caused it. In this example, why did the membrane preparations vary in ATPase activity? The reporting of data relative to a standard value is sometimes informally referred to as *normalization*. (Note that the term *normalization* is also used to describe the process whereby data are transformed into a z-score, which represents the score's position on a Gaussian curve.)

Example 2: Use of ratios to mask or enhance changes

A second problem with data reported as a ratio concerns the size of the denominator, which may either mask or enhance the perception of any changes. To enhance an effect, ratios are calculated with denominators that are as small as possible. For example, suppose that 91% of people were employed and 9% unemployed when an administration took office, but that during that term of office, the numbers changed to 95% employed and 5% unemployed. This change could be expressed either as:

$$\left(\frac{4}{95}\right) \times 100\% = 4.2\%$$

an increase in employment (probably by the opposition), or as:

$$\left(\frac{4}{9}\right) \times 100\% = 44\%$$

a decrease in unemployment (probably by the current administration).

Example 3: Novel indices and cutoff lines

A distressing finding of modern sociology is the ineffectiveness of many social programs. These programs are often very expensive, and justifying their existence on pragmatic (as opposed to moral or ethical) grounds is difficult. One approach to the problem is to devise new indices that make the results look better. Rosenthal and Rubin[11] devised a simple procedure for converting an estimate of effect size into a tabular display (binomial effect size display [BESD]).

Table 13-8 Success rates for dental implant placement for surgeons A and B

Surgeon	Success rate for smokers	No. of implants placed in smokers	Success rate for nonsmokers	No. of implants placed in nonsmokers	Overall success rate
A	80%	1000	95%	100	$\frac{(0.8 \times 1000) + (0.95 \times 100)}{1100} = 81\%$
B	70%	100	85%	1000	$\frac{(0.7 \times 100) + (0.85 \times 1000)}{1100} = 84\%$

Rather than making a statement like, "A special reading program accounts for only 9% of the total variation," we could say of the same data that it "reduced the need for tutoring by almost one half." A reader should always look carefully at novel indices, especially when arbitrary cutoff lines like "responders/nonresponders" or "needs/does not need tutors" are used. Are arbitrary definitions introduced to offer the investigators a means to conclude whatever they want?

Example 4: Ratios of ratios of ratios of . . .

Sometimes investigators normalize data to form a ratio and then compare the ratios. The net effect of all this computation is that the reader ends up so far removed from the original data that the reader becomes confused and accepts the authors' conclusions. For example, a study on the effect of a drug on bone loss in an animal model of periodontal disease compared bone loss by measuring the length of the root surrounded by alveolar bone relative to the total length of the root to give a value of percent bone attachment. This ratio was computed at various times to give a rate that was a ratio of a ratio:

$$\frac{\% \text{ bone loss}}{\text{month}}$$

Then the drug-treated and control groups were compared to give an effectiveness ratio, which is a ratio of a ratio of a ratio:

$$\frac{\text{rate of bone loss with drug treatment}}{\text{rate of bone loss in control}}$$

In this composite value, it is virtually impossible to comprehend what the variation was in the original measurements, or even the actual amount of bone lost.

More on aggregated measurements

The Simpson paradox

A common statistical artifact called the *Simpson paradox* refers to the situation in which the aggregated data actually point in the opposite direction to that of the same data when disaggregated.[12] Consider Table 13-8, which shows the success rates for smokers and nonsmokers for dental implants placed by Surgeons A and B. Both surgeons have lower success rates for smokers than for nonsmokers.

For both smokers and nonsmokers, Surgeon A has a higher success rate—in fact, 10% higher for each. Yet, his overall success rate is less than Surgeon B's. The reason for the difference is that Surgeon B places more implants in nonsmokers than in smokers, whereas Surgeon A's patients are mainly smokers, whose implants are less likely to be successful. In this example, we could conclude that careful case selection (ie, limiting the number of smokers) by surgeons may be more important in perceived overall success rate than surgical skill. But the more general theme is that some misleading conclusions can arise when one aggregates data across subclassifications (in this case, smokers and nonsmokers).

Subgroup analysis

The obverse of the problems posed by the Simpson paradox is the question of when is it legitimate to break down aggregated data into subgroups to determine whether a treatment had an effect on a subgroup. For example, consider a randomized controlled trial, where a drug was given to a group of males and females, and its effects compared with those obtained in a placebo-treated group. Suppose that no statistically significant effect was found; however, close scrutiny of the data and separate examination of the response of males and females might reveal that males benefited but females did not. The first question of interest is whether the results simply occurred by chance. If many possible subgroups (eg, sex, physiologic values) and many possible ways of comparing the subgroups exist, it is likely for some difference to arise by chance in at least one subgroup. The most rigorous approach would be to test the finding in a subsequent experiment. A possibly acceptable approach would be to report the difference, particularly if there was a good explanation for the result that could have been postulated in advance (even though it was not). For example, in a study of the effects of flossing, an investigator could postulate in advance that flossing might be least effective for posterior teeth because they are hard to access. An investigator might not consider that possibility in advance of the experiment, but—confronted by data showing flossing improved oral hygiene markedly in anterior but not posterior teeth—might decide to report it as a statistically significant difference. An unacceptable approach would be to make as many comparisons as possible, in the hope that one might turn out to be statistically significant; at the very least, the statistical test should be modified appropriately (such as with the Bonferroni corrections) to correct for the multiple comparisons being made.

Exploratory data analysis

Subgroup analysis, in which various relationships are considered, is a subset of the larger topic of exploratory data analysis. This analysis is probably as old as science itself, but its legitimization and enrichment is attributable to the statistician Tukey.[13] In explanatory data analysis, an investigator examines the data and looks for patterns. In the breath analysis example given previously, the data were looked at in various ways, such as in ratios or difference from background. As noted in the example, some of these operations can mislead the reader, but they also can provide new insights into the data and show patterns that may not be evident in unprocessed data. Exploratory data analysis is one of the more enjoyable scientific activities, for it enables an investigator to gain new insights and typically involves less grunt work than the collection of data. Indeed, a scientist can even use other people's data, perhaps finding a pattern missed by the original investigators.

Finding unexpected patterns is one of the major paths to discovery. As a simple example of exploratory data analysis, consider the data of Simonton[14] that records the average age at which scientists in various disciplines made their most important contribution. Simonton[15] has published a figure on this (as well as other) data, in which the disciplines are ordered alphabetically (a much simplified version is given in Fig 13-2a). Alphabetical arrangement offers the reader the advantage of ease in finding particular data. However, it does not provide any insight into why the data are what they are—whether some underlying principle or pattern might explain the data.

Seeing the data in Fig 13-2a, and remembering vaguely Lord Bertrand Russell's comment that when he no longer could do mathematics he switched to philosophy, I began to wonder if that pattern also occurred in mathematically based disciplines—ie, is it the case that the more mathematics used in a discipline, the younger the scientists' ages will be at the time of their most important contributions? First, I ranked the disciplines, according to my crude guess, as to how much each discipline, on average, used mathematics. I then redrew the data with the disciplines spread along the x-axis according to my guess and plotted the age at which the best contribution occurred for each (Fig 13-2b). A rough relationship is evident; the more mathematics involved in a discipline, the earlier the scientist "peaked." A serious study would require a lot more work; for example, an investigator might have to look at the work of individual scientists, their ages at the time of their most important contribution, how much mathematics was involved, and so forth. But conducting a preliminary exploration of the data and identifying a pattern provide the seeds for a future investigation.

Moreover, simply looking at the data in detail brings up other issues that it may inform. For example, at my university, there has been a heated debate on the issue of mandatory retirement at age 65. The administration, of course, wanted to make retirement mandatory at age 65, as this gives them flexibility in their planning and also saves costs (as old professors tend to be more expensive than freshly hired young ones). Faculty members, as a general rule, want mandatory retirement to be eliminated, as this gives them more options. Phrases like "distilled experience" are used to justify keeping the elderly professors with all their wisdom on the payroll. When we look at the ordinate of Fig 13-2, however, we realize that for every science, the average age of scientists at the time of their best contributions is younger than 45 years. When we con-

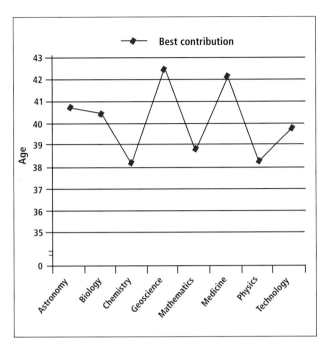

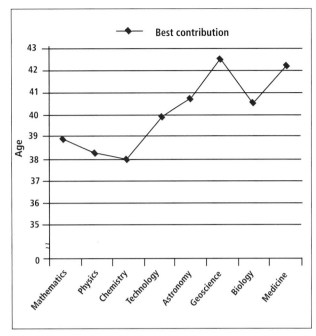

Fig 13-2a Average age at which scientists make their best contribution. Discipline ordered alphabetically. Data from Simonton.[13]

Fig 13-2b Same data as Fig 13-2a. Disciplines are ordered by a crude assessment of the amount of mathematics involved in each field. Data from Simonton.[13]

sider the SDs (not given here), it does not appear likely that professors will make their finest research contributions after age 65.

Wainer[16] makes three points on the use of graphs in exploratory data analysis: *(1)* impact is important. Ideally, a graph should be vivid enough that its primary message is inescapable, but *(2)* understanding a graph is not automatic. A good legend can make a weak graph into a strong one. Wainer believes that a legend should state the point of the graph. Indeed, having to prepare informative legends may reduce the number of pointless graphs in a paper, as it makes the pointlessness of the graph evident. *(3)* A graph can make points that might not have been seen otherwise.

Minimum Requirements for Reporting Data

There are four minimum requirements for reporting data:

1. It should be clear exactly how the measurement was done.
2. There should be some measure of central tendency (eg, mean, median, or mode).
3. There should be some measure of variation (eg, SD, standard error (SE), confidence limits, or range).
4. There should be a statement about the total number of objects studied.

It is difficult to evaluate a study without all of this information. However, even when all these values are reported, the reader might not get an accurate impression of the distribution of the values in the sample. Statistics, like the SD, tell us little about distribution of the values in the sample if the data are not distributed normally. Cleveland[17] notes that the normal distribution is symmetric, but real data are often skewed to the right. The normal distribution does not have wild observations, but real data do. The best way to present some sets of data is to show all the data points.

Measurements of Central Tendency

The term *population* refers to a finite or infinite group of things with common characteristics. The *sample* is the observed part of the population. The purpose of any measure of central tendency of a sample is to represent a group of individual values. The best measure of central tendency depends on the situation being described; the most common measures are the mean, the mode, and the median.

Mean

The arithmetic *mean* is defined as:

$$\text{mean} = \overline{X} = \frac{1}{n}\sum_{i=1}^{n} X_i = \frac{x_1 + x_2 + x_3 + \cdots + x_n}{n}$$

where x_i = value of each measurement, and n = number in sample.

Of the three measures of central tendency, only the mean uses all the actual numerical values of the observations. Moreover, each observation enters into the calculation. The mean uses more of the information in a set of data than either the mode or the median.

The problem with using the mean as an estimate of the average value is that the mean can be unduly influenced by extreme values. For instance, in salary negotiations with school boards, teachers sometimes become upset when the news media report their average salaries as indicated by the mean. The mean salary for professional employees of a school board is a value that is inflated by the high salaries of administrators and principals. Thus, teachers argue, the mean does not reflect the actual money paid to the teachers who face the children in the front lines of the classroom.

Mode

The *mode* is the most frequently occurring value in a set of measurements. In Fig 13-3, the mode corresponds to the peak of the distribution curve. Its use in biologic science is limited, but it can be thought of as being a "typical" example. Although not affected by extreme values, the mode is easily shifted by the accidental accumulation of scores at some point that may be a considerable distance away from the central tendency of the distribution. Occasionally, samples will have two peaks in the frequency-distribution curve. Such a curve is bimodal, and the use of the mode becomes problematic. The data on death by horse kick (see Fig 9-6) provide an example in which the mode describes the distribution quite well. In most years, no one was killed, and this statistic is more readily digested than the parameters of the Poisson distribution. The mode is the only measure of central tendency that makes sense for nominal scale data. It makes sense to state that the modal (most frequent) sex of dental students is male, and that their modal

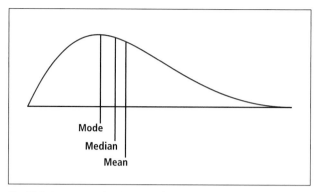

Fig 13-3 Frequency density curve for a moderately skewed distribution in which the three measures of central tendency (mode, median, and mean) occur at different values. For a perfectly symmetrical distribution, they would all coincide.

hair color is brown, but statements about their mean hair color or median sex would be meaningless.

Median

The *median* of a set of n observations is the middle value when the data are arranged in order of increasing size. If the sample has an even number of observations, the median is the average of the two central values. The median is unaffected by extreme values in the sample. The median is useful, because it can be calculated when some values are missing but are known to be above or below a certain level. For example, the median age of death for a group can be determined as soon as 50% of the members have died. Such a situation often arises in tests of cancer therapies. Calculation of the mean would have to wait until all the members had died. Thus, the median is particularly useful in reporting survival of patients or restorations.

Summary

Consider a sample that yielded the values 1, 2, 2, 3, 4, 5, 6:

$$\text{Mean} = \frac{1+2+2+3+4+5+6}{7} = 3.28$$

Mode = 2 (two data points were 2, the rest of the data points occurred only once)

Median = 3

The relationship between three of the measures of central tendency is given in Fig 13-3.

Measures of dispersion

Evaluation of results often concerns not only the average of a sample but also the dispersion, or spread, of the data around the central value. Once again, it is desirable for the value describing the data dispersion to be as representative of the sample as possible. We will examine several measures of dispersion.

Range

The *range* (R) is defined as R = x_{max} – x_{min}, where x_{max} is the highest, and x_{min} is the lowest values in the sample.

The range is an efficient measure of dispersion when there are very few observations in the sample. For this reason, the range has been widely used in quality-control work, where spot checks are made using small samples. The range can be applied to all types of data.

Standard deviation

SD, the square root of variance, is the most common measure of dispersion. The variance of a sample (s^2) is defined as:

$$s^2 = \frac{\sum_{i=1}^{n}\left(x_i - \overline{X}\right)^2}{n-1}$$

where $\overline{X}$ = mean, and n = number in sample.

The number of "independent" observations, represented by n – 1, is called *degrees of freedom* (*df*). The value for the *df* is one less than the total number of observations, because one *df* is lost when the mean is calculated. That is, if the mean and the values of n – 1 of the observations are known, the value of the nth observation can be calculated. The variance for a population, rather than a sample from the population, is given by σ^2, where μ is the true population mean:

$$\sigma^2 = \frac{\sum_{i=1}^{n}\left(x_i - \mu\right)^2}{n}$$

For a sample from the population, the applicable formula for the SD (which is the square root of the variance) is:

$$s = \sqrt{\frac{\sum_{i=1}^{n}\left(x_i - \overline{X}\right)^2}{n-1}}$$

Standard error

A common technique for portraying sample-to-sample variation of a statistic is to graph error bars to portray plus and minus one SE of the statistic, in a way similar to that used when the sample SD is used to summarize the variation of the data.

The formuzla for standard error of the mean (SEM) $s_{\overline{X}}$ follows:

$$s_{\overline{X}} = \frac{s}{\sqrt{n}}$$

A SE of a statistic conveys information about the confidence intervals of the statistic, the mean plus or minus one SE is approximately a 68% confidence interval. Thus, the SEM quantifies uncertainty in the estimate of the mean. Variability in the population, the type of information in which the reader is interested, is not directly demonstrated. Thus, Glantz[18] recommends that data should never be summarized with the SEM. What makes the SE attractive to many authors, however, is that the $s_{\overline{X}}$ is smaller than the SD; thus, the appearance of the variability in the data is reduced, because the error bars are smaller.

Significant Digits: Conventions in Reporting Statistical Data

Published reports often appear to have a spurious degree of precision. Different authorities recommend different conventions. Some believe that, as a general rule, investigators should not pretend to know more than they really do. In this view, they should not report any more digits than can be read, or at least estimated, from the scale that was read. However, the precision of a measurement is given by its SD. Precision is not indicated by the number of significant digits in the result.

The actual number of digits reported is to some extent a question of style. Mainland[19] suggests carrying two more figures than will be required at the end. In the analysis of the data by ANOVA techniques, Pearce[20] recommends expressing the data so that there are three digits that can vary from one to the other. For example, data could take the form: 1.413, 1.536, 1.440, etc, in one case; and 101.413, 101.536, 101.440, etc, in another. In both cases, it is the last three digits that vary among the values. In the ANOVA technique, Pearce advises expressing the summation terms to two decimal places beyond those arising from the act of squaring.

Finally, Gilbert[21] recommends reporting one more decimal place in the SE than in the mean itself, making it possible to be accurate in subsequent calculations (such as confidence limits). However, Gilbert also states that, in biology, it is rarely worth carrying decimals more than three significant digits in any mean. Few would disagree with Gilbert's declaration that if someone claims a duck lays 4.603 eggs on average, the final digit, 3, is almost certainly useless.

Tables

Tables are used to present exact values of numeric data when the amount of data is too extensive to be summarized in the text. Huth[22] recommends that there should be no more than one table or illustration per thousand words of text, and that tables should be used when readers need the exact values of more data than could be summarized in a few sentences of text. Overuse of tables, figures, and illustrations is often symptomatic of an author's desire to disguise dross as gold. Day[23] remarks that:

> Many authors, especially those who are still beginners, think that a table, graph or chart somehow adds importance to the data. Thus, in a search for credibility, there is a tendency to convert a few data elements into an impressive-looking graph or table.

Several commonsense rules are applicable[24]:

1. When four or more items of statistical information or data are to be presented, the material will be clearer in tabular form.
2. Trends in the data should be exploited to coincide with reader expectations. Time series or concentration are examples of data where readers expect data to be presented with the earliest or smaller values first, and later or larger values last. In some instances, authors design tables based on ease of locating particular data entries. For example, if United States income levels were reported by state, the first row would discuss Alabama, and the last row, Wyoming. However, as noted by Wainer,[25] such a

presentation may preclude readers from discerning important patterns.
3. The data should be arranged so that the major comparisons are clear.
4. Inessential data should be omitted.

Data tables can be used deceptively. Occasionally, tables are used where the reader might expect a figure or histogram. On examining the table, the reader sometimes finds an irregular point in the data that does not conform to the general pattern. In general, it is much easier to detect irregularities in a graph or histogram than in sets of written numbers. Hence, tables must be examined closely to check internal consistency.

Illustrations

Illustrations, such as photographs, are necessary when they are the evidence being offered to support a conclusion. Ultrastructural studies provide an example; the electron micrographs are the evidence. In other instances, diagrams or charts summarize and demonstrate the relationship between groups.

The pioneer statistician Fisher[26] viewed diagrams as follows:

> Diagrams prove nothing but bring outstanding features readily to the eye; they are therefore no substitute for such critical tests as may be applied to the data but are valuable in suggesting such tests.

This view was also held by Hill, who wrote, "Graphs should always be regarded as subsidiary aids to the intelligence and not as evidence of associations or trends."[27] Figures and/or illustrations efficiently provide information, and by virtue of their prominence relative to material presented in the text automatically emphasize the points being made.

Understanding presentation techniques

A number of techniques are available to slant illustrations so that they provide support for the author's views. Several of these are graphic analogues of rhetorical techniques.

Selection

The general rule with selection seems to be that authors do not show what they do not want the reader to see. "Warts and all" is not a frequently employed reporting strategy. By selecting the illustrations, authors direct and focus attention on particular aspects of the study. To a certain extent, such focusing is inevitable, for not every observation or detail in a study will be published. The problem arises when the information presented is selectively biased toward a particular interpretation, or when the selection makes the technical aspects of a study appear better than they really are. On a technical level, microscopic fields that exhibit prominent debris or precipitates are seldom shown, as they might lead the reader to think that techniques were applied sloppily. On the issue of representiveness, authors often choose examples that exaggerate effects. For example, if the authors claim that a high percentage of cells stain with a particular antibody, but there is variation in the actual percentage of cells stained in various fields, they would generally choose for publication a field that most strongly demonstrated the conclusion.

Arrows

Typically, authors insert arrows or other markers into micrographs. This stratagem has two strengths: (a) it directs attention to the features that most strongly feature in their interpretation; (b) the marker itself might obscure some feature that the authors do not want to be seen.

Providing context

Authors may or may not provide context for their illustrations. A useful strategy for photomicrographs is to include a figure at lower power magnification, with the area containing the feature of interest shown in higher magnification as an inset or separate figure. In this way, the "big picture," which will necessarily be more representative, can be given along with a detailed view of the feature of interest.

Another means of providing context is the scale or micron bar printed directly on a micrograph. Some journals allow authors to place the magnifications in the figure legend. In theory, either method enables the reader to measure the size of features in a micrograph. However, if only magnifications are given, a reader must measure the feature of interest on the micrograph and divide by the magnification to determine the size of the feature. That takes some mental effort, and readers,

being cognitive misers, will be unlikely to make the effort. So, if authors have something whose size is not what it should be, they would be wise to eschew scale bars and, in their stead, report magnifications.

Context for figures reporting quantitative data are given by the controls. For instance, if the effects of a drug are being studied, the negative control (no drug) will show the basal response of the assay system, and the positive control (eg, a drug known to maximally affect the response) will demonstrate the possible responsiveness of the assay system. Authors may manipulate their choice of controls to suit their interpretive needs. A study touting the effects of a new mouthrinse on breath odor might compare the new product, not with the best available treatment, but rather with a well-known product of marginal effectiveness.

"Persuading with pap"

This phrase, taken from Monmonier's *How to Lie with Maps,*[28] refers to the practice of using highly simplistic maps—or, alternately, maps with irrelevant minutiae; the former persuade readers by reducing complexity, while the latter obscure important or inconvenient points by burying them in a mass of details. In science, schematic diagrams or cartoons suggesting mechanisms or relationships can perform this role. Modern biological and clinical studies are often complex, and interpretations are made based on relationships of varying strength. Readers, who are almost always cognitive misers, like authors to do their thinking for them, so they welcome simplified diagrams that make vague concepts concrete. However, a weak set of data that just reaches statistical significance but shows only a small effect size may become a solid arrow indicating a firm cause-effect relationship in a schematic diagram on mechanism. Similarly, a cartoon illustrating the findings of a study on a drug affecting cell signaling might feature a well-established fact (eg, the structure of a G-linked receptor, with its seven transmembrane components) casting a halo over the less well-established structures and relationships that were actually studied.

Leading the reader

Leading the reader is a particularly useful tactic in figure legends, where authors will effectively tell the reader what to think; that is, they will mix in interpretation with the description of the observations. Being cognitive misers, readers are often not adverse to being led. Figure legends are expected to be brief, so that when interpretation is placed in legends, qualifying words and caveats can be left out without attracting undue attention. Leading the reader is essential in achieving the persuasive intentions of authors; if an interpretation is not given in the figure legend, readers will have to figure it out themselves. In such a situation, three eventualities are possible (two of which, from the author's point of view, should be avoided): *(1)* readers will stumble on the same conclusion as the authors, *(2)* they will reach a different interpretation, or *(3)* they will become confused. The best strategy is to lay out the figure in such a manner that the explanation or interpretations are self-evident. Tufte has given the principles of how this can be done, as well as numerous examples of where it has or has not been done, in a series of insightful books.[1,29,30] The most effective illustration combines the direct visual evidence of images with the explanatory power of honestly conceived diagrams.

Evaluating graphs: Tufte's evaluative ratios

Graphs are often used in place of tables if a pronounced trend or relationship between the variables is plotted. Appearance and clarity of figures are important in determining effectiveness. Guidelines for the visual presentation of charts and graphs in the life sciences have been published by Simmonds and Bragg,[31] in association with the Institute of Medical and Biological Illustration, as well as by Tufte, in his excellent book, *The Visual Display of Quantitative Information.*[29] Tufte has devised several indices to evaluate illustrations. The first two deal largely with the efficiency of information presentation.

Data-ink ratio

Data-ink ratio (DIR) is the proportion of the graphic's ink devoted to the nonredundant display of data:

$$DIR = \frac{data\ ink}{total\ ink\ to\ print\ the\ graph}$$

Tufte advises maximizing the DIR within reason. In practice, this often means eliminating grids, plotting points boldly, and erasing redundant data ink or unnecessary nondata ink, such as redundant labels. For example, there is often no point in presenting both halves of symmetric measures, such as error bars.

Data density index

The *data density index* (DDI) of a graphic measures the amount of data displayed in relation to the graphic's size:

$$DDI = \frac{no.\ of\ entries\ in\ data\ matrix}{area\ of\ graphic}$$

Tufte surveyed a number of scientific journals and computed their median DDI: *Nature* scored 48; *Science,* 21; *New England Journal of Medicine,* 12; and *Scientific American,* 5. He concluded that the average published graphic is pretty thin, that is, it does not illustrate much data for the area it occupies (see Fig 13-8). It will be interesting to see how the advent of electronic publishing affects data density. In standard print journals, the cost of publication is related to the length of the articles. Some journals, such as Quintessence's *International Journal of Oral and Maxillofacial Implants,* ask referees whether any figures or illustrations can be omitted. However, for electronic publications, article length is not a significant factor in cost, and editors will probably be less vigilant in identifying pointless figures.

Lie factor

The *lie factor* (LF) deals with quantifying the distortions present in some figures and is defined as follows:

$$LF = \frac{size\ of\ effect\ shown\ in\ graphic}{size\ of\ effect\ in\ data}$$

The LF will be illustrated later.

Evaluating graphics: Cleveland's hierarchy of graphical perception

By investigating the perception of graphs from the theory of visual perception and by performing experiments in graphical perception, Cleveland[32] was able to assess the accuracies with which readers perform graphical perception tasks. For information to be most accurately interpreted by the reader, data should be displayed so that the reader uses the most accurate processes of graphical perception. The following list presents Cleveland's hierarchy[32] of perception, from the most accurate to the least accurate:

1. Position along a common scale
2. Position along identical, nonaligned scales
3. Length

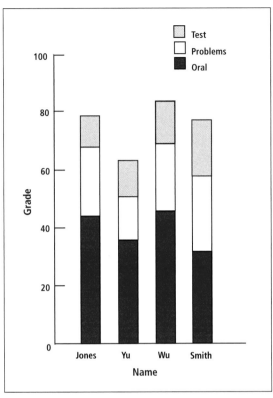 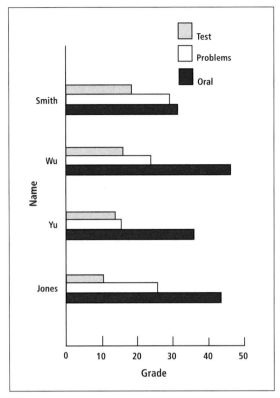

Fig 13-4 The grade data for four students are presented in two graphs to demonstrate Cleveland's hierarchy of perception. *(a)* Stacked bar graph. *(b)* Bar graph; in this configuration, a fourth bar (total grade) could be added for each student, if desired.

4. Angle/slope (Cleveland's data cannot discriminate between these two.)
5. Area
6. Volume
7. Color hue, color saturation, color density

As an illustration of Cleveland's hierarchy, consider Fig 13-4. A student's grade in my undergraduate course ORBI 430 is calculated by the sum of the marks on a test, problem sets, and an oral examination. Figure 13-4a presents the data for four students as a stacked bar graph. Because the oral component has a common baseline, you can compare the grades of the students directly. Comparing the problem-set and test values is difficult, however, because they involve length judgments (ranked 3 on the Cleveland hierarchy), which are not as accurate as position judgments along a common scale (ranked 1). This information

could be presented as a bar graph with a common scale (as shown in Fig 13-4b), which makes it possible to compare all components on a common scale, and, consequently, process the information more accurately. Cleveland believes that it is never necessary to resort to a divided bar chart, because any set of data that can be shown by a divided bar chart can also be shown by a graphical method, which replaces length judgments by position judgments.

Although bar graphs have the advantage of comparing data along a common scale, there is a potential problem in the manner in which the bars are filled. The difference in contrast between the hatchings should not be too dramatic, because it has been found that the eye is drawn to the black areas, making them difficult to compare with unshaded areas.

As another example of applying Cleveland's hierarchy, consider the distribution of the UBC expenditures,

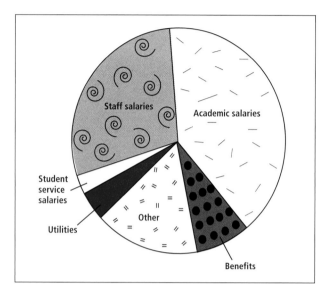

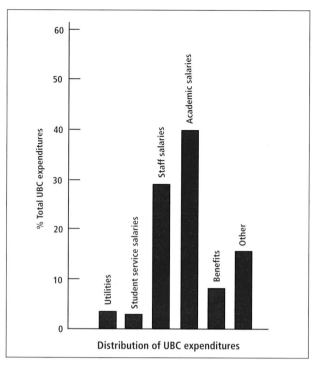

Fig 13-5 The distribution of UBC expenditures is presented in two forms to demonstrate the Cleveland hierarchy of perception. *(a)* Pie chart. *(b)* Bar graph.

presented in Fig 13-5a as a pie chart. Comparing the various components requires the reader to make angle judgments—a task rated fourth in the Cleveland hierarchy. Angles cannot be estimated as accurately as position judgments along a common scale. Thus, Fig 13-5b, a bar chart presenting the same data, enables comparisons between the categories to be made both more accurately and more conveniently than in the pie chart. Although often derided by statisticians and graphic designers, pie charts have been shown by Simken and Hastie[33] to be effective in certain situations. Pie charts are not widely used in scientific graphics, but are common in advertising and other mass-media applications, where they are often tilted and given depth, so they appear like floating platters. These additional manipulations make them even more difficult to interpret.

Students sometimes confuse bar graphs and histograms. A *bar graph* has spaces between the bars and is used when the bars represent discrete factors, such as exposure to some treatment or data obtained from different species. A *histogram* has no spaces between the individual columns and is used when the columns represent a variable that can be varied continuously. Histograms reveal the distribution of a variable.

The art of deception as applied to graphs and figures

Good graphics display data accurately and clearly. With the advent of computer graphics, a large amount of data can be presented clearly in a small amount of space. However, a clear, accurate representation of all the data does not always serve authors' interests in demonstrating their arguments, and some authors, knowingly or unknowingly, stoop to the art of deception.

Our concern in this section is how graphs can be presented so that they appear to strengthen arguments. Elements of the art of deception have been practiced for some time. Huff's[34] 1954 classic *How to Lie with Statistics* dealt with the topic that has been updated by the more recent *How to Display Data Badly* by Wainer.[35] Cleveland's[32] landmark book *The Elements of Graphing Data* presents the current standards and rationale for presenting data clearly.

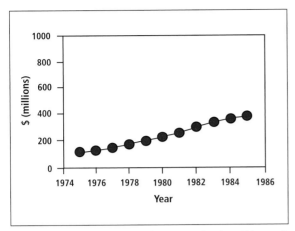

Fig 13-6a Plot of BC's expenditures on dentists. This graph uses large units on the ordinate.

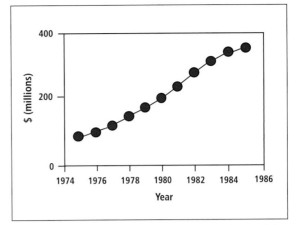

Fig 13-6b Plot of BC's expenditures on dentists. This graph has obvious extrapolation difficulties.

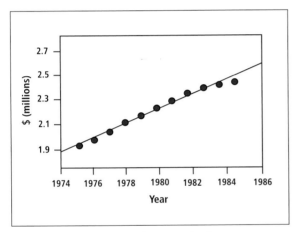

Fig 13-6c Log of BC's expenditures on dentists.

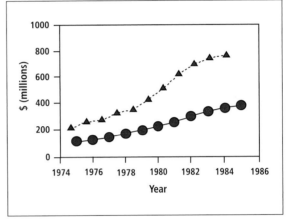

Fig 13-6d Plot of BC's expenditures on dentists *(circles)* and physicians *(triangles)*.

Use of scales

Consider the graphs presented in Fig 13-6, which plot expenditures of the province of British Columbia (BC) on dentists.

The increase in expenditure seems more rapid in Fig 13-6b than in Fig 13-6a, solely because of the scale of presentation. It should be pointed out that Fig 13-6a is a poor graph, because the scale units on the ordinate are too large (the general rule is that they should be selected so that the curve at least roughly extends over about two thirds the range of both ordinate and abscissa). Cleveland[32] advises that scales be chosen so the data fill up as much of the data region as possible, but insists that authors should always be willing to forego this fill principle to achieve an effective comparison. In particular, comparing a number of panels in a single figure will generally work better if all panels have the same scale, so that comparisons can be made between panels, even if the individual panels are not filled. Fig 13-6b is clearly better, but it also has problems. Using this curve makes it difficult to predict what the expenditure will be in the future (all things being equal), because the form of the curve is difficult to extrapolate. This can be solved by plotting the log of expenditures, as shown in Fig 13-6c. Because this curve is fitted to a smooth curve, it is easier to extrapolate. Of course, such an extrapolation will not necessarily yield the right prediction, because conditions might develop that destroy the assumption that the past pattern applies to the future. For instance, the onset of a recession might affect expenditures on dentistry substantially.

Logarithmic scales are useful when it is important to understand percent change or multiplicative factors. The most common is a *semi-log plot*, in which the log of the dependent variable is plotted against linear scale. On a semi-log plot, percents and factors are easier to judge, because equal multiplicative factors and percentages result in equal distances throughout the entire scale. That is, when the slope of a semi-log plot is straight, the rate of relative change is constant.

Semi-log plots are often used in growth curves, where cell number is increasing exponentially, and the plot of cell number with time on a semi-log plot will be linear. Similarly, dose-response curves can be plotted using a semi-log plot, because dose can be logarithmically related to the number of receptors stimulated. Like any curve-fitting procedure, the presence of a straight line does not uniquely identify any particular process, so that the straight line semi-log plot found for expenditures in dentistry could result from: *(a)* dentists increasing their fee schedule guide by the same percentage per year while the number of procedures remains constant; *(b)* dentists charging the same for procedures while the number of procedures grows by the same rate every year; or *(c)* a combination of such factors.

In any case, each of the three curves gives a different impression about consumer spending. Figure 13-6a could be used by a dental association to show that consumer spending on dentistry is rising slowly; Fig 13-6b, by a consumer association to prove that dental expenditures are rising too rapidly; and Fig 13-6c, by the government to estimate the taxes they will receive from dentists.

Scales can be used to affect the perception of variation in individual data points. A log scale, for example, will compress the apparent amount of variation. An advantage of taking logs, however, is that the overlap caused by positively skewed data will often be alleviated, and the resolution of the graph will be improved. Thus, there are many valid reasons why data should be transformed and various rules that should be applied.[36] In summary, the scale used affects our perception of the data. If a reader is suspicious about a scale, the best thing to do is to replot the data in a more suitable form and see how it looks.

Suppress the baseline

Another trick in the art of deception (used in bar graphs, histograms, as well as graphs) is simply to exclude the zero value of the ordinate (Fig 13-7) and to expand the scale. An obvious advantage for the author is that baseline suppression magnifies any differences between the groups. However, including zero in every graph makes no sense if it makes the ordinate axis so large that the resolution of the graph is destroyed; thus, zero should be included in the scale if it does not

waste undue space or seriously degrade the comparisons being made. If zero is not included, a break in the ordinal scale or a note in the legend should indicate its absence.

Hype a small amount of data

Figure 13-8, redrawn from the feminist magazine *A Room of One's Own,*[37] illustrates the tactic of data hype. The amount of information presented is small, comprising only six pieces of data in an area of approximately 20 cm: the percentage of individual grants awarded to men and women, the percentage of grant monies awarded to men and women, and the amounts of money awarded to men and women. Moreover, because—for either grants or money—the percentages allocated to men and women must add up to 100%, there are actually only three pieces of information: the total amount of money, the ratio of money granted to men and women, and the ratio of men to women receiving grants. Tufte's data density index can be calculated as follows:

$$DDI = \frac{3}{20} = 0.15$$

Wainer[35] reported that the DDI for popular and technical media ranged from 0.1 to 362. Clearly, this illustration falls in the lowest strata.

Hiding the data

Omit essential data
Figure 13-8 also omits important data. To assess these data, you need to know the distribution of men and women applying for grants. If equal numbers of men and women applied, there would be reason to consider that there might be some discrimination against women. But if the ratio of men to women applying for money was 2:1, there would be no evidence for bias.

Odious comparisons
Most observers would agree that Fig 13-6a looks wrong because there is too much blank space. Readers might question the scale and figure out that the chosen scale makes the increases look small. To banish such thoughts, the author might include another line on the graph. In Fig 13-6d, data on spending on physicians has been added to the graph. The scale is legitimized by this second curve. The expenditure on dentists' services looks small relative to the increased expenditures on physicians.

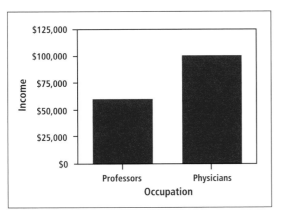

Fig 13-7a Bar graph with zero value included in ordinate (income).

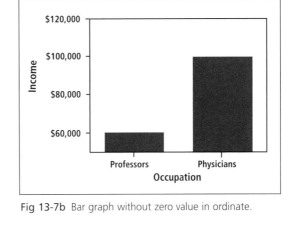

Fig 13-7b Bar graph without zero value in ordinate.

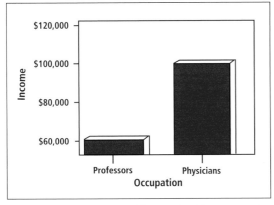

Fig 13-7c Three-dimensional bar graph without zero value in ordinate.

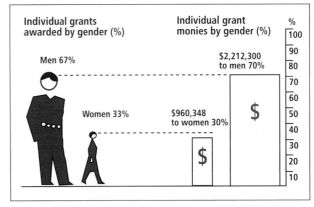

Fig 13-8 Example of magnifying a small amount of data. Total number of grants awarded to individuals in all categories by theatre section of the Canada Council between 1972 and 1981 was 996. Total monies disbursed was $3,172,648. (Redrawn with permission from Fraticelli.[37])

Using areas or volumes to represent unidimensional data

Figure 13-8 also illustrates this principle. Note that the two parts of the illustration cite percentages, a linear quantity. Yet, these percent values are represented by pictures of dollar bills and people. Because the width of the dollar bill is proportioned to its height, the original ratio of $ male/$ female of 7:3, appears, by comparing areas, to be 6:1. We can calculate the lie factor, Tufte's measure of distortion, as follows:

$$LF = \frac{\text{size of effect shown in graphic}}{\text{size of effect in data}}$$

size of effect in data = 2.3
size of effect in graphic = 6

$$Lie\ factor = \frac{6}{2.3} = 2.6$$

Lie factors greater than 1.05 or less than 0.95 indicate substantial distortion, far beyond minor innaccuracies in plotting.[29]

However, Cleveland[30] has found that when people are shown two areas whose magnitudes are a_1 and a_2 and are asked to judge the ratio of a_1 to a_2, most will judge the ratio on a scale:

$$\left[\frac{a_1}{a_2}\right]^{\beta}$$

where β would typically have a value of 0.7.

Thus, in this example, the perceived size of the effect in the graphic equals $(7/3)^{0.7} = 3.5$, and the perceived lie factor is probably closer to a value of 1.5, which still indicates substantial distortion.

Until recently, the use of three-dimensional figures to illustrate unidimensional values in scientific presentations has been infrequent. However, many computer graphic programs now offer the option of adding depth to bar graphs. Figure 13-7c shows how this tactic can be used to hype the professor/physician comparison, by presenting volumes to magnify the effect. It is difficult to determine the actual values of these three-dimensional bar graphs. In *SYGRAPH: The System for Graphics,* Wilkinson[38] describes the addition of a third dimension as "perspective mania," and notes that he cannot think of a single instance in which a perspective bar graph should be used. However, the *SYGRAPH* application offers a full assortment of three-dimensional graphs. Why? "We had to make some concession to the marketplace."[38] Thus, it appears that some users of *SYGRAPH,* despite explicit advice to do otherwise, produce misleading graphics. Such behavior, like other examples in this chapter, may be further evidence for the doctrine of original sin.

References

1. Tufte ER. Beautiful Evidence. Cheshire, CT: Graphics Press, 2006:9.
2. Tufte ER. Beautiful Evidence. Cheshire, CT: Graphics Press, 2006.
3. Kemp M. A perfect and faithful record: Mind and body in medical photography before 1900. In: Thomas A, Braun M (eds). Beauty of Another Order: Photography in Science. New Haven, CT: Yale Univ Press, in association with the National Gallery of Canada, 1997:120–149.
4. Judson HF. The Great Betrayal: Fraud in Science. Orlando: Harcourt, 2004:61–64.
5. Godfrey E. By Reason of Doubt: The Belshaw Case. Halifax, Nova Scotia: Goodread Biographies, 1984.
6. Medawar P. The Strange Case of Spotted Mice: And Other Classic Essays on Science. Oxford: Oxford Univ Press, 1996:132–143.
7. Gould SJ. The Mismeasure of Man. New York: WW Norton, 1981:92.
8. Purves D, Williams SM. Neuroscience, ed 2. Sunderland, MA: Sinauer Associates, 2001.
9. Lawson D. Photomicrography. London: Academic Press, 972:310–313.
10. Tufte ER. Beautiful Evidence. Cheshire, CT: Graphics Press, 2006:13.
11. Rosenthal R, Rubin DB. A simple, general purpose display of magnitude of experimental effect. J Educ Psychol 1982;74:166–169.
12. Wainer H. Graphic Discovery. Princeton: Princeton Univ Press, 2005:63–67.
13. Wainer H. Graphic Discovery. Princeton: Princeton Univ Press, 2005:117–124.
14. Simonton DK. Career landmarks in science: Individual differences and interdisciplinary contrasts. Dev Psychol 1991;27:119–130.
15. Simonton DK. Creativity in Science. Cambridge: Cambridge Univ Press, 2004:69.
16. Wainer H. Graphic Discovery. Princeton: Princeton Univ Press, 2005:122–124.
17. Cleveland WS. The Elements of Graphing Data. Monterey, CA: Wordsworth, 1985:84.
18. Glantz SA. Primer of Biostatistics, ed 2. New York: McGraw-Hill, 1987:26–29.
19. Mainland D. Elementary Medical Statistics, ed 2. Philadelphia: Saunders, 1963:168–170.
20. Pearce SC. Biological Statistics: An Introduction. New York: McGraw-Hill, 1965:10.
21. Gilbert N. Biometrical Interpretation. Oxford: Clarendon Press, 1973:23.
22. Huth EJ. How to Write and Publish Papers in the Medical Sciences. Philadelphia: ISI Press, 1982:124–126.
23. Day RA. How to Write and Publish a Scientific Paper. Philadelphia: ISI Press, 1979:49.
24. Weisman HM. Technical Report Writing. Columbus, OH: Merrill, 1975:104.
25. Wainer H. Graphic Discovery. Princeton: Princeton Univ Press, 2005.
26. Mainland D. Elementary Medical Statistics, ed 2. Philadelphia: Saunders, 1963:170.
27. Hill AB, Hill ID. Bradford Hill's Principle's of Medical Statistics, ed 12. London: Edward Arnold, 1991:53.
28. Monmonier M. How to Lie with Maps, ed 2. Chicago: Univ of Chicago Press, 1996:79.
29. Tufte ER. The Visual Display of Quantitative Information. Cheshire, CT: Graphics Press, 1983:57,161–169.
30. Tufte ER. Envisioning Information. Cheshire, CT: Graphics Press, 1990.
31. Simmonds D, Bragg G. Charts and Graphs. Lancaster: MTP Press, in association with the Institute of Medical and Biological Illustration, 1980.
32. Cleveland WS. The Elements of Graphing Data. Monterey, CA: Wadsworth Advanced Books and Software, 1985:229–294.
33. Simkin D, Hastie R. An information-processing analysis of graph perception. J Am Stat Assoc 1987;82:42.
34. Huff D. How to Lie with Statistics. New York: Norton, 1954:39–73.
35. Wainer H. How to display data badly. Am Stat 1984;38:137.
36. Zar JH. Biostatistical Analysis, ed 2. Englewood Cliffs, NJ: Prentice Hall, 1984:236–242.
37. Fraticelli R. "Any black crippled woman can!" or a feminist's notes from outside the sheltered workshop. A Room of One's Own 1983;8.2:10.
38. Wilkinson L. SYGRAPH: The System for Graphics. Evanston, IL: SYSTAT, 1989:54.

14 Diagnostic Tests and Measurements in Clinical Practice

Carol Oakley, DDS, MSC, PhD
Donald M. Brunette, PhD

Principles of Diagnosis

First-year medical and dental students tend to misdiagnose common conditions in favor of exotic ailments that reflect their most recent lecture topics. These students fail to heed the commonsense adage: "If it looks like a duck, quacks and waddles like a duck, then it probably is a duck!" The unfortunate problem with "common" sense is that it is not very common. Nevertheless, common things do occur commonly, and this phenomenon is the basis for the adage, "When you hear hoofbeats, think of horses and not zebras." Of course, the correct application of this adage depends upon whether the hoofbeats are heard on the plains of North America or on the plains of the Serengeti in Africa. These adages respectively illustrate two concepts: the principle of pattern recognition and the effect of prevalence. Both principles are important components of the diagnostic process.

Dentistry has been chided for failing to emphasize the diagnostic process in favor of merging diagnosis with treatment planning.[1] However, in 1988, a conference of public health dentists predicted that by 2025, the person dealing with oral health problems would not be known as a "dentist" but rather as an "oral physician" or some similar title.[2] Like other physicians, the oral physician should be able to evaluate and interpret measurements and tests to provide a diagnosis indicating the presence or absence of a disease. In turn, this diagnosis is expected to direct a subsequent course of management or treatment.

Arriving at differential diagnoses and treatment plans require an organized approach. One method used to facilitate the gathering/documentation of information and to generate diagnoses and treatment plans is the SOAP format. *SOAP* is an abbreviation for:

> Subjective information
> Objective information
> Assessment
> Plan

Subjective information is the information provided by the patient, what the patient tells the clinician:

• Chief complaint
• Medical history
• Dental history
• Social/work/family history
• Symptoms
• Stated preferences for treatment, nontreatment, etc

Objective information is the observations and findings of the clinician:

• Patient's vital signs
• Clinical findings (signs)
• Radiographic findings
• Any diagnostic test results

Assessment is the clinician's interpretation of the objective information:

• Diagnosis via differential diagnosis
• Etiology
• Prognosis

The *plan* is the course of action or treatment/management proposed by and/or performed by the clinician, based on the objective findings and assessment above:

• Treatment options (there may be more than one)
• Documentation that the treatment options were presented and discussed with the patient

- Cost estimates
- Details of actual treatment delivered

The subjective and objective information may collectively be considered diagnostic tools, because both information sources are used to generate a diagnosis.[1] The fundamental purpose of a diagnosis is to either rule in or rule out the presence of a particular disease or condition, so that individuals with the condition can be distinguished from those without the condition. This diagnostic process demands the application of exact criteria to define the condition that is the target of the process. In general, clinicians, researchers, and patients agree that the presence of disease indicates a change in anatomy, physiology, biochemistry, or psychology, but they are less likely to agree on the exact criteria that define a particular condition.[3]

Two major principles of disease are described by Wulff[4]: *(1)* the *nominalistic* or *patient-oriented* principle, and *(2)* the *essentialistic* principle, which emphasizes disease as an independent entity.

In the patient-oriented nominalistic approach, disease classification concerns the classification of sick patients. Disease is not considered to exist as an independent entity, and a particular disease is defined by the group of characteristics that occur more often in "patients" with the disease than in other people. Patients demonstrate a pattern of similar symptoms and signs, as well as similar prognoses and responses to treatments. Moreover, the nominalistic approach does not require a definition of "normalcy" and acknowledges that definitions of disease may vary between different societies.[4]

The essentialistic view[4] is closely related to a more contemporary principle of disease termed *biochemical fundamentalism*,[5] which is based on biochemistry and molecular biology. Once the underlying biochemical events are understood, the course of a disease can be predicted theoretically, because diseases are assumed to follow regular patterns. Definition of the "normal" state is avoided; biotechnology and statistical concepts define the disease state in terms of both the distribution of specified features in a specific population and the extent to which that distribution differs from a similar assessment of a group the investigators consider "not diseased."[4,5] In fact, this statistical approach forms the basis for utilizing biomarkers as diagnostic or screening tests.

Irrespective of the approach, essential prerequisites in arriving at a diagnosis should ideally include a clear, unambiguous definition and an understanding of the natural history of the particular disease being investigated. Definitions of a specific disease

may change over time, and specified criteria may be limited to specified populations at specified time periods. Testing protocols/conditions for the disease may also be specified. These concepts are illustrated below using the example of diagnosis of hypertension.

Test data may be divided into different categories of "disease." For ease of discussion, this chapter focuses primarily on dichotomous data divided arbitrarily into two mutually exclusive categories: *positive* or *negative.* The results of a pregnancy test are either positive or negative; it is not possible to be "a little bit pregnant." In contrast, some tests, such as blood pressure (BP) measurements for assessment of hypertension, may indicate several levels of *abnormality* (see below). Nevertheless, precise definitions can be crucial in making literal life-and-death decisions, such as decisions about organ donation.

Diagnostic data (ie, symptoms, signs, and test results) may be applied at three levels: screening, confirmation, and exclusion. The focus of screening procedures is the early detection of disease, before symptoms become apparent. Screening tests are conducted on individuals without symptoms associated with the condition for which screening is being performed. Screening tests help to classify individuals with respect to their likelihood of having a particular disease, but they cannot diagnose disease. For individuals with a positive screening test result, subsequent evaluation with additional tests to rule in or rule out the presence of the disease must be performed[3,6] (see also the section on screening and decision making later in the chapter).

The diagnosis of hypertension illustrates these testing concepts. Most adults have had their BP measured in their physician's office. Dentists also measure patients' BP as part of baseline vital signs obtained during the examination and also to screen for hypertension. Additionally, many individuals may measure their BP at home or at pharmacy booths. In May 2003, the Joint National Committee (JNC) on Prevention, Detection, Evaluation, and Treatment of High Blood Pressure[7] published new guidelines regarding hypertension.

✓ The population is defined: classification of BP is for adults ages 18 and older.
✓ The time period is defined: May 2003 (JNC7) onward; the new classification replaces JNC6 (1997).
✓ The methods of testing are operationally specified: "The classification is based on the average of two or more properly measured, seated BP readings on each of two or more office visits."[7]

Box 14-1 Principles of diagnostic decision analysis

Principle 1: Clinicians should not consider patients as absolutely having a disease, but rather as having only the probability of disease. The probability of disease is based on the prevalence of the disease, the patient's history (including risk factors, symptoms, signs, and previous test results), and the clinician's previous experience with similar situations.

Principle 2: Clinicians use diagnostic tests to improve their estimate of the probability of disease, and the estimate following the test may be lower or higher than the probability before the test. Tests should be selected by their ability or power to revise the initial probability of disease.

Principle 3: The probability that disease is actually present, following a positive or negative test result, should be calculated before the test is performed. Application of this principle results in fewer useless tests being performed.

Principle 4: A diagnostic test should revise the initial probability of disease. However, if the revision in the probability of disease does not alter the planned course of management/treatment, then the use of the test should be reexamined. Unless the test provides information desired for an unrelated problem, there is no sense in performing tests that will not alter the planned course of management/treatment.

- The auscultatory method of BP measurement should be used.
- The operator should be trained and regularly retrained in the standardized technique.
- The patient must be properly prepared and positioned, and persons should be seated quietly for at least 5 minutes in a chair (rather than on an examination table), with feet on the floor, and arm supported at heart level.
- Caffeine, exercise, and smoking should be avoided for at least 30 minutes before measurement.
- An appropriately sized cuff should be used for accuracy (cuff bladder encircling at least 80% of the arm).
- At least two measurements should be made and the average recorded. The BP measurement may be verified in the contralateral arm.
- Systolic BP (SBP) is the point at which the first of two or more Korotkoff sounds is heard (onset of phase 1) and the disappearance of korotkoff sound (onset of phase 5) is used to define diastolic BP (DBP).
- Ambulatory BP monitoring is indicated for evaluation of "white-coat" hypertension.

✓ In contrast with the JNC6 (1997) classification, JNC7 (2003) introduced a new category designated *prehypertension* (SBP 120–139/DBP 80–89 mm Hg), and JNC6 hypertension stages 2 and 3 were combined into JNC7 stage 2 hypertension. Initiation of drug therapy is recommended at JNC7 stage 1 hypertension (SBP 140–159/DBP 90–99 mm Hg). "Normal" BP cutoffs were reduced from SBP <130 mm Hg and DBP <85 mm Hg (JNC6) to SBP <120 mm Hg and DBP <80 mm Hg (JNC7).[7–9]

At any specified time, a specified population can be considered to comprise three populations: (1) nonpatients, asymptomatic individuals; (2) patients who have positive results for the disease of interest; or (3) patients with similar conditions but who do not have the disease of interest. The clinician's objective is to correctly classify individuals into the appropriate category. As noted above, this process is initiated with the patient's chief complaint(s) and history (the symptoms), followed by the clinical examination (signs) and perhaps additional diagnostic tests. The typical dental clinical examination may include recording a patient's vital signs; assessing facial profile/symmetry; palpating the cervical/submandibular nodes, muscles of mastication, and lateral condylar poles; listening for temporomandibular joint (TMJ) noises; recording mandibular excursions; examining oral soft tissues; employing dental explorers, periodontal probes, electric pulp testers, or ice; and prescribing dental radiographs.

Principles of Decision Analysis

Both clinicians and patients expect that the information gleaned from these investigations is truthful, reliable, and useful for providing a diagnosis that will direct a subsequent course of management. Interpreting the data in order to arrive at a diagnosis should be guided by four principles of decision analysis (Box 14-1).[10–12]

Principle 1 states that in the diagnostic context, patients have a *probability* or *risk* of disease; they *do not have a disease*. The initial probability or risk of a partic-

Box 14-2 Definitions of and calculations for test characteristics

Accuracy
- the overall agreement between the test and the gold standard
- may be calculated from a 2 × 2 contingency table, as shown in Fig 14-4 by the formula
$$\frac{a+d}{a+b+c+d}$$

Sensitivity
- the proportion of diseased individuals correctly identified by the test
- also known as the *true-positive rate*
- calculated from a 2 × 2 contingency table, as shown in Fig 14-4 by the formula
$$\frac{a}{a+c}$$

Specificity
- the proportion of nondiseased individuals correctly identified by the test
- also known as the *true-negative rate*
- calculated from a 2 × 2 contingency table, as shown in Fig 14-4 by the formula
$$\frac{d}{b+d}$$

Prevalence
- the overall probability or risk that the disease is present prior to the test
- also known as the *pretest likelihood*
- the proportion of individuals in a population who have the disease at a specific point in time; prevalence in a specified population may change over time, and prevalence may change if the definition of the disease changes
- calculated from a 2 × 2 contingency table, as shown in Fig 14-4 by the formula
$$\frac{a+c}{a+b+c+d}$$

PTL(+)
- posttest likelihood of a positive test result
- also known as the *positive predictive value*
- for an individual with a positive test result, PTL(+) is the probability that the disease is actually present
- calculated from a 2 × 2 contingency table, as shown in Fig 14-4 by the formula
$$\frac{a}{a+b}$$

When the sensitivity, specificity, and prevalance or pretest likelihood are known, PTL(+) may be calculated by the formula

$$PTL(+) = \frac{P \times LR+}{(1.0-P)+P \times LR+} \qquad where\ LR+ = \frac{true\ positive}{false\ positive} = \frac{sensitivity}{1.0 - specificity}$$

PTL(–)
- posttest likelihood of a negative test result
- for an individual with a negative test result, PTL(–) is the probability that the disease is actually present
- calculated from a 2 × 2 contingency table, as shown in Fig 14-4 by the formula
$$\frac{c}{c+d}$$

When the sensitivity, specificity, and prevalence or pretest likelihood are known, PTL(–) may be calculated by the formula

$$PTL(-) = \frac{P \times LR-}{(1.0-P)+P \times LR-} \qquad where\ LR- = \frac{false\ negative}{true\ negative} = \frac{1.0 - sensitivity}{specificity}$$

NPV
- negative predictive value
- for an individual with a negative test result, NPV is the probability that disease is really absent
- calculated from a 2 × 2 contingency table, as shown in Fig 14-4 by the formula
$$\frac{d}{c+d}$$

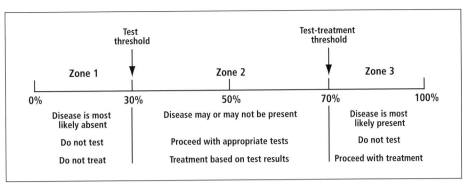

Fig 14-1 Threshold approach to decision analysis.

ular disease being present is equivalent to the *prevalence* (Box 14-2) of that particular disease in a specified population at a specified period of time. This initial probability (prevalence) may then be revised upward or downward, depending on the patient's symptoms, signs from the examination, and previous test results as well as the clinician's previous clinical experience with similar situations. The probability or risk of disease is increased if the patient has one or more risk factors for the disease. Hence, the patient is assigned an initial or *pretest probability*, or likelihood of disease being present.

After completing the patient history and clinical examination, the clinician may be confident that a particular disease is present. Therefore, further investigation or testing for diagnostic purposes is not required, and the appropriate management should proceed without delay. In similar fashion, if the clinician is confident that a particular disease is not present, then further testing is not warranted.

However, the clinician may remain undecided as to the presence or absence of a particular disease. As per principle 2, diagnostic tests may now be considered to revise, either upward or downward, the initial pretest probability. However, the measurements, assays, and/or diagnostic test results *cannot confer 100% certainty as to the presence (ie, positive result) or absence (ie, negative result) of disease, and there is a risk of false-positive and false-negative results.* Hence, test results (either positive or negative) can only revise (upward or downward) the pretest probability, and the decision whether a test provides useful information is *independent* of the actual result.

Once a test result is obtained, both clinician and patient must accept and deal with the result; "cherry-picking" the desired result would facilitate personal bias and reinforce preconceived notions, thus violating the principle of objective testing.

The threshold approach is used in decision analysis (Fig 14-1):

1. For each particular disease or condition, the clinician sets a threshold for testing, known as the *test threshold*.
2. The clinician sets a second threshold for treatment, known as the *test-treatment threshold*. These thresholds represent cutoff probabilities for ruling in or ruling out a particular disease. The threshold values depend on the disease and the subsequent consequences/course of management related to either ruling in or ruling out the disease. False-positive and false-negative results have consequences that must be weighed in each individual's case. The test should not be performed if it is not powerful enough to revise the pretest probability, so that either a positive or negative result would alter the pretest-planned course of action.
3. When the pretest probability falls between the test threshold and test-treatment threshold, then testing is indicated and treatment should proceed on the basis of the test results. In general, diagnostic tests are most useful when the pretest probability falls roughly between 30% and 70%.[13-15]

The threshold approach to decision analysis is illustrated by the following examples for the disease of pulpal pathology and the test of periapical radiograph. In zone 1 (see Fig 14-1), the pretest probability of disease is below the test threshold. The patient describes the sudden onset of pain to cold, sweet, or sour foods and beverages. These symptoms involve the maxillary anterior teeth, and the patient expresses concern about the need for root canal treatments. The patient denies a history of trauma but reports the occasional use of an orthodontic retainer and the recent application of at-home tooth-whitening products daily over the past week. Examination reveals an unrestored dentition with localized facial cervical recession. At this time, root sensitivity caused by recent application of bleaching products to exposed dentin is the most probable diagnosis. Pulpal pathology is most likely absent. Information obtained from a periapical radiograph would not alter the diagnosis or alter the course of management (topical application of desensitizing agents). Even a positive test result (eg, widened periodontal ligament space around the root apex) would not alter the posttest probability to a level that would justify endodontic treatment. Hence, neither endodontic treatment nor further testing should proceed.

In zone 2 (see Fig 14-1), the patient presents with complaints of intermittent pain and gingival swelling along the facial aspect of the mandibular right central incisor. Examination reveals a well-maintained dentition and a fistula with obliteration of the mucobuccal fold adjacent to the incisor, which has a large cervical restoration. Periodontal probing around the incisor range from 2 to 6 mm, but it is not possible to probe the sulcus/pockets and communicate directly with the fistula. The patient reports pain to percussion and reports delayed and mild sensation to cold stimulation. A necrotic pulp and/or periodontal abscess may be present. A radiograph with a gutta percha point inserted into the fistula is warranted, because it may provide useful information for diagnosis and further management.

In zone 3 (see Fig 14-1), the patient denies current complaints involving the mandibular left first molar but reports a history of "toothache that stopped after the tooth broke." Examination reveals that the molar has fractured lingual cusps, with visible gross caries involving the pulp chamber. The patient denies sensation to cold stimulation. Caries, tooth fracture, and necrotic pulp are diagnosed without the need for radiographs. However, a radiograph is required to guide prognosis and further treatment, either extraction or endodontic therapy.

Reliability of Measurements

As noted previously, patients and clinicians have the reasonable expectation that measurements are reliable. *Reliability* refers to the reproducibility or ability to obtain the same measurement consistently over sequential measures. The most direct way to determine reliability is to measure the same things with same device several times and compare the results. Note that in our example of measuring BP the "classification is based on the average of two or more properly measured, seated BP readings on each of two or more office visits."[7]

A measure is *reliable* when the variation or random fluctuation due to errors in measurement is small. Measurements are *not reliable* when there are extraneous factors that may be unknown or difficult to control. Reliability of a measurement may be affected by three sources of variability: *(1)* the system or phenomenon being measured; *(2)* the examination itself, such as the examination environment, equipment, or instruments; or *(3)* the examiners.

Consider a student's performance in examinations. There is probably some true score that accurately indicates a student's knowledge of the course's content, but the actual grade received depends on:

1. Variations in performance during the test period (eg, some students might get tired during the test)
2. Variations in performance from day to day (the student might be sick, hungover, etc)
3. Variations in the conditions under which the examination is administered (eg, time of day, room ventilation)
4. Sample of test items used (eg, all the questions could be on areas the student has not studied)

These factors lead to the examination grade not reflecting the student's knowledge, and can be considered sources of error in the estimation of the student's knowledge. The larger these factors are, the less reliable the examination grade is as a measure.

Variation in the system or phenomenon being measured

The phenomenon being measured may exhibit normal biological variability. For example, throughout the day and under different circumstances (eg, body position, stress, and exercise), BP and pulse rate fluctuate and diurnal and menstrual cycles cause hormonal fluctuations. Moreover, the very act of measurement may influence or alter the phenomenon being measured so that repeated measurements (test and retest) are not reproducible (not reliable). When patients are asked to open their mouth as wide as possible, they may not be able to at first. After several attempts, the inter-incisal distance may increase, or even decrease, due to fatigue. The act of repeated mandibular movements may also affect other clinical variables for assessment of temporomandibular disorders (TMDs) such as tenderness to muscle palpation and assessment of TMJ sounds so that findings may not be stable in either the short or long term.[16] Some phenomena, such as BP, will demonstrate "regression toward the mean," by returning to usual levels over time.[17] Therefore, some phenomena require repeated evaluations over time before a diagnosis is finalized. In fact, the inherent variability of physical attributes associated with many dental conditions is responsible for the inability to attain higher reliability scores.

Variability from examination equipment and environment

Laboratories often assess the precision of their methods by running repeated determinations on the same sample. If the method destroys the sample, the sample can be split, and measurements can be made on the subsamples. For example, the mass NB10 at the American National Bureau of Standards is supposed to weigh exactly 10 g. Eleven determinations of the weight of NB10 gave a value of 9.9995982 g, with 95% confidence limits of ±0.0000023.[18] We can see that the reliability of weight determination is very high. This is expected, because elaborate instrumentation for weighing objects has been developed, and the observations are performed under well-specified conditions. Typically, the results are expressed as a standard deviation (SD) of the individual values or as a confidence interval around the calculated mean.

The incorrect function or use of measuring devices or instruments may also be a source of variability. Reliable recording of BP depends not only on a calibrated sphygmomanometer but also on correct positioning of an appropriate-sized cuff onto the arm, and proper inflation of the cuff.

Coefficient of variation

In some instances, it is of interest to express the variability of the measurement relative to the size of the quantity being measured. In such cases, the coefficient of variation (CV) is used, which is defined as:

$$CV = \frac{s}{\bar{X}}$$

It is often expressed as a percentage, ie,

$$CV = \frac{s}{\bar{X}} \times 100\%$$

where s = SD of the measurements, and $\bar{X}$ = mean of the measurements.

We can see from the formula that CV is a measure of the relative variability of a sample. Because s and $\bar{X}$ have the same units, the ratio (ie, CV) has no units at all. The CV may only be calculated for ratio-scale data.

Precision

It is important to distinguish the precision of a measurement from the reliability of the measurement. The *precision* of a measurement refers to the exactness or degree of refinement with which a measurement is stated. Clinicians may measure the anatomic root length on a radiograph to the nearest half millimeter with a Boley gauge. This measurement could be made electronically, using tools with more precision and measurements to the nearest hundredth millimeter. However, the use of higher precision would likely not translate to higher reliability scores and may not be clinically relevant or necessary. Precision does not confer reliability.

Variability of the examiner(s)

Biologic variation among examiners accounts for variable acuity of their senses (eg, sight, touch, hearing), which may be further affected by their mood and sleep status. Examiners may be inexperienced or incompetent. They may replace evidence by inference, which can close a clinician's mind to other diagnoses.[3] Consider a patient who describes difficulty in opening her mouth and swelling and pain along the right side of her face, which began several hours after a forceps extraction of an erupted carious maxillary right third molar. The dentist suspects an infection and pre-

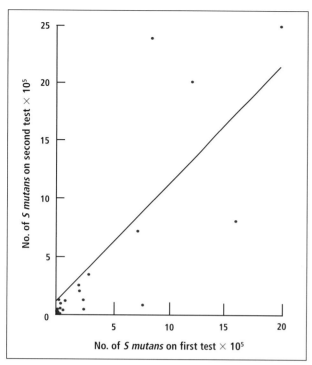

Fig 14-2 Pearson autocorrelation of *Streptococcus mutans* counts in the saliva of third-year dental students on 2 successive weeks. Slope ≈ 1; intercept ≈ 1.5; correlation coefficient ≈ 0.65.

croscope stage, the suspicion of malignancy would be raised.[20-22] In such instances, the pathologist may unconsciously grade the dysplasia or carcinoma as more severe than if the clinical information were not available to the pathologist.[19]

Measurements of examiner agreement

For conditions such as a TMD, biologic assays do not exist, and/or criteria for the condition may not be very specific. In these instances, the best course is to determine if the investigators are consistent in their judgments. There are several approaches to evaluate the reliability of such measurements. For any approach, however, a distinction is made between the situation in which the same person examines the same subjects more than once, called an *intra-examiner* (or *within examiner* or *intrarater*) *comparison,* and the contrasting comparison, the *interexaminer* (or *between examiners* or *interrater*) *comparison,* which occurs when the scores assigned by different examiners to the same subjects are correlated.

Calculation of the correlation coefficient

In this approach, the scores given by one examiner are plotted against the scores given by another examiner (if an interexaminer comparison is being made), or by the same examiner at a different time (if an intra-examiner comparison is desired), and the correlation coefficient is calculated. Streiner and Norman[23] note that the Pearson correlation coefficient is an inappropriate and liberal measure of reliability that usually overestimates the true reliability. Nevertheless, although theoretically weak, it is widely understood and commonly used.

In brief, obtaining a Pearson correlation coefficient involves measuring a number of objects by the same technique at different times and is best used if the data are in the form of continuous measurements rather than categorical judgments. This approach is based on regression analysis and gives the extent to which the relationship between two variables can be described by a straight line. The correlation coefficient r has a value of –1 (perfect negative correlation) to +1 (perfect positive correlation). A value of 0 indicates no relationship. The square of the correlation coefficient (r^2) represents the proportion of the variance of values of the dependent variable (y), which can be accounted for by the values of the independent variable (x). An example of a correlational approach is given in Fig 14-2.

In this example, individual dental students were assessed for the number of *Streptococcus mutans* in their

scribes powerful antibiotics. Unfortunately, the symptoms do not resolve, and, after 3 days, the patient reports bruising along the right side of her face and persistent discomfort to opening her mouth. A hematoma developed from injection of local anesthetic, and wide opening during extraction resulted in trismus of the masticatory muscles. In this example, the clinician has jumped to the conclusion that the initial symptoms were caused by bacterial infection and failed to consider the not-uncommon alternatives of hematoma and TMD.

Clinicians also tend to diagnose what they expect or hope to find[3]; hence, a clinician's mind-set may affect the diagnosis. For example, in addition to the histomorphology of the tissue on the slide, pathologists may be influenced by other factors when arriving at a diagnosis. The clinical data may be incorrectly weighted or "double counted" in the pathologist's diagnosis, if the pathologist has knowledge of the patient's clinical presentation.[19] If a pathologist is informed that a biopsy specimen was obtained from the mouth of a heavy smoker and alcohol drinker and from an area of erythroleukoplakia in the mandibular retromolar region, even before the slide is placed on the mi-

saliva on 2 successive weeks. The data are presented as a scattergram in which the number of colony-forming units/milliliter of saliva of each student on the first test is plotted against the number found on the second test. The best straight line for these points has been calculated by the least squares method (explained in detail in Box et al,[24] see chapter 12). The correlation coefficient calculated for these data is 0.65. The square of the correlation coefficient indicates the proportion of the variability that can be explained by the correlation. That is, in this instance, $0.65 \times 0.65 = 0.42 = 42\%$. Thus, 42% of the variability in the data can be explained by differences in individuals' saliva, and the other 58% must be explained by other effects, such as differences in saliva with time, laboratory technique, or sampling variations.

Indices of agreement

A problem with the use of the correlation coefficient is that two examiners could have a perfect correlation if one consistently scored the same amount higher or lower than the other. A number of indices have been devised to counteract this problem. Some researchers prefer to use some estimate of consistency in which the proportion of judgments that are the same is estimated. This approach is commonly used when there are only two categories, such as the presence or absence of a particular sign or symptom.

Proportion agreement

Proportion agreement reports the proportion of times that examiners are in complete agreement divided by the number of instances examined. When this ratio is multiplied by 100, it is called *percent agreement*. If the comparison is made between the observations of one examiner at different times, proportion agreement has been called the *repeatability index*, ie, the ability of an examiner to repeat the observations. It should be noted that, if there is a limited number of categories, this index would be expected to be relatively high. Gingival scores, where there are only three possible choices (0, 1, and 2), would be expected to agree one third of the time because of chance alone, if the three conditions were equally represented in the sample studied. Accordingly, techniques such as the Kappa statistic have been developed to adjust for the contribution of chance to agreement.

Kappa

Fleiss and Chilton[25] have introduced the Kappa statistic into dental measurements as a more appropriate

means to evaluate reliability, because it adjusts for the degree of agreement expected purely by chance. Kappa values below 0.4 indicate poor agreement; between 0.4 and 0.75, fair agreement; and values from 0.75 to the maximum of 1, excellent agreement. In studies of the reliability of many kinds of clinical variables in medicine, Koran[26] found most of the values to be below 0.35. Fleiss et al [27] found Kappa to be 0.80 or higher for dental caries.

The effect of method of calculation: An example from caries research

The method of calculation can emphasize the differences or agreement between different examinations of the same subject, as can be exemplified from caries research where various indices have been used. For illustration, we will consider a situation in which two investigators independently evaluate the same teeth in different individuals. Three numbers result from such a study: a = number of teeth (or sites) in which the examiners disagreed as to carious status; b = number of teeth (or sites) consistently diagnosed as carious; and c = number of teeth consistently diagnosed as sound.

Suppose that in a study of 200 teeth, the investigators agreed that 100 teeth were sound. Another 100 teeth were classed by at least one investigator as carious. The investigators agreed on 95 teeth and disagreed on 5. Therefore, in this example, a = 5, b = 95, and c = 100. Various indices can be calculated from such data.

The reproducibility ratio:

$$r = \frac{a}{b} \qquad \text{example: } \frac{5}{95} = 0.053$$

Ideally, r should be as close to zero or as low a value as possible.

Percent reproducibility:

$$r\% = \frac{a}{a+b} \qquad \text{example: } \frac{5}{5+95} \times 100 = 5\%$$

Both these indices emphasize diagnostic variability, because they focus only on the teeth diagnosed as carious. Shaw and Murray[28] have proposed the use of a modified reproducibility index r' defined below:

$$r^1 = \frac{a}{b+c} \qquad \text{example: } \frac{5}{100+95} = 0.026$$

This index considers all the teeth, both sound and carious. For many populations, such as those living in affluent areas, the large number of easily diagnosed sound teeth would make this index low, and results would appear quite reproducible. This example illustrates that reproducibility is influenced by the population of objects considered.

The analysis of variance approach to estimating reliability: The intraclass correlation coefficient

In this approach, the variance in a population of measurements is partitioned into the effects of the various components of the process including—for example, in the instance that different observers were scoring patients—the effects of patients, observers, and random error. The calculation of the error term involves determining how much each individual score deviates from its expected value. The *reliability coefficient* is defined as the ratio of variance among patients of the total of error variance plus variance among patients (for an example, see Fleiss and Kingman[29]):

$$R = \frac{\sigma^2 \text{ patients}}{\sigma^2 \text{ patients} + \sigma^2 \text{ error}}$$

Notice that if the error variance equals 0, the reliability coefficient is 1, and the measurement perfectly reflects the true values for the patients. The previous formula assumes that the scores can be corrected for the effects of different observers. If this is not the case, the appropriate formula would be:

$$R = \frac{\sigma^2 \text{ patients}}{\sigma^2 \text{ patients} + \sigma^2 \text{ observers} + \sigma^2 \text{ error}}$$

In interpreting reliability coefficients, it should be remembered that, because the coefficient is the ratio of subject variability to total variability, tests conducted on heterogeneous populations, which have high variability, will tend to give high reliability values. An extensive discussion of reliability measures is given in Streiner and Norman.[30]

Relationship of the standard error of the measurement to reliability

As mentioned in chapter 11, we can consider measured values as: Observed Value = True Value + Error. Just as the arithmetic mean of several measurements gives a more precise estimate of the population mean than a single measurement, so the mean of several replicate measurements on a subject or specimen is more reliable than a single measurement.

The standard error of measurement (SEMt) is equal to the SD of the error components in a set of observed values. If the reliability of the measurement were perfect, then there would be no error component, and the SEMt would equal zero. If the measurement were completely unreliable, the observed values would reflect only the error, and the SEMt would equal the SD of the observed values. Thus, there is a relationship between reliability and the SEMt, which is shown by the formula:

$$SEMt = s\sqrt{(1 - R)}$$

where s is the SD, and R is the reliability, which can take values from 0 to 1.

A number of strategies can improve reliability. The first strategy, *replication*, is to increase the number of measurements on each patient or specimen. In the instance when more than one examiner or rater is used, it may be advantageous to retrain or drop a deviant rater or stratify later in the analysis. Fleiss[31] discusses these strategies and other aspects of reliability.

Table 14-1 summarizes some of the reliability values found in various measurements in dentistry. The values would depend on exactly how the measurements were done. In a sophisticated study, Abbas et al[41] used analysis of variance to analyze data on the effect of training and probing force on the reproducibility of interproximal-probing measurements made by three different examiners. The training consisted of a video program, which demonstrated how to use the probe on a standardized spot and a standardized direction of insertion into the pocket. The study also compared a probe that delivered a constant probing force and a standard Merritt-B probe. The results showed that both training and a pressure probe were required to eliminate significant differences among examiners. Moreover, only nonbleeding pockets gave reproducible measurements.

Kappa values for various measures in periodontics are given in Table 14-1. With the exception of probing depth and gingival inflammation, the values of Kappa compare favorably with those found for clinical measurements in medicine. However, there is enough variability that further research in developing diagnostic criteria for periodontal disease is warranted.

Table 14-1 Reliability values for measurements in dentistry

Test	Correlation coefficient		Kappa value		Percent agreement	
	Inter	Intra	Inter	Intra	Inter	Intra
Periodontics						
Gingival redness[32]	0.61					
Plaque[32]	0.81	0.32	0.22[*]		44%	47.5%
BOP[34]						64%
Lack of BOP[34]						78%
Probing depth, general	0.63[+]	0.72[+]	0.26[#]		69%[+]	81.2%[‡]
Dental radiographs						
Vital/nonvital[36]					43%	72%
Caries, calibrated rater[37]			0.73	0.80		
Periodontal disease, calibrated[37]			0.80	0.79		
Interdental bone loss/gain						
Conventional method[38]					38.3%	60.9%
Periapical condition						
Normal[39]					37%	81.5%
Widening of periodontal ligament[39]					9%	40.2%
Periapical radiolucency[39]					27%	76.2%
Orthodontics						
Need for orthodontic treatment[38]	0.81					
Occlusal stability[38]	0.56					
Dental-facial attractiveness[38]	0.88					
Masticatory function[38]	0.72					
Dysfunction index[40]	0.84	0.92				
Palpation index[40]	0.87	0.86				
Craniomandibular index[40]	0.95	0.96				

[*]Data also from Haffajee et al.[33]
[+]Data from Clemmer et al.[32]
[#]Data from Fleiss and Chilton.[25]
[‡]Data from Smith et al.[35]
BOP = bleeding on probing.

Validity of Measurements and Tests

Diagnostic tests involve measurements of a criterion known to be altered by the presence of the disease of interest. Chapter 11 discusses measurement validity as the ability to determine the truthfulness of a measurement technique—that is, whether the technique actually measures what it intends to measure. Validity involves comparisons with measures already accepted as "true," for instance, by such organizations as the National Institute of Standards and Technology.

The relationship between validity and reliability is complex (Fig 14-3). Typically, if a test is valid, it is also reliable, for the test would be unlikely to register well on measures of validity if it fluctuated wildly when measuring the same conditions. Reliability can be identical to validity in instances where the reference test is in agreement among observers.

Similarly to measurements, diagnostic tests must be valid. A major issue with any new test is its validity: Does the test really measure what it claims? Answering this question often requires comparing a new test with a reference test, called the *gold standard*. The gold standard has been accepted as "true" and as the acknowledged standard for the definitive diagnosis of

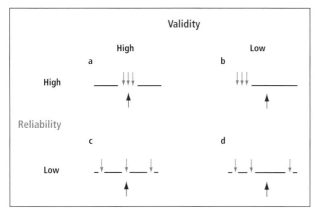

Fig 14-3 The complex relationship between validity and reliability. *(a)* High validity and high reliability: eg, a calibrated digital ruler used by calibrated, trained examiners to measure root length of an incisor on a periapical radiograph obtained using the parallel technique. *(b)* Low validity and high reliability: eg, a calibrated digital ruler used by calibrated, trained examiners to measure the root length of an incisor on a periapical radiograph obtained using the bisecting angle technique. *(c)* High validity and low reliability: eg, a calibrated digital ruler used by calibrated, trained examiners to measure dimensions of a block of dry ice at room temperature. *(d)* Low validity and low reliability: eg, a group of untrained examiners use their fingers' widths to determine a patient's maximal interincisal opening over repeated jaw openings.

New diagnostic test results	Gold standard test results: Positive (patient really has disease)	Gold standard test results: Negative (patient really does not have disease)	
Positive (patient appears to have disease)	a True positives	b False positives	a + b
Negative (patient appears not to have disease)	c False negatives	d True negatives	c + d
	a + c	b + d	a + b + c + d

Fig 14-4 Contingency table showing comparison between gold standard (GS) and a new test (NT). For instance, for the disease of caries, the GS is histologic examination, and an NT for diagnosis of caries may be a laser device. Positive result with GS means the patient really has disease. Negative result with GS means the patient really does not have disease. Positive result with NT means the patient appears to have disease. Negative result with NT means the patient appears to not have disease.

the specified disease. Be aware that even if a measurement is highly reliable (reproducible), the measurement has no diagnostic value if it is not valid and does not accurately reflect the characteristic of interest. For example, a clinician may reliably measure the root length of an incisor on a periapical radiograph. However, if the bisecting angle technique rather than the parallel radiographic technique is employed, the measured root length may not be a true or valid representation of the anatomic root length.

The traditional classification of disease is based on pathologic anatomy obtained through biopsy, surgery, or autopsy. However, these invasive procedures are not always feasible and are risky, expensive, and often impossible to perform in a timely manner. Therefore, surrogate parameters such as biologic assays (eg, blood tests) and imaging (eg, radiographs, magnetic resonance imaging) are employed.

A particular problem in dentistry is that the major methods of evaluating oral conditions—namely, the decayed, missing, or filled teeth (DMFT), and probing depth (or other indicators of the tooth's relationship with its supporting structures)—are *cumulative indices*. Therefore, the value obtained in measurement reflects the individual's history up to that point in time, and may not accurately portray what is happening at the time of measurement. Thus, loss of attachment indicates that destruction of periodontal tissue has occurred but does not necessarily indicate that tissue destruction is currently taking place.

Thus, there is a great deal of interest in developing new measures of disease activity, so that the clinician can appropriately treat a patient's present condition. If future laboratory findings can be linked to certain conditions, such as active attachment loss, TMD, or fibromyalgia, then the new measurement must be assessed for its validity. That is, the new test is compared with the existing gold standard. If the new test proves to have test characteristics superior to the gold standard, then the superior method would be regarded as the new reference (gold) standard.

By using a 2 × 2 contingency table (Fig 14-4), a direct comparison between the new test and the reference (gold) standard is made, and characteristics or parameters of the new test are calculated. The test characteristics (sensitivity, specificity, and predictive values) are mathematical probabilities that provide a general impression of the diagnostic strength of a test. However, these characteristics cannot assure the usefulness or utility of the test for a particular application.

Reference tests have a number of problems. First, in some instances, there may be no real gold standard. At this time, biologic assays for conditions such as fibromyalgia and TMDs do not exist, and there is no gold standard for active periodontal disease. In such cases, arbitrary standards for disease progression must be used to approximate the true definition of disease[42]; changes over time in key clinical diagnostic features are employed to provide a general nominalistic impression of the "diseased" condition.

Second, an investigator might question the point of using another test when a gold standard is available. Unfortunately, the gold standard may give an answer too late to be of use, and clinical decisions often call for immediate action. For active periodontal disease, the usual reference used as a gold standard is attachment loss over time, but the answer provided by this standard would come too late to help the patient.

Third, without access to a gold standard, sometimes investigators attempt to assess the sensitivity and specificity of a new test indirectly, by using a test with a known or unknown relationship to a gold standard as a reference. Such indirect assessment is, by its very nature, less powerful than a direct comparison (see Fig 14-4).

Test validity: Sensitivity and specificity

Sensitivity and *specificity* are important characteristics of a test, but they are commonly misunderstood or misused. A study of the literature on diagnostic tests revealed that 74% of the studies failed to demonstrate more than four of seven methodologic criteria for the appropriate use of these terms.[43] This section will outline the concepts of sensitivity and specificity and their application to dentistry.

Consider the following, in which a new test for diagnosing disease is compared with a gold standard (see Fig 14-4 and Box 14-2):

a = Number of true-positive results; the patient is found to have the disease with the gold standard, and the new test also has positive results.
b = Number of false-positive results; the new test has positive results, whereas the gold standard is negative.
c = Number of false-negative results; the results for the new test are negative and for the gold standard are positive.
d = Number of true-negative results; results of both tests are negative.

Table 14-2 Radiographic and visual appearance of surface caries on extracted teeth*

Radiograph (NT)	Visual (GS) Positive	Negative	Marginal total
Positive	127[a]	16[b]	143
Negative	122[c]	130[d]	252
Marginal total	249	146	395

*Data from Marthaler and Germann.[44]
[a]True-positive results.
[b]False-positive results.
[c]False-negative results.
[d]True-negative results.
NT = new test; GS = gold standard.

To illustrate this example, consider the data from Marthaler and Germann's[44] work comparing the radiographic and visual appearance of small smooth surface caries lesions on extracted teeth (Table 14-2). In this instance, visual screening will serve as the gold standard, because radiographs do not detect lesions in which a portion of mineral has been removed. A pure gold standard for caries used in experimental studies includes microradiography or histologic studies of sectioned teeth, but these obviously involve more work and were not required for the purposes of the study.

For simplicity, the data have been reduced to lesions being either present or absent, and only the data from premolars and molars have been used. *Sensitivity* is defined as the proportion of those with true disease that is diagnosed with the new test as having the disease. That is, sensitivity is the proportion of diseased people that is identified correctly by the test. Sensitivity is also known as the *true-positive rate* (see Box 14-2).

The formula indicates that a high value for sensitivity can be obtained only if the number of false-negative results (c) is low. It follows that when a test with high sensitivity yields a negative result (ie, indicates the absence of disease), there is a high probability that the disease is really absent, because false-negative results are rare. Thus, tests with high sensitivity are particularly useful for ruling out the presence of disease.

In this example,

$$\text{Sensitivity} = \frac{a}{a + c}$$

$$\text{Sensitivity of radiograph} = \frac{127}{249} = 51\%$$

As predicted from physical principles, radiographs are not a sensitive method of detecting caries.

Specificity is defined as the ability of a diagnostic test to correctly identify the absence of disease. That is, specificity is the proportion of nondiseased people that is identified correctly by the test. Specificity is also known as the *true-negative rate.*

The formula indicates that a high value for specificity can only be achieved if the number of false-positive results (b) is low. It follows that when a test with a high specificity yields a positive result (ie, indicates the presence of a disease), there is a high probability that the disease is really present, because false-positive results are rare with a high-specificity test. Thus, tests with high specificities are particularly useful for ruling in the presence of disease. For example, a certain protocol using bleeding on probing as a diagnostic test has a low sensitivity but a high specificity. Lang[42] suggests that the absence of bleeding on probing is an excellent diagnostic test to verify clinically healthy periodontal conditions.

$$\text{Specificity} = \frac{d}{b + d}$$

In our example:

$$\text{Specificity of radiographs} = \frac{130}{146} = 89\%$$

Note that sensitivity and specificity are typically calculated in defined populations in which only the extremes of disease are represented. The reference (gold) standard has already confirmed an individual's disease status as either healthy (very healthy) or diseased (very diseased). However, in the typical situation, the clinician is confronted with equivocal cases among a population of diseased and healthy individuals. If the clinician was already confident of the disease status of a patient, there would be no need for further investigation (see discussion regarding threshold approach to decision analysis).

Specificity and sensitivity are measures of how a test correctly identifies diseased and healthy individuals, respectively. Sensitivity and specificity are stable properties of a test, because they do not change when different proportions of diseased and nondiseased (healthy) patients are tested. However, these measures provide no information to the clinician as to how the test will perform on individuals whose disease status is not known (the equivocal cases).

Predictive values provide information about how often a test will yield a correct diagnosis in a mixed population of healthy, equivocal, and diseased individ-uals. Predictive values are not stable properties of a test, because they vary widely as prevalence of the disease changes.

The *positive predictive value*, also known as the *posttest probability of a positive test* (PTL[+]), tells a clinician the proportion of patients with a positive test result correctly identified by the new test as having disease. For a patient with a positive test result, the positive predictive value is the probability that the disease is actually present.

$$\text{Positive predictive value} = \frac{a}{a + b} = \frac{127}{127 + 16} = 89\%$$

The *negative predictive value* indicates the proportion of patients with a negative test result correctly identified by the test as not having disease. For a patient with a negative test result, the negative predictive value is the probability that the disease is absent.

$$\text{Negative predictive value} = \frac{d}{c + d} = \frac{130}{122 + 130} = 52\%$$

However, although the test result is negative, the clinician needs to know the probability that the disease is actually present. Therefore, the *posttest likelihood of a negative test* (PTL[–]) is used in lieu of the negative predictive value. For a patient with a negative test result, PTL[–] is the probability that the disease is actually present. A negative result will reduce the probability of disease being present, but it will not completely eliminate this possibility.

$$\text{PTL}(-) = \frac{c}{c + d}$$

Accuracy is the proportion of results in agreement with the gold standard.

$$\text{Accuracy} = \frac{a + d}{a + b + c + d} = \frac{127 + 130}{127 + 16 + 122 + 130} = 65\%$$

Do not be misled by a high accuracy value; accuracy is not the sole measure or guarantee of a test's clinical usefulness.

Prevalence is the proportion of subjects with the disease. Prevalence is also known as the *pretest likelihood* and is the overall probability that the disease is present prior to the test. Prevalence is defined in a specified population and can change over time and may change if the definition of the disease changes.

$$\text{Prevalence} = \frac{a + c}{a + b + c + d} = \frac{249}{395} = 63\%$$

Predictive values and accuracy

Often, diagnostic tests are developed in settings such as university hospitals where the prevalence of disease is high. When a diagnostic test developed among patients with a high prevalence of the target disorder is applied to patients with a lower prevalence of the disorder, the positive predictive value falls, and the negative predictive value rises. The teeth examined by Marthaler and Germann[35] had a high prevalence of caries ($\approx 1/2$). Suppose the study had dealt with a less acute situation, where only $\approx 1/10$ of the teeth had caries. In the same-sized sample of 395 teeth, we would expect ≈ 40 lesions. Because the sensitivity of the test remains the same, 51% of the 40 lesions (ie, $\approx$ 20 teeth) would be correctly identified on radiographs as carious (ie, a = 20); the other 20 would be false-negative results (ie, c = 20).

Because the specificity of the test is also constant (ie, a stable property of the test), 89% of the 355 ($\approx$ 316) sound teeth would be correctly identified as sound (ie, d = 316), and 11% would be false-positive results, (ie, b = 39). Using these new values drawn from a group with a lower prevalence of caries, we can construct the following:

$$\text{Positive predictive value} = \frac{a}{a+b} = \frac{20}{59} = 34\%$$

$$\text{Negative predictive value} = \frac{d}{c+d} = \frac{316}{336} = 94\%$$

$$\text{Accuracy} = \frac{a+d}{a+b+c+d} = \frac{336}{395} = 85\%$$

Notice that all these values differ from the values obtained for the sample with the high prevalence of caries. The overall accuracy of the test improved from 65% to 85%. Thus, in considering radiographic data from surveys, we could be more confident in the accuracy of the data taken from populations with a low incidence of caries.

Spectrum of severity and variability

Because the most severe cases of diseases are generally the easiest to identify, the population used in a test should mimic the target population in the spectrum of disease severity. Moreover, the population studied should contain individuals with different but commonly confused conditions in appropriate propor-

tion to the general population.[45] So, in the study of caries diagnosis, the sample should replicate the target population in terms of the distribution of smooth surface, pits, and approximal caries.

Screening and decision making

The dependence of positive and negative predictive values on the population studied can cause interesting dilemmas in the application of diagnostic tests to population screening and decision making. Initially, an investigator might think that a test with high sensitivity would be useful for screening if the probability of the disease is low and the purpose of the test is to detect the disease. However, in the examination of large numbers of people, even if the highly sensitive test is highly specific, it will generate a large number of false-positive results. For example, a test with a specificity of 0.95 applied to a population of 1 million would generate 50,000 false-positive results. Indeed, the number of false-positive results will outnumber the true-positive results, if the prevalence of the disease is less than 1 – specificity. In certain situations, such as cancer screening, false-positive results can cause considerable emotional trauma. Another assumption about disease screening is that identifying a disease early enables a significantly improved outcome through appropriate intervention, but this is not always the case. There has been considerable debate on the appropriateness of mammography in the early identification of breast cancer. The issue is whether early diagnoses do, in fact, increase the lifespans of those with true-positive results to a degree that compensates for the emotional trauma and biopsies endured by those with false-positive results, as well as the psychological problems faced by those with true-positive results who live longer with the knowledge that they have cancer. Skrabanek and McCormick[46] claim that mammography is a poor screening test, because its positive predictive value in asymptomatic populations is between 5% and 10%. This means that only 5 to 10 positive mammogram results out of 100 are truly positive. However, that conclusion could be rendered obsolete by refinements in instrumentation that change the specificity and sensitivity values.

Similarly, in dental science Mileman and coworkers[47] have applied decision-making methods to analyze the effectiveness of diagnostic techniques for approximal caries. Assuming, not unreasonably, a sensitivity of 35% and a specificity of 95% in the clini-

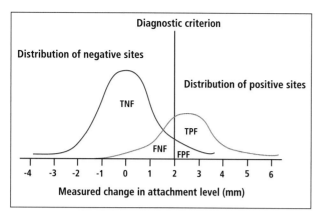

Fig 14-5 Differential criteria yield different estimates of sensitivity and specificity. TNF = true-negative fraction; FNF = false-negative fraction; TPF = true-positive fraction; FPF = false-positive fraction. (Redrawn with permission from Ralls and Cohen.[49])

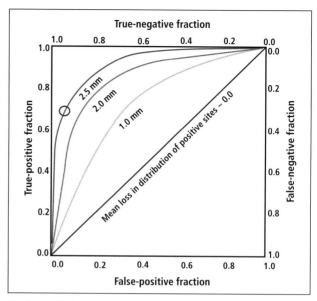

Fig 14-6 ROC curve from data in Fig 14-5.

cal environment (the procedure would probably yield higher values for sensitivity if it were applied by clinical investigators in research institutions), the probe-and-look method was found to be counterproductive in populations with low caries prevalence (eg, 0.05). Under these conditions, the number of sound surfaces diagnosed incorrectly with dentinal caries would actually exceed the number of surfaces in which dentinal caries was correctly diagnosed.

In summary, the actual clinical use of sensitivity and specificity values of measurements depends on factors such as prevalence and availability of effective therapeutic procedures. A detailed look at these and other issues is given by Sackett et al.[48]

Receiver operating characteristic analysis

In discussing sensitivity and specificity in the previous section, we assumed that results would fall neatly into the discrete categories of *positive* or *negative*. Many tests, however, yield data with more than two outcomes (see hypertension discussion earlier in the chapter). For example, in assessing whether active periodontal disease is present, changes in attachment level could be set at 1, 2, or 3 mm. In deciding when disease is present, one clinician might decide that disease was

present when the attachment loss was 1 mm or greater. Another clinician might be more concerned with the variations caused by measurement error and decide with certainty that disease was present only with a loss of 2 mm or greater. These differing criteria applied to the same population of patients would yield different estimates of the sensitivity and specificity of the attachment-loss assay for periodontal disease. This situation is illustrated in Fig 14-5, which plots the frequency distribution of positive (active disease) and negative sites against measured change in attachment level. In this example, it is assumed that the true-positive sites have a mean attachment loss of 2.5 mm, and the true-negative sites have a mean attachment loss of 0 mm. The variability of scores within the distributions is assumed to be a function solely of random error (ie, the actual loss is either 0.0 or 2.5). These assumptions are obviously simplistic; in a real population, there would be positive sites that vary in attachment losses.

The SD of both distributions is 1 mm, which is close to the measurement error observed in many studies. The diagnostic criterion is represented as a vertical line drawn at an attachment level, and it determines the fraction of true-positive, false-positive, true-negative, and false-negative results. If we adopted a diagnostic criterion of 4.0 mm loss before diagnosing disease, we could see that, by drawing a vertical line in Fig 14-5 at 4 mm, the number of false-positive results would be

Table 14-3 Sensitivities, specificities, and likelihood ratios of some diagnostic tests used in dentistry

Test	Sensitivity	Specificity	LR+*	LR–+
Caries				
Clinical examination[49]	0.13	0.94	2.2	0.93
Bite-wing radiographs[47]	0.73	0.97	24.3	0.28
Periodontics				
Bone loss (subtraction radiography)[51]	0.91	0.96	22.8	0.09
Gingival redness[33]	0.27	0.67	0.82	1.09
Plaque[33]	0.47	0.65	1.3	0.82
Bleeding on probing (2 mm, 5/6 threshold)[41]	0.29	0.88	2.4	0.81
TMDs				
TMJ sounds (manual palpation, single click)[52]	0.43	0.75	1.7	0.76
Disk displacement (MRI, sagittal)[53]	0.86	0.63	2.3	0.22
Degenerative changes (tomography, sagittal)[54]	0.47	0.94	7.8	0.56

*LR+ is calculated by $\dfrac{\text{sensitivity}}{1.0 - \text{specificity}}$ +LR– is calculated by $\dfrac{1.0 - \text{sensitivity}}{\text{specificity}}$

zero, but the number of false-negative results would be very high.

In recent years, this problem of establishing diagnostic criteria has been tackled by receiver operating characteristic (ROC) analysis, an approach originating in statistical decision theory and electronic signal detection. In dental research, ROC has been applied to periodontal diagnosis[49] and caries detection.[50] ROC enables the comparison of tests without any selection of upper or lower reference limits or any particular sensitivity and specificity. An ROC graph plots the true-positive fraction (TPF) as a function of the false-positive fraction (FPF). TPF is equivalent to sensitivity, and FPF is equivalent to 1 – specificity. Each diagnostic criterion gives rise to a single point on the ROC curve. When probability fractions are used in ROC analysis, the curves are independent of disease prevalence, thus reflecting the performance of the diagnostic system per se. The data from Fig 14-5, in which the mean attachment loss is 2.5 mm, are replotted as an ROC curve in Fig 14-6. The point representing the 2.0-mm attachment level diagnostic criterion is circled.

Figure 14-6 also gives the curves that would be obtained if the mean loss were 0.0 mm and 1.0 mm. The area (Az) under the diagonal (when the average loss is 0.0 mm) equals 0.5 (ie, Az = 0.5) and represents the value for chance alone. Discriminatory ability above the level of chance for diagnostic accuracy is indicated by Az values between 0.5 and 1.0. Obviously, as the size of the attachment loss becomes bigger, the decision between positive and negative sites becomes easier to make accurately; this is shown in the ROC analysis by greater area under the curve.

Clinical measurements: Some sensitivities/specificities of measurements in dentistry

A sample of the sensitivities and specificities of some diagnostic tests in dentistry are given in Table 14-3. No attempt has been made to review comprehensively the studies in this area. Moreover, the studies differ in the type of patients, criteria for gold standards, and the time spans over which measurements were made. Thus, direct comparisons between methods cannot necessarily be made, and this table merely indicates the general range in which the measurements fall.

The rather mediocre performance of common methods of caries detection has led to the development of alternative approaches. Several methods for diagnosing small occlusal caries lesions have been developed, including laser fluorescence (ie, DIAGNO-Dent, KaVo Dental), fiberoptic transillumination, fissure discoloration, electrical-resistance measurement, and ratings of fissure morphology. Of the more novel

Table 14-4 The effect of prevalence on the predictive value of an excellent sign, symptom, or laboratory test[*10]

	Prevalence[+] (%)														
	99	95	90	80	70	60	50	40	30	20	10	5	1	0.5	0.1
Predictive value of a positive test for disease[#] (%)	99.9	99.7	99.4	99	98	97	95	93	89	83	68	50	16	9	2
Predictive value of a negative test for no disease[‡] (%)	16	50	68	83	89	93	95	97	98	99	99.4	99.7	99.9	99.97	99.99
Predictive value of a negative test for disease[§] (%)	84	50	32	17	11	7	5	3	2	1	0.6	0.3	0.1	0.03	0.01

[*]Both sensitivity and specificity equal 95% is every case.
[+]Pretest likelihood or prior probability of disease.
[#]Posterior probability of disease following a positive test result.
[‡]Posterior probability of no disease following a negative test result.
[§]Posterior probability of disease following a negative test result.

diagnostic systems, only electrical-resistance measurement with a sensitivity of 0.96 and a specificity of 0.71 had an acceptable performance.[55–59]

Utility of a Diagnostic Test

High sensitivity and high specificity are desirable qualities of a test, but these characteristics alone do not determine whether a test is useful in a particular clinical situation. Recall that the information provided by posttest likelihoods (ie, PTL[+], PTL[–]) is required by the clinician faced with providing diagnosis of an equivocal case (ie, pretest probability in the 40% to 60% range).

Posttest likelihoods are strongly affected by prevalence, and this is illustrated in Table 14-4. Note that for each pretest probability (prevalence 99% to 0.1%), the same test is applied. This test appears to be excellent, as both the sensitivity and specificity are 95%. As the pretest probability (prevalence) decreases, the positive predictive value (PTL[+]; see Box 14-2) also decreases. In turn, the posttest probability of having the disease following a negative result (PTL[–]) must increase! Notice that even an excellent test (95% sensitivity and specificity) effects only minor changes in posttest probabilities at either end of the prevalence scale. As prevalence falls, more information is provided by a negative result (ie, the absence of a symptom or sign) than from a positive result or presence of a sign or symptom. The greatest increase or decrease from pretest to posttest probability of disease occurs when the pretest probability ranges from 40% to 60%.

Now refer back to principle 3 and principle 4 of the diagnostic decision analysis in Box 14-1. These principles require that interpretation of possible test outcomes precede the actual ordering/application of the test, and that testing should proceed only if the test outcome will direct a change in the subsequent management of the case. How may this be accomplished?

Recall that the prevalence of the condition in a specified population is assigned as the initial pretest probability, which may then be revised upward or downward, based on the relevant patient history, signs, and symptoms. If the sensitivity and specificity of a particular test are known, then it is possible to calculate the posttest likelihoods of a positive and negative test result (see Box 14-2).

Calculations for PTL(+) and PTL(–) utilize *likelihood ratios* (LRs), which "express the odds that a given level of a diagnostic test result would be expected in a patient with (as opposed to one without) the target disorder."[6] Recall that sensitivity and specificity are probability statements that may be converted to odds ratios. Although conveyed differently, probabilities and odds ratios contain the same information. Thus, even money odds ratios of 1:1 means a probability of 50%.

$$LR+ = \frac{\text{true positive}}{\text{false positive}} = \frac{\text{sensitivity}}{1.0 - \text{specificity}}$$

$$LR- = \frac{\text{false negative}}{\text{true negative}} = \frac{1.0 - \text{sensitivity}}{\text{specificity}}$$

LRs are easy to calculate (see Box 14-2), and they provide a measure of a test's ability or power to revise the pretest probabilities. As a general rule, tests powerful enough to revise pretest probabilities of disease have LR+ with values greater than 10 and LR– less than 0.1. As a rule of thumb, if the sum of test's sensitivity and specificity is unity (1.0), then the LRs of the test are also unity (1.0), and the test is useless, because it has no power to revise the pretest probability. Compared with sensitivity and specificity, LRs are less susceptible to changes in prevalence or pretest probabilities.

Likelihood ratios and nomograms

In the clinical setting, a more efficient method than the formulae in Box 14-2 for calculating posttest likelihoods is required, and a *nomogram* (Fig 14-7) offers a convenient and fast alternative. Table 14-3 illustrates the sensitivities, specificities, and LRs of some diagnostic tests used in dentistry.

Figure 14-8 demonstrates use of the nomogram in the diagnostic decisions for three patients with potential interproximal caries (the disease) and use of DIAGNODent laser device (the test). For the detection of approximal caries, the DIAGNODent device has a reported sensitivity of 0.75 and a specificity of 0.96.[50,58,59] From the formulae in Box 14-2, LR+ is calculated as 18.75; LR– is 0.26.

In each case, the clinician detects a small area of discoloration on the distal aspect of the mandibular first premolar, but the clinician is not able to engage the explorer interproximally. For the disease of caries, the clinician has assigned a test threshold of 30% and a test-treatment threshold of 65% (see Figs 14-1).

Patient A (see Fig 14-8) is an adolescent female with an unrestored permanent dentition, who practices excellent oral hygiene and is very compliant with twice-yearly prophylaxis appointments. Bitewing radiographs taken 1 year ago at the completion of orthodontic treatment do not reveal any abnormalities. The clinician assigns a pretest probability for caries of 1%. The clinician's pretest probability is located well below the test threshold of 30%; therefore, application of the DIAGNODent is not indicated. In the event that the test (DIAGNODent) yielded a positive test result, the probability of caries (PTL[+]) can be calculated by aligning the straightedge at 1% in the pretest probability column with ≈ 20 (18.75) in the LR column. The posttest probability of caries is raised to ≈ 15%. Despite this positive test result, no further

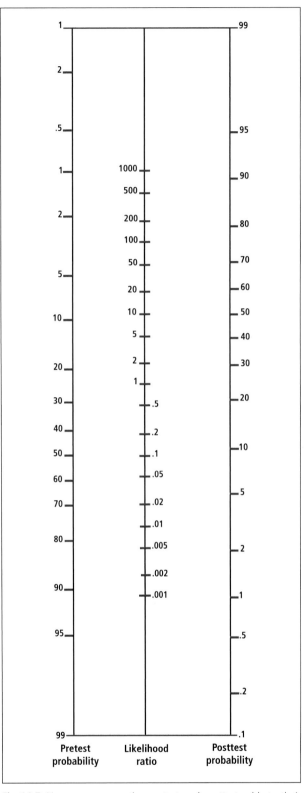

Fig 14-7 Nomogram converting pretest and posttest odds to their corresponding probabilities. To use the nomogram, a straightedge must align with the pretest probability (left-hand column) with the LR (center column) of the test being used. The posttest probability is revealed by reading across the straightedge to the right-hand column on the nomogram. (Reprinted with permission from Sackett et al.[60])

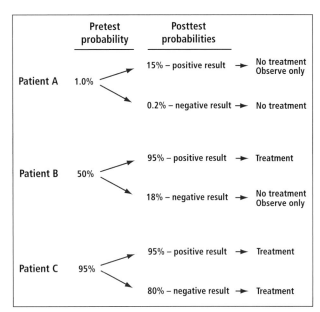

Fig 14-8 Use of LRs and the nomogram in diagnostic decisions for three patients with possible caries who have undergone a DIAGNO-Dent laser test.

tests or restoration would be indicated, because this probability—although higher than the pretest probability of 1%—is still much lower than the test threshold of 30%. If the test results were negative, then PTL(–) can be calculated, using the LR of 0.26, to be ≈ 0.2%, effectively ruling out the presence of caries.

Patient B (see Fig 14-8) is a young adult with a moderately restored posterior dentition, who has been traveling the world for several years and demonstrates poor oral hygiene and poor compliance with recommended dental recall and prophylaxis appointments. The patient was last seen 3 years ago, when bitewing radiographs revealed three sites of interproximal caries. The clinician assigns a pretest probability of 50% to the presence of caries. This pretest probability is located between the test and test-treatment thresholds; therefore, additional information (testing) is indicated. With a positive test result (PTL[+] is ≈ 95%), treatment is indicated, but a negative test result (PTL[–] ≈ 18%) rules out the disease and treatment.

Patient C (see Fig 14-8) is an elderly patient with a heavily restored dentition and recent history of recurrent and new caries. The patient is being treated for depression, and the medication has caused xerostomia; although she is a compliant patient, Patient C demonstrates poor oral hygiene. The clinician assigns a pretest probability for caries at 95%, and treatment is indicated without further diagnostic testing. That is, in this case, DIAGNODent is not required to establish

the diagnosis of caries, although radiographs may provide useful information to guide treatment of the caries or diagnosis/treatment of other pathologies. For Patient C, even a negative test result would still result in ≈ 80% posttest probability of caries being present and requiring treatment. This case illustrates that when the probability of disease is high, clinicians must be careful not to overestimate the meaning of negative test results.

Summary

It is clear that many dental measurements, as commonly practiced, are not highly reproducible, but at least the reproducibility of clinical measurements in dentistry compares favorably with many of the measurements made in medicine. This lack of reproducibility in the measurements is probably one of the factors that explains disagreement between clinical studies.

This chapter has also presented an evidence-based approach to the application of diagnostic data and tests. In themselves, positive or negative test results are meaningless unless applied correctly within the clinical context and to the initial probability of disease being present. Be aware that, while test characteristics can identify a good test, the particular circumstances in which the test is applied (prevalence, test-treatment thresholds) will determine whether a particular test can be useful (utility) in the clinical setting. Hence, the reader may become not only a more discriminating clinician but also a more discriminating consumer of tests prescribed by the medical profession and, increasingly, by the pharmaceutical industry.

References

1. Beck JD. Issues in assessment of diagnostic tests and risk for periodontal diseases. Periodontol 2000 1995;7:100–198.
2. Barnes DE. Implications for public health planning of the ability to predict high and low risk groups for dental caries. In: Johnson NW (ed). Risk Markers for Oral Diseases. Vol 1: Dental Caries. Cambridge: Cambridge Univ Press, 1991:482.
3. Sackett DL, Haynes RB, Tugwell P. Clinical Epidemiology. A Basic Science for Clinical Medicine, ed 2. Boston: Little, Brown, 1991:3–170.
4. Wulff HR. Rational Diagnosis and Treatment. Oxford: Blackwell, 1976.

5. Dabelsteen E, Mackenzie IC. The scientific basis for oral diagnosis. In: Mackenzie IC, Squier CA, Dabelsteen E (eds). Oral Mucosal Diseases: Biology, Etiology and Therapy. Copenhagen: Laegeforeningens Forlag, 1987:99–102.

6. Hennekens, CH, Buring JE. Screening. In: Mayrent SL (ed). Epidemiology in Medicine. Boston: Little, Brown, 1987: 327–347.

7. The Seventh Report of the Joint National Committee on Prevention, Detection, Evaluation, and Treatment of High Blood Pressure (JNC 7). US Department of Health and Human Services, National Institute of Health. Available at http://www.nhlbi.nih.gov/guidelines/hypertension/jnc7full.pdf. Accessed June 27, 2007.

8. National High Blood Pressure Education Program Coordinating Committee. Seventh Report of the Joint National Committee on Prevention, Detection, Evaluation, and Treatment of High Blood Pressure (JNC 7). National Institutes of Health Publication No. 04-5230. Rockville, MD. US Department of Health and Human Services; August 2004.

9. Chobanian AV, Bakris GL, Black HR, et al. Seventh report on the Joint National Committee on Prevention, Detection, Evaluation, and Treatment of High Blood Pressure: The JNC 7 (Express) Report. JAMA 2003;289:2560–2572.

10. Sackett DL, Richardson WS, Rosenberg W, Haynes RB. Evidence-Based Medicine: How to Practice and Teach EBM. New York, Churchill Livingstone, 1997:127.

11. Schechter MT, Sheps SB. Diagnostic testing revisited: Pathways through uncertainty. Can Med Assoc J 1985;132: 755–759.

12. Oakley C, Brunette DM. The use of diagnostic data in clinical dental practice. Dent Clin North Am 2002;46:87–115.

13. Choi BC, Jokovic A. Diagnostic tests. J Can Dent Assoc 1996;62:6–7.

14. Matthews DC, Banting DW. Authors' response. J Can Dent Assoc 1996;62:7.

15. Matthews DC, Banting DW, Bohay RN. The use of diagnostic tests to aid clinical diagnosis. J Can Dent Assoc 1995; 61:785–791.

16. Widmer CG. Physical characteristics associated with temporomandibular disorders. In: Sessle BJ, Bryant PS, Dionne RA (eds). Temporomandibular Disorders and Related Pain Conditions. Seattle: IASP Press, 1995:161–174.

17. Tversky A, Kahneman D. Judgement under certainty: Heuristics and biases. Science 1974;185:1124.

18. Moore DS. Statistics: Concepts and Controversies. San Francisco: Freeman, 1979:106–108.

19. Schwartz WB, Wolfe HJ, Pauker SG. Pathology and probabilities: A new approach to interpreting and reporting biopsies. N Eng J Med 1981;305:917–913.

20. Ephros H, Samit A. Leukoplakia and malignant transformation. Oral Surg Oral Med Oral Pathol Oral Radiol Endod 1997;83:187.

21. Kramer IRH. Basic histopathological features of oral premalignant lesions. In: Mackenzie IC, Dabelsteen E, Squier CA (eds). Oral Premalignancy. Iowa City: Univ of Iowa Press, 1980,23–34.

22. Kramer IRH. Prognosis from features observable by conventional histopahtological examination. In: Mackenzie IC, Dabelsteen E, Squier CA (eds). Oral Premalignancy. Iowa City: Univ of Iowa Press, 1980:304–311.

23. Streiner DL, Norman GR. Health Measurement Scales. Oxford: Oxford Univ Press, 1989:79–95.

24. Box GEP, Hunter WG, Hunter JS. Statistics for Experimenters. New York: Wiley, 1978:453–509.

25. Fleiss JL, Chilton NW. The measurement of interexaminer agreement and periodontal disease. J Periodontal Res 1983;18:601.

26. Koran LM. The reliability of clinical methods, data and judgments. N Engl J Med 1975;293(pt 1):642, (pt 2):695.

27. Fleiss JL, Fischman SL, Chilton NW, Park MH. Reliability of discrete measurements in caries trials. Caries Res 1979;13:23.

28. Shaw L, Murray JJ. Inter-examiner and intra-examiner reproducibility in clinical and radiographic diagnosis. Int Dent J 1975;25:280.

29. Fleiss JL, Kingman A. Statistical management of data in clinical research. Crit Rev Oral Biol Med 1990;1:55.

30. Streiner DL, Norman GR. Health Measurement Scales. Oxford: Oxford Univ Press, 1989:79–96.

31. Fleiss JL. The Design and Analysis of Clinical Experiments. New York: Wiley, 1986:1–32.

32. Clemmer BA, Barbano JP. Reproductability of periodontal scores in clinical trals. J Periodontal Res Suppl 1974;9: 188–128.

33. Haffajee AD, Socransky SS, Goodson JM. Clinical parameters as predictors of destructive periodontal disease activity. J Clin Periodontol 1983;10:257–265.

34. Janssen PT, Faber JA, van Palenstein Helderman WH. Reproducibility of bleeding tendency measurements and the reproducibility of mouth bleeding scores for the individual patient. J Periodont Res 1986;21:653–659.

35. Smith LW, Suomi JD, Greene JC, Barbano JP. A study of intra-examiner variation in scoring oral hygiene status, gingival inflammation and epithelial attachment level. J Periodontol 1970;41:671.

36. Abdel Wahab MH, Greenfield TA, Swallow JN. Interpretation of intraoral periapical radiographs. J Dent 1984;12: 302–313.

37. Valachovic RW, Douglass CW, Berkey CS, McNeil BJ, Chauncey HH. Examiner reliability in dental radiography. J Dent Res 1986;65:432–436.

38. Grondahl K, Grondahl HG, Wennstrom J, Heijl L. Examiner agreement in estimating changes in periodontal bone from conventional and subtraction radiographs. J Clin Periodontol 1987;14:74–79.

39. Reit C, Hollender L. Radiographic evaluation of endodontic therapy and the influence of observer variation. Scand J Dent Res 1983;91:205–212.

40. Fricton JR, Schiffman EL. Reliability of a craniomandibular index. J Dent Res 1986;65:1359–1364.

41. Abbas F, Hart AAM, Oosting J, Van der Velden U. Effects of training and probing force on the reproducibility of pocket depth measurements. J Periodontal Res 1982;17: 226.

42. Lang NP. Clinical markers of active periodontal disease. In: Johnson NW (ed). Risk Markers for Oral Diseases. Vol 3: Periodontal Disease: Markers of Disease Susceptibility and Activity. Cambridge: Cambridge Univ Press, 1991:179.

43. Sheps SB, Schechter MT. The assessment of diagnostic tests: A survey of current medical research. JAMA 1984;252:2418.

44. Marthaler HM, Germann M. Radiographic and visual appearance of small smooth surface caries lesions studied on extracted teeth. Caries Res 1970;4:224.

45. Manji F, Fejerskov O, Baelum V, Luan W-M, Chan X. The epidemiological features of dental caries in African and Chinese populations: Implications for risk assessment. In: Johnson NW (ed). Dental Caries: Markers of High and Low Risk Groups and Individuals. Cambridge: Cambridge Univ Press, 1991:62.

46. Skrabanek P, McCormick J. Follies and Fallacies in Medicine. Buffalo, NY: Prometheus, 1990:94–96.

47. Mileman PA, Vissers T, Purdell-Lewis DJ. The application of decision making analysis to the diagnosis of approximal caries. Community Dent Health 1986;3:65.

48. Sackett DL, Haynes RB, Tugwell P. Clinical Epidemiology: A Basic Science for Clinical Medicine, ed 1. Boston: Little, Brown, 1985:59–138.

49. Ralls SA, Cohen ME. Problems in identifying "bursts" of periodontal attachment loss. J Periodontol 1986;57:746.

50. Verdonschot EH, Bronkhorst EM, Burgersdijk RCW, Konig KG, Schaeken MJM, Truin GJ. Performance of some diagnostic systems in examinations for small occlusal carious lesions. Caries Res 1992;26:59–64.

51. Jeffcoat MK, Reddy M. Progression of probing attachment loss in adult periodontitis. J Periodontol 1991;62:185.

52. Dworkin SF, LeResche L, DeRouen T, Von Korff M. Assessing clinical signs of temporomandibular disorders: Reliability of clinical examiners. J Prosthet Dent 1990;63:574–579.

53. Westesson PL, Katzberg RW, Tallents RH, Sanchez-Woodworth RE, Svensson SA, Espeland MA. Temporomandibular joint: Comparison of MR images with crysosectional anatomy. Radiology 1987;164:59–64.

54. Tanimoto K, Petersson A, Rohlin M, Hansson LG, Johansen CC. Comparison of computed with conventional tomography in the evaluation of temporomandibular joint disease: A study of autopsy specimens. Dentomaxillofac Radiol 1990;19:21–27.

55. Pretty IA, Maupome G. A closer look at diagnosis in clinical dental practice, Pt 5: Emerging technologies for caries detection and diagnosis. J Can Dent Assoc 2004;70:540.

56. Tranaeus S, Shi XQ, Angmar-Mansson B. Caries risk assessment: Methods available to clinicians for caries detection. Community Dent Oral Epidemiol 2005;33:265–73.

57. Tam LE, McComb D. Diagnosis of occlusal caries, Pt 2: Recent diagnostic technologies. J Can Dent Assoc 2001;67:459–63.

58. Alwas-Danowska HM, Plasschaert AJ, Suliborski S, Verdonschot EH. Reliability and validity issues of laser fluorescence measurements in occlusal caries diagnosis. J Dent 2002;30:129–134.

59. Shi XQ, Tranaeus S, Angmar-Mansson B. Comparison of QLF and DIAGNOdent for quantification of smooth surface caries. Caries Res 2001;35:21–6.

60. Sackett DL, Haynes RB, Tugwell P. Clinical Epidemiology. A Basic Science for Clinical Medicine, ed 2. Boston: Little, Brown, 1991:120.

15 | Research Strategies and Threats to Validity

> *Scientific principles and laws do not lie on the surface of nature. They are hidden, and must be wrested from nature by an active and elaborate technique of inquiry.*
>
> —John Dewey[1]

Constraints, Purposes, and Objectives

In many ways, the strategies involved in scientific research resemble those used in everyday problem solving. The amount of effort expended relates to the scope of the problem and the importance of the solution. Studies are performed against a background of constraints, such as funding, the investigator's available time for research, the research niche involving accessibility of materials or subjects and competitors, as well as the need to comply with bureaucracies (eg, ethics review boards or animal care committees). In this chapter, I outline considerations common to most research strategies and introduce some basic concepts of clinical research. (More detailed information is given in chapters 16 to 19 and includes examples of the kinds of statistical tools used in analysis and interpretation.)

Funding

Research requires funding. The successful research strategy can be pragmatically defined as that which results in an operating grant. But, faced with a paucity

of funds and an abundance of applicants, granting agencies adopt rigorous criteria for research funding, often using peer-review mechanisms. Meeting these criteria is itself a science; the science of "grantsmanship" has been the subject of numerous articles and books.[2–4] Scientists spend a depressing amount of time preparing grant applications and reviewing others' applications. Recent grant success rates at the Canadian Institutes of Health Research hover around 15%—that is, roughly only one of seven grant applications is funded, and each one probably takes about 2 months to prepare. As a result, investigators must come up with imaginative approaches to finding funds from diverse sources and must choose topics amenable to small-scale studies. Dentistry is rich in this tradition, because some kinds of study, such as comparisons of materials, can attract support from industry and can ethically be incorporated into ongoing treatment protocols in the clinic.

Although the specifics of evaluating proposals differ from topic to topic, much of the advice boils down to DeBakey's[5] four criteria for a publishable paper: The proposed research must be new, true, important, and comprehensible. Meador[6] recalls Edison's statement that genius is 1% inspiration and 99% perspiration, commenting that the 1% is indispensable. The important aims of the proposal should be emphasized.[2–4] Mackenzie[7] notes that neophyte grant writers use ex-

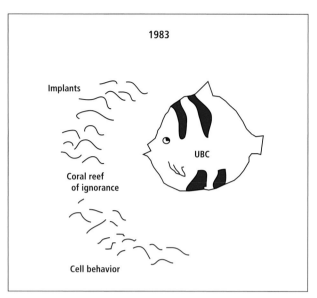

Fig 15-1a Investigative niche for micropatterned and micromachined surfaces in 1983. UBC = University of British Columbia.

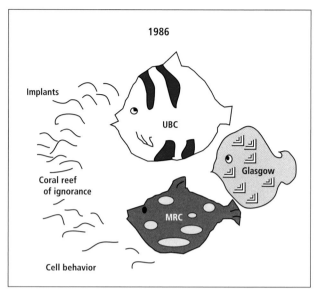

Fig 15-1b Investigative niche for micropatterned and micromachined surfaces in 1986. UBC = University of British Columbia; MRC = Medical Research Council (United Kingdom).

cessive wordiness, compromising comprehensibility. Reviewers likely will believe that poorly expressed ideas are equally poorly understood by the writer. DeBakey and DeBakey[8] stress the need to avoid jargon and to practice good exposition comprising clarity, conciseness, continuity, consistency, simplicity, logical transition, and readability.

Proposals can be deficient in many ways. A review of three studies of shortcomings of rejected or poorly rated applications identified the following three types of deficiency as being most prevalent[9]:

• Shortcomings in the problem: 18% to 58%. Problems often had insufficient importance or were nebulous, unduly complex, or were premature (ie, required a pilot study first).
• Shortcomings in the approach: 73% to 99%. Issues included unsound methods, neglect of statistical issues, lack of imagination, or use of methods unsuited to the objectives of the study.
• Weaknesses in the qualifications of the investigator: 38% to 60%.

Mackenzie[7] has devised a *detailed* checklist for proposal writing for dental faculty. But, before any actual writing is done, an investigator must consider some big-picture issues.

Time Available for Research

A problem plaguing dental research is the busyness of dental academics. A dental clinician on faculty at a dental school must teach not only in the lecture hall but also in the clinic, serve on university committees, and participate in the activities of organized dentistry by providing expert advice to local regulatory bodies or dental associations. Because meetings occur at definite times (whereas research is a moveable feast), research can sometimes disappear from the dental academic's agenda. I recently had the opportunity to review the research activities of a dental school. The modal proportional time commitment for research was only 10%; it was not surprising that little research was being produced.

Niche

To make progress in research, investigators must find a niche where they have a selective advantage. Life among academics circling a research topic can be likened to the competition among species that occurs near a coral reef. Figure 15-1 shows the niche that I occupied starting around 1983. For a while, I (represented as an angelfish labeled *UBC*) was the only in-

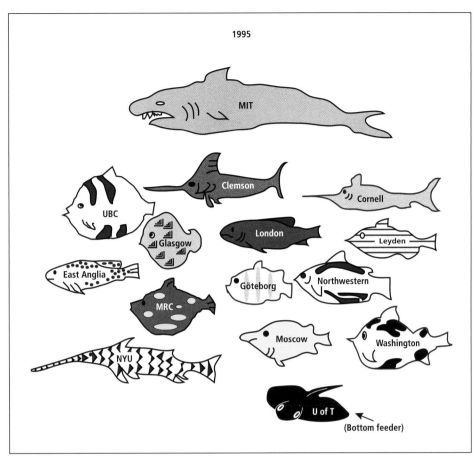

Fig 15-1c Investigative niche for micropatterned and micromachined surfaces in 1995. UBC = University of British Columbia; MRC = Medical Research Council (United Kingdom); U of T = University of Toronto.

vestigator using microfabricated surfaces to study cell behavior (see Fig 15-1a). I had the whole coral reef of ignorance of effects of microfabricated surface topographies on cell behavior to explore. By 1986, investigators from the United Kingdom had moved into my reef, and I had to adjust to their activities by avoiding experiments that I could do less efficiently than they (see Fig 15-1b). For example, they might have developed methods to culture a particular type of cell with which I had no experience, so that avenue of development was closed off. By 1995, a number of American, Canadian, and European laboratories—with more resources than those available to me—were using microfabricated surfaces (see Fig 15-1c). To survive among the sharks and rays, I had to devise experiments that were either novel or that entailed use of systems where the University of British Columbia (UBC) had a competitive edge. Eventually, as the ques-

tions became more sophisticated, the available resources at UBC proved insufficient, and the only way to compete was to forge collaborations with laboratories in other universities (such as the Laboratory for Surface Science Technology at the Swiss Federal Institute of Technology) to gain access to equipment and insights unavailable at UBC. The net effect of all this activity (both mine and my competitors) was that the coral reef of ignorance slowly was eaten away, and, as it eroded, new surfaces were exposed that initiated new research questions. The problem for little fish inhabiting some niches is Darwin's "survival of the fittest." Some investigators dropped out after few contributions; others have survived for decades. Niches come in various forms—competence in technique, availability of specific patient populations, collaboration with industry or other university laboratories, or superior organizational arrangements.

Demonstration vs discovery

Investigators vary in personality, from stamp collectors to wide-eyed dreamers; different types of investigation attract different styles of investigators. The *randomized controlled trial* (RCT; also called *randomized clinical trial* and *randomized control trial*) has—at least potentially—the power to give firm actionable conclusions and has a definite attraction for clinical investigators who want to improve current practice in their own working lifetimes. Systematic reviews of such trials can yield a gold standard for treatment, but such reviews often have limitations—because of heterogeneity in patients, techniques, timing of observations, and choice of outcome variables—that may obviate combining studies. Some of these problems can be minimized by increasing study size and standardizing methods across studies. But increasing the scale of the study entails costs (eg, statisticians, elaborate software for managing patients, and sufficient support staff). The high cost results in such studies being undertaken only when the risk of failure is low—a situation that often exists when an investigator is making only incremental changes (eg, variations in structure of a drug family that has already exhibited some success). Complex studies, such as multicenter trials, succeed because of the organizational and problem-solving abilities of the investigators, who must ensure that high-quality data are collected under well-defined conditions. But doing such studies is not necessarily a creative endeavor, because, in essence, the goal is that of demonstration—showing that a particular treatment, often previously tested in smaller-scale studies—has a high probability of success under a wider range of conditions.

Discovery-based strategies typically occur on a smaller scale and could involve just a single investigator. The cost is low, but the risk of failure to come to a definitive conclusion may be high. The conclusion of the study might not widely affect clinical practice, because clinicians might be skeptical of trying treatments that have not had wide exposure. Nevertheless, this more risky approach is most likely to seed exciting new developments.

Focus

In writing grant proposals, it is common to speculate on the significance of the work, often with respect to a particular practical end. The purposes of scientific papers, which often center on just one specific aim of the proposal, are typically more limited. Experience has shown that research is most likely to be successful when it is purposeful, that is, when it is designed to yield information in discrete, concrete packages. Well-designed studies propose a significant question and answer it well. Writers of manuals on grantsmanship counsel grant writers to focus on specific aspects of problems, making sure that the problem is not overstated, contains concrete and attainable objectives, and concentrates on specific topics.

In clinical research, a lack of focus often results when investigators try to answer too many questions with one piece of research. The available subjects become split into groups too small to provide statistical power for any one aspect of the investigation. However, calculations for statistical power require information on the size of the expected effect and the variability in the data. Often this information can be gathered only through pilot studies. In requesting funds for a project, applicants must demonstrate that the proposal will successfully produce interpretable results.

Classification of research strategies and the certainty of their conclusions

A common classification of research designs follows (see also Frey[10]).

Non-experimental designs involve just one group of subjects (or, more broadly, observational units), be they people or animals, such as might occur in determining the prevalence of caries in a community. The simplest form would be purely descriptive and involve only summarizing the data by categories. Alternatively, a relationship between measured variables (such as a weight-height relationship) may be quantified. Such studies do not provide evidence of cause and effect, but, nevertheless, they may provide clues. For example, Jenner[11] noted correlation between occupation (milk maid) and decreased susceptibility to disease (smallpox), leading him to conduct more definitive studies that led to the use of vaccinations.

Pre-experimental designs also usually involve one group, but more measurements are involved over time to determine whether changes have occurred. This type of design is used in dental practices, as dentists try to optimize their procedures. For example, a dentist may treat a group of patients using a new material in their restorations, then may follow-up with them to determine time required before the restorations need to be replaced. A comparison would be made to the dentist's expectations of lifetime for the material currently used—an informal type of historical control. Alternatively, a practitioner might make a set of measurements on patients, then introduce a treatment and make subsequent measurements. For example, a dental hygienist might measure plaque scores on patients, instruct them in oral hygiene, and follow-up on their progress to assess how knowledge of proper technique influenced their plaque scores. Such a study would not be definitive in establishing a cause-effect relationship, because there would be other confounding variables that might influence the outcome. For example, the patients might change their eating behavior because they knew that their plaque scores were being monitored over time.

Quasi-experimental designs involve a comparison group, but, typically, subjects are not assigned to the treated or control group randomly. On occasion, the lack of random assignment occurs because the formation of groups was outside the investigators' control (as can happen because of referral patterns or patient selection of treatment). Without random assignment, the two groups may well differ in a number of measured or unmeasured variables that might influence the results of the study.

True experimental designs include appropriate comparison groups, and subjects are assigned to the groups randomly—a procedure that enables investigators to assume that the groups are equal on unmeasured variables and, thus, would not contribute to any effects observed as a result of the experimental manipulation.

A question of current debate is the certainty of the conclusions of various types of design. Early estimates, such as those attributed to Sackett,[12] suggested that RCTs give around 90% certainty, whereas a *cohort analytic study* is around 20%; a *case-control study,* about 12%; a *before-after study,* around 6%; and a *descriptive study,* about 2%. A landmark paper by Sacks et al[13] later found that the percentage of trials in which the agent being tested was found to be effective depended on the design of the investigation. Only 20% of papers using RCT claimed the agent was effective, whereas almost 80% of *historical-controlled trials* claimed effectiveness. Bias in patient selection was posited as the prime cause of the difference. More recently, Concato et al[14] have undertaken comparisons of the results of RCTs with well-designed *observational studies* (cohort and case-control) and have found that the latter did not overestimate treatment effectiveness. Moreover, the observational

studies were less prone to *heterogeneity* (defined as variability in point estimates of treatment effectiveness among studies). Concato et al[14] argue that the observational studies are likely to include a broader representation of the at-risk population. Perhaps the situation is best summed up by Grossman and Mackenzie,[15] who posit that studies should be evaluated by appropriate criteria for particular applications, and not according to a simplistic RCT/non-RCT dichotomy.

Study design: Sampling and time's arrow

Studies differ in how the sample is selected and in the relationship of the observations to time's arrow.

Cohort studies have groups that are selected on the basis of exposure; a *cohort* is simply a group of individuals who share certain characteristics.

The *prospective cohort study* goes forward with time; groups selected on the basis of exposure to a risk factor are compared with a control group that is not exposed. Observations are made over a period of time, and an outcome of interest—be it disease incidence or lifetime of a restoration—is determined. Comparison is made with a concurrent control group that may or may not be matched on various characteristics.

The *retrospective cohort study* examines data that have already been collected. Groups are formed based on exposure at a given point in time and are followed from that time forward to the present.

Cross-sectional designs occur when all of the information is related to the point in time when the data are collected.

Intervention designs are prospective and involve assignment of the exposure.

Case-control designs are sampled according to outcome. Persons with the disease or other outcome of interest are compared with people without the disease or outcome to determine which factors may have played a role in developing the disease or outcome of interest. Case-control designs are always retrospective or cross-sectional, because the outcome (ie, the case) is the basis of the selection into groups.

Surveys sample a defined population to determine the prevalence of a condition, as well as to assess associations such as physical activity and weight. Because they cannot determine the sequence of the association (ie, whether the putative cause preceded the effect), surveys do not speak directly to cause-effect relationships, but they can provide clues.

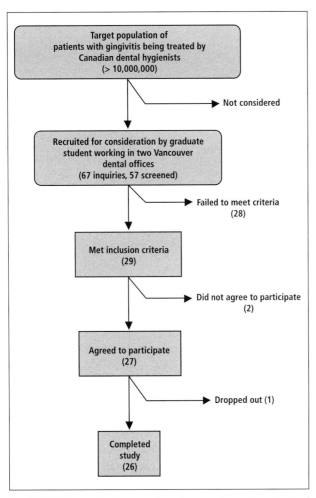

Fig 15-2 Subject selection and flow for a study on the effects of chlorhexidine-soaked dental floss funded by the Canadian Dental Hygiene Association Fund for Research and Education.

Subject selection

Studies actually include only a few of the many people to whom the investigator hopes the results apply. The selection of subjects has the inevitable side effect of limiting, at least to some degree, the interpretation. Figure 15-2 presents the subject-selection process of a study conducted by my graduate student, Pauline Imai. Because the study was funded by the Canadian Dental Hygiene Association Fund for Research and Education, our patron hoped the results would refer to the target population of the patients with gingivitis of Canadian dental hygienists. Notice that each step in the selection introduces a possibility of bias. We worked in two practices in Vancouver, so the extent to which the study population represented all Canadian patients with gingivitis is unknown; however, considering the heterogeneity of the larger population, the study group likely was not highly representative. In addition, people who agree to participate in studies may well differ in a number of properties from the less altruistic masses. Small-scale studies like this are sometimes referred to as *explanatory trials*; their intent is to determine whether a treatment works under certain well-specified conditions. These studies stand in contradistinction to *pragmatic trials*, which seek to determine whether a treatment works under real-world conditions.

Thus, a consequence of the selection procedure is that often the participants in a study are not broadly representative of the target population. Because studies on the same topic conducted in different locations may experience different influences in selecting study participants, there may be markedly different types of subjects, and results may vary. Consider the difference between the likely participants in a study on guided tissue regeneration done in a private practice limited to periodontics vs study participants recruited from patients being treated at a dental school. The two sets of subjects would probably differ in social and economic status, knowledge of oral hygiene procedures, and motivation. For example, if the treatment was sensitive to the oral hygiene practices of the participants, there might be a difference in outcome, even if the intervention was applied equally well in both locations. Selection bias, which can affect both the external and internal validity of a study, is discussed in more detail later in this chapter.

The Concept of Validity

An important issue in research design is the validity of the study. The term *validity* is used somewhat differently when discussing a study than when discussing a measurement (as was done in chapter 11). For a study, a distinction is made between *internal* and *external validity*. *Internal validity* refers to the extent that the data support the hypothesis. A study is internally valid when conclusions about the hypothesis can be inferred from the data and there are no plausible alternative explanations. An investigator must understand the threats to internal validity.

Campbell and Stanley's threats to internal validity

Chapter 7, on inductive logic, emphasized that the logical criticism of inductive arguments often depends on constructing alternative hypotheses that can also explain the results. Proposing alternative hypotheses can require detailed specialized knowledge about the topic under investigation. But often in clinical research, certain factors that lead to alternative hypotheses occur so frequently that they merit special consideration. These factors (commonly called *threats to validity*) were first explicitly outlined for educational research by Campbell and Stanley.[16]

Campbell and Stanley also introduced a shorthand notation for describing common investigation strategies that is briefly outlined here, as it aids description of the research strategies to be described later. Typically, a study begins with identifying eligible subjects (or other experimental units, such as animals or cell cultures). Then these may be exposed to the following operations:

> R = Randomized. Randomization must be done by a specific procedure, such as use of a random-number table; it is not synonymous with *haphazard allocation*. The purpose of such random allocation is to ensure that the groups are comparable before any manipulations or treatments are performed.
>
> O = Observed. In some cases, several observations will be made successively, and these are designated as O1, O2, O3 . . . .
>
> X = Treated. In some research strategies, a treatment will be applied to the group.

This list, although not exhaustive, covers several of the most important factors in interpreting research. The factors were originally identified from studies of education but have found wide applicability in other fields. Although each is discussed separately, interactions can occur. The list is presented here because it will enable us to consider how each of the research strategies may be affected by these factors. Appendix 5, abbreviated from Campbell and Stanley, lists the possible deficiencies in various experimental and quasi-experimental designs. But the possibility of a given threat to validity does not indicate that the threat is probable or that it constitutes a plausible explanation of the data. In naturalistic observation, for example, the effect of time is often a threat to validity, but it may not be a significant effect if the interval between observations is short or if the process itself is time invariant. Thus, in evaluating the influence of these threats to validity, the goal is not only to determine whether they might occur but also the magnitude of their influence.

History

Consider the following types of investigation. A given Group A (eg, the population of Toronto) is observed for some property, such as the prevalence of tooth decay. Conclusions might be reached about the group by itself; the data might indicate that caries prevalence decreased with time, or the data might be compared with another Group, B, where observations were made at the same time or at different times. However, during the elapsed interval, many events can occur, and these can interfere with the study. For example, the analysis of the incidence of tooth decay for a given region would be complicated by factors that altered the amount of fluoride ingested.

Another problem related to history is that often the investigator does not know exactly the factors to which the group was exposed, and these factors may differ between groups. This problem can be controlled by designing a *longitudinal study*, in which the groups are selected in the present and examined in the future. In this prospective design, the groups will be exposed to the same historical factors concurrently as the groups age together. A methodologic problem with longitudinal studies is sample shrinkage. For example, in studying dental health in the elderly population, an investigator could lose many in the sample, as they might die before the study is completed (see discussion on mortality later in this chapter).

The effects of history become particularly important in situations where the observations are made over an extended period. One of the problems in the study of environmental carcinogenesis is that the time required for the tumors to develop can be long, and, consequently, the subjects get exposed to many chemical compounds. In surgical research, Spitzer[17] notes that you should always approach research dependent on historical controls with a great deal of constructive skepticism. Clinical science advances in general, and it would be easy to attribute improvement to a particular surgical (or dental) procedure when the benefit could be due to the array of accompanying interventions used in the total treatment of the patient.

Maturation

There are many changes associated with aging. A number of longitudinal observational studies, such as those that report the natural history of periodontal disease, have been designed to assess these changes. When experiments run for a long period, it is difficult to separate the effects of aging from the effects of treatment. Spontaneous remissions can be considered another effect of maturation. Maturation can account for the supposed efficacy of quack remedies. "The art of medicine," Voltaire tells us, "consists of amusing the patient while nature cures the disease."

At first glance, it appears that maturation could be studied by simply observing individuals of various ages. In this approach, called a *cross-sectional study,* an investigator slices, as it were, the population into sections based on age and observes some property. The advantage of this method is that it enables an investigator to get all of the information at once and to obtain as large a sample as desired. The difficulty is that the effects of maturation are confounded with the effects of history. An individual who is now 60 years old not only would be 40 years older than an individual who is 20, but also would have lived his earlier years in an environment when nutritional and other health-related practices differed from those experienced by the 20-year-old patient.

Reaction

When we measure something, we alter it. The alteration may be slight, but it can be large. For example, gingival crevicular fluid flow is measured by placing paper strips in the crevice. But the mechanical irritation caused by the filter paper increases vascular permeability and fluid flow.[18]

Selection

When subjects are grouped, there is the chance that a selection process is operative that makes the experimental and control groups different even before the treatment is applied. For example, we might want to justify periodontal surgical therapy by designing a study to compare the periodontal health of a group of people who elected to take surgical treatment in a prominent periodontal practice with a group who decided against surgical treatment. After a number of years, the group that opted for treatment might enjoy better periodontal health. However, it is not difficult to imagine that the two groups would differ in many as-

pects besides the fact that one group was treated. The individuals who chose treatment would likely be wealthier or more highly motivated with respect to dental hygiene. For such selection-biased studies, we must ask what caused the differences—the way the groups were selected or the treatment itself?

Mortality

As a study progresses, subjects are often lost from the various comparison groups. This loss of subjects is particularly noticeable in some long-term studies in which the subjects are treated at dental schools, where it seems difficult to get the patients to return for reexamination or observation. The question that arises is: Are the patients who returned different from the ones who did not? The reasons the patients stayed away may be relevant to the experiment (eg, the treatment did not work, and they went elsewhere), or they may be trivial (eg, the patient moved and could not be located). Nevertheless, the experiment can be compromised if there is a large mortality of subjects in the study and/or the groups in the study are affected differently by mortality.

Instrumentation

A measuring instrument may change during the course of an experiment, so that the results obtained at the beginning of a study are different from those that are obtained at the end. While it is unlikely that the markings on a periodontal probe will change, the person using it may change his or her technique over time. This problem is generally handled by calibrating instruments and observers. More reliable measurements of student performance on restorative dental procedures can be obtained when the evaluators have undergone some sort of calibration procedure.

Regression

Have you ever wondered why instructors are reluctant to offer praise? They may be victims of statistical regression. We can think of a student's performance as being influenced by a number of factors, some of which are random. Sometimes, albeit rarely, all random factors occur in such a way that they produce a product that is better than average. Let us suppose that the instructor praises the student when the student demonstrates such excellence. However, on the next procedure this unlikely combination of factors will not occur; the product will be worse, and the instructor will conclude that praise has a bad effect on performance.

Unfortunately, if the random factors all conspire against the student and he or she produces a bad product, the instructor will berate the student, and, in all probability, the student will do better the next time. The instructor will conclude that the tongue-lashing worked. The phenomenon at work is called *statistical regression*. It is most important in experiments where subjects are selected into groups on the basis of extreme scores on characteristics measured by an imprecise procedure (ie, has a large standard deviation), because extreme measurements tend to regress toward the mean, regardless of any treatment.

Dental students and their instructors are not the only victims of statistical regression; the phenomenon has been documented for flight instructors and their students. Tversky and Kahneman[19] concluded that:

> By regression alone, therefore, behavior is most likely to improve after punishment and most likely to deteriorate after reward. Consequently the human condition is such that, by chance alone, one is most often rewarded by punishing others and most often punished by rewarding them.

Regression toward the mean can be a potential problem in any study that entails repeat measurements. Gunsolley et al[20] found that the majority of perceived loss of attachment due to scaling at sites of minimal probing depth that have been reported in many studies may be caused by the statistical phenomenon of regression toward the mean.

External Validity

External validity refers to the extent to which findings of a particular study can be generalized to other conditions or populations. It should be noted that external validity is a secondary consideration; it is relevant only when a study has internal validity. If there are many ways of interpreting the data (ie, low internal validity), nothing is established, and there is no point in extrapolating the findings to other conditions. Evaluating external validity requires clinical—and not statistical—expertise. Checklists for the evaluation of papers often mention external validity only briefly and do not give specific procedures. One widely available checklist focuses on two questions involving locality

and available evidence. With respect to locality, can the results be applied to the local population that the physician is treating? Clinicians are urged to consider whether the subjects covered in the study could be sufficiently different from the ones they treat to cause concern and whether the local setting differs from that of the study. The second question deals with the issue of whether the results of the study agree with other available evidence. The vague guidelines illustrate the current situation; although internal validity can be fairly rigorously evaluated, assessing external validity is much more subjective. Although difficult to fix, problems with external validity are often easy to spot, sometimes just by comparing the title of the study with the sample actually studied. Sechrest and Hannah[21] note that every sample can be considered a *convenience sample*, because investigators can only study what is available to them. Nevertheless, some investigators work hard to obtain samples representative of the population to which they intend to refer their findings.

It would seem that evaluating external validity requires detailed examination of the population or variables used in the study and of the patients of a particular practice to whom the treatment might be applied. Detailed information on both groups is seldom available, but, on occasion, large obvious differences are evident. We can easily imagine that a study on oral hygiene using dental students as subjects may not extrapolate well to the general population, who have less knowledge of oral hygiene and its importance to health. Another test of external validity is whether the relationship between the variables in the study agrees with other research on the topic. That is, if many studies in different settings agree, it seems likely that the effect is large enough to overcome local differences in population and facilities.

As noted earlier, selection criteria for inclusion into a study exert a major effect on external validity, because, strictly speaking, they effectively define and thereby constrict the target population. Nevertheless, it is possible that the findings of a study apply more widely; that is, they are not limited to the particular group specified by the inclusion and exclusion criteria, or to other specifics of the study (such as where it was done). The best answer to a criticism of external validity is to repeat the study in other contexts with different patient groups in other medical/dental centers. This approach is one rationale for the use of multicenter trials. Another approach is to make a case for the results applying more generally by arguing the similarity in relevant properties of the expanded target

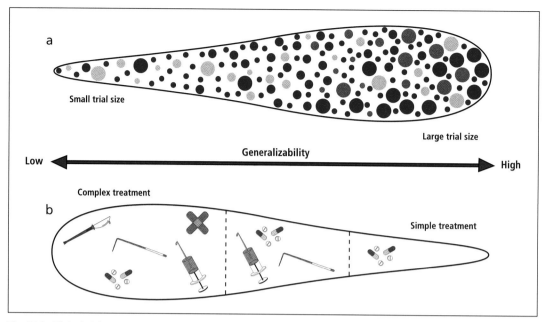

Fig 15-3 Clinical trials are more generalizable when they are large and involve simple treatments. *(a)* A larger sample benefits both the statistical generalizability (ie, more precise estimates of a population parameter) as well as the scientific generalizability (ie, applicability to another target population, because a large trial size will tend to select a more diverse population that may contain elements similar to other populations. *(b)* A simple treatment also benefits generalizability. This is illustrated by a treatment in which one procedure with a probability of success of 90% is required; success will occur 90% of the time. However, if three procedures are required, each with a probability of success of 90%, success will occur 70% (ie, 0.9^3) of the time. If five procedures, each with a probability of success of 90%, are required, success will occur only 59% (ie, 0.9^5) of the time.

population and the original target population, specified by the inclusion and exclusion criteria. However, because there are so many known and unknown factors that could influence any given result, determining similarity between any two populations (such as a study population and the patients in any given practice) has the potential to be problematic and uncertain.

After reviewing some of the issues involved in determining external validity of RCTs, Rothwell[22] delivered a somewhat pessimistic report:

1. Differences exist between countries in the time after diagnosis to treatment, and very different treatment effects can be observed.
2. Eligibility criteria are often poorly reported even in large RCTs; moreover, sometimes subjects are selected after "run-in" periods, where poorly compliant subjects are excluded. On occasion, patients who have previously been demonstrated to respond to related drugs are selected, leading to an "enriched" subject population.
3. Characteristics of randomized patients who are recruited are found to differ from the general pool of

those who are eligible, even in large trials. Recruitment of less than 10% of potentially eligible patients is common.
4. Trials may have protocols that differ from those in usual clinical practice. Consider the original implant studies of Brånemark, in which patients benefited from much more expert scrutiny than would be possible in a private practice.
5. Outcome measures used in clinical trials may be surrogates for the clinically relevant variables.
6. Adverse effects of treatment are poorly reported.

Rothwell[22] concluded that some trials have excellent external validity, but many do not, particularly some of those performed by the pharmaceutical industry.

A more positive view was taken in a recent informal review[23] that concluded that generalizing results from well-conducted trials to clinical practice can mostly be carried out with confidence, especially for simple therapies. More complex therapies require careful consideration. Based, in part, on studies reporting the outcome of complex surgeries, the authors suggested the relationship illustrated in Fig 15-3. Simply put, the larger a study's sample size and the simpler the treatment, the more confident a reader becomes in extrapolating from the study to other populations. We can see how surgery, in particular, might be chosen as the example, because the success of surgical procedures relies to a large extent on the personal technical skills of the surgeon. For example, readers of the dental research literature may have no way of assessing the technical competence of the individuals performing the procedures and, because of the typical brevity of the materials and methods section, may have little idea of how difficult some procedures are to accomplish.

Categories and Prevalence of Problems

Sechrest and Hannah[21] reviewed 100 predominantly non-experimental studies (99%), including descriptive studies, relational studies (often for the purpose of predicting some outcome), and quasi-experimental studies (defined as two or more groups compared prospectively or retrospectively with respect to some characteristic, with the intention of inferring differences between the populations from which the groups were drawn). The problems were classified as:

- *Sampling:* Low response rate (< 25%), failure to describe the basic characteristics, and unacknowledged bias in the sample; 50% of the studies had sampling problems.
- *Measurement:* Failure to mention reliability and validity of measurement, and low reliability coefficients, probable bias due to recall ineffectiveness and self-report; 60% of the studies had measurement problems.
- *External validity:* Errors occurred in many instances when data collected on narrow or convenience bases were extrapolated to dissimilar populations; 58% of the studies had problems with external validity.
- *Internal validity:* Failure to rule out likely threats to internal validity, such as selection; 19% of the studies had problems with internal validity
- *Construct validity:* Failure to provide a precise explanation of the concepts. Lack of precision in concept gives investigators too much latitude in the operationalization of manipulations and measures; 25% of the studies had problems with construct validity.

- *Statistical problems:* Liberally using multiple univariate tests without adjustment for inflation of type I error rate (ie, failing to provide a Bonferroni adjustment), failing to report intercorrelations among independent or dependent variables, stating results to be significantly different without appropriate tests, and attributing importance to statistically significant but relatively meaningless outcomes; 46% had problems with the validity of their statistical conclusions.
- *Unjustified conclusions:* Often *causal* conclusions, or claiming unjustified differences between groups and changes over time; 33% of the studies had unjustified conclusions.

References

1. Dewey J. Reconstruction in philosophy. Minola, NY: Dover Publications, 2004:18–20.
2. Hetenyi G. Features of a successful grant application. Address presented at: the College of Medicine, University of Saskatchewan; April 29, 1991; Saskatoon, Canada.
3. Reif-Lehrer L (ed). Writing a Successful Grant Application. Boston: Science Books International, 1982.
4. Dingle JT (ed). How to Obtain Biomedical Research Funding. New York: Elsevier, 1986.
5. DeBakey L. The Scientific Journal: Editorial Policies and Practices: Guidelines for Editors, Reviewers, and Authors. St Louis: Mosby, 1976:1–3.
6. Meador R. Guidelines for Preparing Proposals. Chelsea, MI: Lewis Publishers, 1986:47.
7. Mackenzie RS. Grant writing and review for dental faculty. J Dent Educ 1986;50:180.
8. DeBakey L, DeBakey S. The art of persuasion: Logic and language in proposal writing. Grants Magazine 1978;1:43.
9. Cuca JM. NIH Grant Applications for clinical research: Reasons for poor ratings or disapproval. Clin Res 1983;31: 453–461.
10. Frey B. Statistics Hacks. Sebastopol, CA: O'Reilly, 2006:33.
11. Jenner E. An inquiry into the causes and effects of the Variole Vaccinae, a disease discovered in some of the Western counties, particularly Gloucestershire and known by the name of smallpox. London: DN Shury, 1801.
12. Cited in Helewa A, Walker JM. Critical Evaluation of Research in Physical Rehabilitation. Philadelphia: Saunders, 2000:15.
13. Sacks H, Chalmers TC, Smith H Jr. Randomized versus historical controls for clinical trials. Am J Med 1982;72:233–240.
14. Concato J, Shah N, Horwitz RI. Randomized controlled trials, observational studies, and the hierarchy of research designs. N Engl J Med 2000;342:1887–1892.
15. Grossman J, Mackenzie FJ. The randomized controlled trial: Gold standard, or merely standard? Perspect Biol Med 2005;48:516–534.

16. Campbell DT, Stanley JC. Experimental and Quasi-Experimental Designs for Research. Chicago: Rand McNally, 1963:5–6.
17. Spitzer WO. Selected nonexperimental methods. In: Troidl H et al (ed). Principles and Practice of Research: Strategies for Surgical Investigators. Berlin: Springer-Verlag, 1991:222.
18. Cimasoni G. The Crevicular Fluid, No. 12, Monographs in Oral Science Series. Basel, NY: Karger, 1974:94–95.
19. Tversky A, Kahneman D. Judgment under certainty: Heuristics and biases. Science 1974;185:1124.
20. Gunsolley JC, Yeung GM, Butler JH, Waldrop TC. Is loss of attachment due to root planing and scaling in sites with minimal probing depths a statistical or real occurrence? J Periodontol 2001;72:349–353.
21. Sechrest L, Hannah M. The critical importance of nonexperimental data. In: Sechrest L, Perrin E, Bunker JP (eds). Research Methodology: Strengthening Causal Interpretations of Nonexperimental Data: Conference Proceedings. Rockville, MD: US Department of Health and Human Services, Public Health Service, Agency for Health Care Policy, 1990:1–7.
22. Rothwell PM. Factors that can affect the external validity of randomised controlled trials. PLoS Clin Trials 2006;1:e9.
23. Flather M, Delahunty N, Collinson J. Generalizing results of randomized trials to clinical practice: Reliability and cautions. Clin Trials 2006;3:508–512.

16 | Observation

> *It is the theory that decides what we can observe.*
>
> —Albert Einstein[1]

The strength of studies using naturalistic observation is that they apply directly to the real world. These studies are not burdened by the gap often found in experimentation in which the artificial environment of the laboratory differs from real field conditions. In naturalistic observation, no attempt is made to intervene in the course of nature, but considerable skill may be required to contrive conditions whereby observations can be made and data collected.

Observation-Description Strategy

According to Beveridge,[2] more discoveries have arisen from intense observation of very limited material than from statistics applied to large groups. Darwin's *The Origin of Species* is perhaps the greatest scientific work based almost wholly on observation. Observation is still a useful strategy. Although the effect of fluoride has been documented with sophisticated laboratory techniques and elaborate epidemiologic surveys, the initial findings were based on detailed and careful naturalistic observation.[3] The Audubon Society's Christ-

mas Bird Count continues the tradition; more than 50,000 members gather data on the locales of over a thousand species in the Western hemisphere. Between 1954 and 1989, some 100 papers in refereed journals used Christmas Bird Count data.[4]

Classical epidemiology represents a use of the observation-description strategy, for it is concerned with three major variables that describe the distribution of disease or condition: *person, place,* and *time.* Typical data from classical epidemiologic studies include data on the *prevalence* and *incidence* of disease:

$$\text{Prevalence} = \frac{\text{no. of people with the disease}}{\text{no. of people at risk}}$$

Incidence is determined over a specified period and is defined as follows:

$$\text{Incidence} = \frac{\text{no. of new cases in a fixed time period}}{\text{no. of people at risk}}$$

Prevalence and incidence are linked by the formula:

$$\text{Prevalence} = \text{incidence} \times \text{average duration (of disease)}$$

This formula demonstrates that chronic diseases, because they last a long time, tend to produce high prevalence values.

Operational considerations

People notice things that they expect or wish to see. As is demonstrated in the courts, where eyewitnesses often disagree, people do not necessarily observe or remember events accurately. The observation-description strategy requires that, in order to be of value, observations be detailed, systematic, and recorded as soon as possible after the event. The observations should be objective, that is, they must reflect reality rather than the observer's preconceptions or biases. Because it is difficult to be completely objective, an approach to this problem is to have multiple observers make multiple observations. In this way, the observers can check each other's observations and agree on what occurred. In dental research, it is not uncommon to confirm observations either by repeated measurements made by the same clinician or by having different clinicians examine the same patient. Another approach, not often possible in clinical research, is to use naive observers, that is, individuals who, by virtue of their lack of training or interest in a topic, have no preconceived notions of what to expect. In some psychological experiments (the ethics of which are debatable), observers or participants have been misled so that their behavior or observations will not be biased.

Central to the observation-description strategy is the classification of observations, which imposes or perhaps invents the order or pattern of relationships between the classes. The ideal is for the categories not to overlap yet to accommodate all possible observations. Classification systems are driven by the theories used in their construction. For example, bacteria traditionally have been classified by their shape, nutritional requirements, and staining properties, as these properties enabled many bacteria to be classified unambiguously into families that made sense. With the advent of modern methods of DNA analysis, taxonomic relationships are now often determined by the homology of the organisms' DNA, a much more fundamental property, which has led to the discovery of unsuspected relationships between apparently disparate species. The new technology and theories has led to the reworking of some bacterial family trees.

Advantages

Practical and ethical considerations may determine that naturalistic observation is the only feasible strategy. Our knowledge of the growth and development of humans is based largely on material obtained from spontaneous abortions or accidental deaths. Discovering this information by experiment would require the execution of individuals at various times after conception and would obviously be unacceptable on ethical grounds. Another advantage of the observation-description strategy is that it can be inexpensive, because elaborate equipment to control the environment is not required. Thus, many people, such as amateur bird watchers, are able to pursue this approach to scientific investigation.

Weaknesses

There are several weaknesses associated with a straight descriptive study:

1. Comparison is made between observations made at different times. Because the observations are not simultaneous, there are more opportunities for other circumstances as well as conditions of interest to the investigator to be altered. If an investigator were making observations on dental disease in children in Canada during the past 40 years, comparisons would be clouded by factors such as the introduction or removal of fluoride in some communities, changes in ethnic composition, and any other social or economic changes that might affect dental health.

2. As discussed in chapter 12, many techniques of observation alter the observations themselves. For example, the preparation of tissues for microscopic examination involves a number of steps, and each step has the potential to produce some alteration of biologic structure. Similarly, psychological observations are complicated by interactions between the interviewer and the subject. This problem, called *observational reactivity*, also occurs in experimentation. However, an investigator can include simultaneous controls in an experiment to lessen the effect of observational reactivity.

3. In contrast to experimentation, naturalistic observations can be made under only a limited number of conditions. For example, to assess the carcinogenicity of chemical compounds, laboratory animals are exposed to concentrations of chemicals that are much higher than any they would encounter in their natural environments. These high doses enable effects to be seen that would not be observed in nature.

4. The selection of observations is a complex problem involving both sampling and method. In some in-

stances, it may be possible to get complete (100%) coverage of the population of interest, but, more commonly, a sample must be selected. In that event, the investigator must decide who will select the sample, what tests or measures will be used as criteria for inclusion or exclusion of subjects or objects, and how a random selection of the sample can be obtained. The selection of the sample can be biased in various ways so that it does not represent the parent population.

The selection of the observations to be made is crucial to the observation-description approach. There are so many possible things to observe that observations, by necessity, are restricted to those believed to be most relevant to the question of interest. The questions posed by investigators are influenced by their training, which, in turn, is influenced by the prevailing concepts accepted in their subject disciplines. This can be seen in periodontal research in the "bug-of-the-month club." As research implicates different microorganisms in the pathogenesis of periodontal disease, subsequent investigations in the microbiology of periodontal disease often include the new putative pathogens among the microorganisms studied.

The background of the research worker who asks the question will affect the type of observation that is made. Despite the pain-alleviating measures available to dentists, many patients still harbor anxiety about dental treatment. Investigation of the anxiety could be legitimately undertaken by investigators with different backgrounds, who would make different types of observations. A psychiatrist might investigate anxious patients' attitudes to authority or their experiences with weaning and toilet training, whereas a behavioral psychologist might use a polygraph to measure physiologic parameters during dental visits. The psychiatrists and psychologists would interpret their findings in very different manners based on the prevailing theories of their respective disciplines. The point here is that their backgrounds determine what observations they make.

The sophistication of an observation-description study can be judged by the refinement of the observational tools. Bird watchers can wander around, making random observations and disturbing the birds, or—in a more sophisticated study—they can hide in blinds, making observations at specific locations in a defined sequence. Moreover, the observation-description strategy can be driven by refinements in technology, because these make more detailed observations possible, or enable previously inaccessible observations to be made. The Hubble Space Telescope can make observations that cannot be made on earth. New methods of the assessment of oral disease will probably make it possible to assess oral health in areas of the world where this was previously not feasible.

Characteristics of real-world research

Real world research, sometimes called *naturalistic inquiry,* is the only possible approach to gain insight into the complex, messy, and poorly controlled situations that are nonetheless central to understanding the oral health (or lack thereof) of populations. *Case study* is "the strategy for doing research which involves an empirical investigation of particular contemporary phenomenon within its real life context using multiple sources of evidence."[5] The case is studied in its own right and may yield results that do not necessarily generalize to a larger target population. Real-world research tends to emphasize solving problems and predicting effects, rather than finding causes and quantitative relationships and developing theories.[5]

Naturalistic inquiry has the following characteristics[5,6]:

- Data are collected in a natural setting, and humans are the primary data-gathering instruments.
- Investigators collect qualitative data, and collection can be sensitive, flexible, and adaptable. Data collection often employs open questions. This approach ensures that there is no need to push square observational pegs into round classification holes—as can happen with survey-based research.
- Naturalistic inquiry emphasizes full descriptions and interactions between the investigator and the respondents; analysis can be secondary.
- Use of tacit (intuitive or felt) knowledge is considered legitimate. The investigator's personal experiences and insights are part of the investigation.
- Sampling is often purposive rather than random, because purposive sampling allows the widest range of data to be collected, and it can be adapted as hypotheses emerge from the observations. Investigators accept that one cost of purposive sampling is that standard statistical methodologies used to generalize to target populations cannot be applied to the data. Instead, there is often a tentativeness in generalizing the data.
- Data are analyzed inductively. Specific responses and interactions are examined closely to discover important categories and relationships.

- A *grounded theory,* in which the theory emerges from (ie, is grounded in) the data, may be used, rather than deductively determining whether some principle or law is being followed.
- The focus of questions may change as more information becomes available during a study—a process sometimes called *emergent design.*
- Negotiated outcomes are common, as credibility generally requires that the participants agree with the investigator's interpretation; meanings are often explicitly negotiated with respondents.
- Idiographic interpretation is necessary, as data are interpreted in terms of the particulars of the case, rather than conformance with laws.
- Focus-determined boundaries are observed.
- Special criteria for trustworthiness are devised that are appropriate to the form of the inquiry.

Table 16-1 Criteria for judging quantitative research and qualitative research[6]	
Quantitative research	**Qualitative research**
Internal validity	Credibility
External validity	Transferability
Reliability	Dependability
Objectivity	Confirmability

Naturalistic inquiry often uses *qualitative methods,* but *quantitative methods* may also be involved. Although qualitative and quantitative data are often described as if there were an unbridgeable dichotomous divide between them, Trochim[7] has argued that there is really little difference, as all qualitative data can be coded quantitatively and all quantitative data are based on qualitative judgment. Qualitative data come from various sources, including in-depth interviews; direct observation analogous to that used in studying animal behavior, where one observes but does not question the subject; and analysis of documents or other cultural artifacts. Trochim[7] suggests that criteria different from those used in quantitative research should be applied for evaluating qualitative research studies (Table 16-1).

Credibility relates to the requirement of the researcher to provide sufficient information on the methods used and their justification. Moreover, as the objective of qualitative research is often to provide a description or understanding of phenomena from the subjects' perspective, the subjects are in the best position to make this judgment and should be consulted.

"Transferability refers to the degree to which results of qualitative research can be generalized or transferred to other contexts or settings."[7] As noted above, transferability requires methods that differ from those used in producing statistical generalizations. One approach is to describe the assumptions and contexts in detail so that others can determine how well they relate to other situations of interest. Another is "making the case," where persuasive techniques are used to argue that it is reasonable to generalize.

Dependability, Trochim[7] argues, emphasizes the need for the researcher to account for the context in which the research is done and how it can change findings. Although perfect replication of conditions is generally not possible, dependability is most directly demonstrated by doing another study in another setting and coming to similar conclusions.

Confirmability relates to the question of whether other investigators can confirm the findings.

In naturalistic inquiry, a wide variety of strategy types are used, including the following[5-7]:

- *Endogenous research:* Conducted by "insiders" of a culture using their own epistemology and structure of relevance.
- *Participatory action research:* Participants contribute to formulation of the research question, study design, and analysis.
- *Critical theory:* An epistemology (ie, study of knowledge and how it is justified) that often involves concepts concerning social justice and social change.
- *Phenomenology:* Uncovers meaning of how humans experience phenomena through descriptions of individual experiences.
- *Heuristic design:* Immersion of an investigator into a problem and self-reflection of investigator's personal experience.
- *Life history:* Involves eliciting life experiences and how they are interpreted.
- *Ethnography:* Description and interpretation of cultural patterns of groups (anthropology).
- *Grounded theory:* Generation of theory by inductive process of constant comparison.

Analysis and interpretation of qualitative research

Qualitative research shares many of the characteristics of quantitative research; there has to be clear thinking to determine what is at issue, what other relevant studies bear on the problem, and what are the factors that threaten the validity of the conclusions. As in any logical processing of thought, there should be balance, some consideration of facts that do not fit the interpretation, and revision of explanations when unsupportive data are found. Chronology is important in suggesting possible cause-effect relationships, and various means, such as triangulation, are used to determine the reliability of the data. Greenhalgh and Taylor[8] suggest that a good qualitative study will address a problem through a clearly formulated question. Quoting Nicky Britten, they state that there is a real danger that "the flexibility of the iterative approach will slide into sloppiness as the researcher ceases to be clear about what it is (s)he is investigating."[8] Qualitative data—like quantitative data—must be analyzed systematically, and there is a need to identify, locate, and explore examples that contradict the emergent hypothesis. As with quantitative methods, analysis of qualitative data should be done using explicit, systematic, and reproducible methods. Quality controls can be introduced into qualitative research. Researchers generally agree that the validity (closeness to the truth) of qualitative research benefits by having different researchers independently analyze the data (one form of triangulation). It would be of interest for qualitative investigators to determine interobserver agreement or disagreement, as this would test the assumption sometimes made that the interpretation of subject meanings is self-evident.

However, quantitative data has a way of imposing its own discipline in demonstrating conclusions. In determining whether the difference between groups could be explained by chance, there is a set of statistical conventions that, more or less, must be obeyed to avoid censure. The fact that some of the assumptions in the analysis may not hold for the collected data can be disturbing, but the presentation of the data and the interpretation of differences tend to be standard. In contrast, authors of reports using qualitative data remind me in some ways of scientist-essayists such as Francis Bacon, Lewis Thomas, and Stephen Jay Gould. The author considers various interpretations of the data and argues for the most likely. The essayist has considerable latitude on the aspects that will be emphasized and the rhetorical techniques that will be brought into play. Among the more common approaches taken by writers of case studies are consideration of the characteristics of language (as qualitative data are words, and there is a focus on word choices), discovery of regularities in participants' views, close examination of the texts' meanings, and extensive reflection.[5] The conclusions might or might not be related to a theoretical framework; sometimes pure description might be adequate. Logical argument is employed to demonstrate the plausibility of the conclusions. Relative to quantitative research, writing and rhetorical skills assume increased importance, because they may have to bear more of the load in the demonstration of qualitative research conclusions than they bear in quantitative research, where the data can sometimes speak for themselves.

Perhaps the stickiest question faced by qualitative investigators is the issue of *generalizability*. On the one hand, qualitative researchers tend to argue for the importance of subjectivity and the particulars of the case. On the other hand, qualitative researchers—like quantitative researchers—need money to pursue their projects. Information that can be generalized to other settings is obviously more attractive to funding agencies than are pure descriptive studies. Thus, qualitative researchers claim that generalization is beside the point, but circumstances sometimes dictate that they must generalize anyway. Paley[9] describes their dilemma as follows:

> Like other researchers, they want to talk in generalizable terms about reality; they want to be objective, they want to do theory. But they are saddled with a philosophy that is disabling, because they can only talk about perceptions, and meanings and uniqueness.

Some naturalist observers are acutely aware of the difficulty in selling qualitative research to granting agencies that want a well-defined outcome. Sandelowski et al[10] note that qualitative researchers employing emergent research design must "negotiate the paradox of planning what should not be planned in advance." Their advice to dealing with this paradox is not unlike that given to quantitative investigators: Provide a rationale for your decisions. For example, when purposive sampling is employed, they advise researchers to identify the purpose of sampling, determine the first subject to be examined, describe focal and comparison subject groups, specify the rules governing how sampling decisions will be made, and clarify that no claim should be made that the selected sample can be used for statistical calculations that assume random probability sampling. Similarly, procedures should be specified for data collection, management, and verification.

The Value of Qualitative Methods in Dental Research

Increasingly, qualitative methods are being used in research, education, and policy related to oral health. Table 16-2, taken from Gift,[11] contrasts the qualitative and quantitative research methods in terms of *purpose, function,* and *findings.* In general terms, qualitative research deals with the subjective world of individuals as they describe it, directly and indirectly. While quantitative research can assess outcomes such as decayed, missing, and filled teeth or periodontal status, qualitative research can give insight into why the data are what they are, by exploring such aspects as an individual's motivations, life history, and perceptions. Qualitative approaches can help develop concepts, suggest hypotheses, and identify problems, which might be used in subsequent studies that could include quantitative measures. If researchers using qualitative measures are sometime criticized for inappropriate generalizations, investigators using quantitative measures are probably equally culpable of going beyond their numbers and forming conclusions about subjective perceptions of their subjects. Three examples of how qualitative methods can be used in dental research follow.

Problem identification

When I was 8 years old, I noticed that a friend of my grandmother, Mrs Winpenny, who worked in the local bakery, had beautiful white teeth. When I mentioned this to my mother, she replied, "Well, they're false, of course." She then told me that Mrs Winpenny had wanted white teeth all her life, and when she finally needed a complete set of dentures, she had fought her dentist tooth and nail to get dentures that, to adults, looked like a set of "Chicklets" but that, to a child, looked wonderful. Later, as a young man, I recall being disappointed that my teeth were not any whiter after

Table 16-2 Comparison of qualitative and quantitative research methods in terms of purpose, function, and findings[10]

Approach	Qualitative	Quantitative
Purpose		
Exploratory	Ideal	Suitable
Descriptive	Suitable	Ideal
Function		
Causal	Inappropriate	Ideal
Understanding, depth	Ideal	Inappropriate
Hypothetical, interpretive	Ideal	Suitable
Empirical, statistical	Inappropriate	Ideal
Prediction, accuracy, breadth	Inappropriate	Ideal
Findings		
Implications, problem identification	Ideal	Suitable
Projections	Inappropriate	Ideal

I had them cleaned. Thus, I had both personal and interpersonal evidence that people preferred bright white teeth, even though the dental profession largely ignored their desires and promoted a more natural-looking esthetic. My qualitative approach to discovering this insight might be classified as "life history."

To broaden my base of inference, I could easily have adopted an "ethnographic" approach by looking at the social context of toothpaste advertisements and discovering the Pepsodent commercial dating back many years that assured consumers, "You'll wonder where the yellow went, when you brush your teeth with Pepsodent." To broaden my base of inference further, I might well have embarked on purposive sampling, by asking those friends whose teeth did not exactly sparkle, "Yo, yellow fang, do you wish your teeth were whiter after you visited the dentist?" Or perhaps more diplomatically and in the qualitative research tradition, I could have asked the more open-ended, neutral question, "What do you think about the teeth-cleaning services provided by your dentist?"

A more commercial-oriented mind might have taken this insight on unmet need that was developed by qualitative methods and worked on developing and marketing tooth-whitening products. Before taking out a mortgage on my home to embark on this career, it probably would have been wise to conduct a survey to determine quantitatively the prevalence of people who would pay for tooth whitening. Such action would have illustrated the principle that the insights arising from qualitative studies can lead to quantitative studies with appropriately focused questions.

As it happened, I did not do any of these things, and this is one reason that today I am an impecunious penny-a-word author of a Quintessence book. Although the development of tooth-whitening systems has subsequently happened in spades, the opportunity was open for quite a long time. I would think that qualitative research methods could still be employed to discern consumer preferences that are not expressed, or at least not appreciated, by the dental profession.

Identifying perceptions that affect the delivery of oral health services

One example of qualitative research that produced interesting results, which could not have been found by quantitative methods, is the study of MacEntee et al.[12] By asking older adults the open-ended question "What is the significance of oral health in the lives of older adults?" and by collecting and analyzing their unrestricted responses, the investigators identified three prominent themes: *comfort, hygiene,* and *health.* They found that older patients recognized the need to adapt but did not complain that oral health was a cause of social embarrassment. The subjects' beliefs about the need for treatment did not always agree with the recommendations of health professionals, and home remedies were used to explain why dental visits were unnecessary. Overall, it was clear that the subjects had a rather different view of the maintenance of their oral health than that typical of dentists. Indeed, the investigators concluded that most oral disorders can be managed so that the impact on quality of life is within the adaptive capacity of aging adults—a finding that recommends offering different approaches of oral health care delivery to this group than those currently being applied most commonly.

Supplementing and complementing quantitative approaches

Typically, qualitative research examines relatively few subjects, as the investigators must explore the words and perceptions of their subjects in detail. But it is clearly inappropriate to generalize from close observations of a few subjects to the general population. One method of avoiding this problem is to combine qualitative and quantitative approaches to a single problem. For example, Moore[13] combined qualitative and quantitative approaches to the study of pain by *triangulation,* ie, a process of verifying the same phenomenon using different measures. Moore combined interview, observation, and focus group data with short surveys to gain insight into the perception of pain by different ethnic groups. In addition, there were ethnic differences in the use of local anesthetic for tooth drilling. Different conceptions of ethnic groups on the nature of pain led to differences in how the pain was managed, a finding that introduces a new consideration into chairside care.

Observation-Description Strategy in Clinical Interventions

The closest approach to the observation-description strategy in clinical investigation occurs in those instances where the investigator desires to provide some documentation and publication of clinical experience. It is normally understood that, although such studies may not be definitive, they represent the starting point for explanations. This type of study occurs in a number of formats.

The case study

$$S \rightarrow Tx \xrightarrow{t} O_1 \rightarrow O_2 \rightarrow \ldots O_n$$

where S = pool of eligible subjects, Tx = treatment, and O = observations.

In a *case study*, subjects are treated and carefully observed. Inferences are made on the basis of historical controls, that is, what would have been expected if treatment had not taken place or if a standard treatment had been used. Historical controls are generally regarded as less than ideal, because time and history can play important roles, such as the incremental improvements in dental equipment, materials, and techniques, which would be expected to improve outcomes.

The case study is not an example of the observation-description study in the purest sense, because a treatment is applied. However, in some instances, the treatment is traditional or unproven and could be dealt with as observation on an individual encountering natural hazards. The case study could be considered a quasi-experimental design, but it is not a true experiment, because the subject (the patient) is not selected randomly and there is no control group. It resembles an experiment, in that a treatment is applied, and the subjects are observed closely. Regardless of its exact location in the investigational design taxonomy, the case study is worth discussing here.

The case study is almost universally reviled in books on experiment design primarily because, without a control group, it is impossible to tell what would have occurred without treatment. This defect cannot be remedied by the investigator collecting an increasing number of successful outcomes. Streiner et al[14] noted that case reports involving a total of about 1,500 patients indicated that gastric freezing would cure gastric ulcers. Subsequent properly controlled clinical trials demonstrated that the procedure was useless.

Nevertheless, we could argue that, were it to be present, a truly dramatic treatment effect could likely be observed. Moreover, it must be admitted that this approach is most often used in everyday problem solving, and, to a certain extent, under some conditions, it works. It works best when the effects of the treatment are large and easily observed and occur quickly. Under these conditions, some of the major problems of the design, such as the effects of time and subjective assessment, are less likely to confuse the results. To do a case study is obviously better than refusing to investigate at all, because there is at least some chance that new information will be gained, and it does encourage close observation. This design is most effective if the sequence of events in the absence of treatment is absolutely predictable. Observations from case studies have led to true experimental studies being carried out, and it is generally true that it is better to light one candle than to curse the darkness. Nevertheless, Huth[15] believes that only three types of case report merit publication:

1. *The unique case*: Such a case occurs when a patient exhibits disease manifestations so extraordinary that they cannot be accounted for by known diseases or syndromes.
2. *The case of unexpected association*: When two relatively uncommon diseases are found in one patient, it is possible that their association indicates some kind of causal relationship. There may be some underlying mechanism—for example, a deficiency in the immune system—that explains both.
3. *The case of unexpected events*: An unexpected event may provide a clue to new information. A drug might appear to cause some unexpected benefit or some previously unsuspected adverse effect. If the author wishes to claim a causal relationship, the author must exclude plausible alternative explanations.

Improvements of the case study design by multiple observations

A significant problem of the case study design is that the patient might have improved without treatment. It would be worthwhile for the investigator to determine that the conditions would remain the same in the absence of treatment. For conditions in which there is no urgency for treatment, stability may be established by measuring the baseline; that is, by making multiple observations before treatment and then multiple observations after the treatment. A shorthand description for this design is:

$$S \rightarrow O_1 \overset{t}{\rightarrow} O_2 \rightarrow O_3 \rightarrow Tx \rightarrow O_4 \overset{t}{\rightarrow} O_5 \rightarrow O_6$$

The pattern of observations O_1, O_2, O_3 is compared with the pattern of O_4, O_5, O_6. If the baseline O_1, O_2, O_3 is reasonably stable or has a constant slope, it may be possible to see the changes after the treatment and to be more confident that these changes were brought about by treatment, although other explanations would still be possible, because other effects such as maturation and history are not controlled in this design.

For treatments that are reversible, a further refinement is possible of discontinuing the treatment to allow sufficient time for the baseline values to be established again and to reapply the treatment, that is:

$$S \rightarrow O_1 \xrightarrow{t} O_2 \rightarrow O_3 \rightarrow Tx \rightarrow O_4 \rightarrow O_5 \xrightarrow{t} O_6 \rightarrow \text{Recovery time} \rightarrow O_7 \rightarrow O_8 \rightarrow O_9 \rightarrow Tx \rightarrow O_{10} \rightarrow O_{11} \rightarrow O_{12}$$

The basic advantage of this design is that the effect of the treatment can be replicated. Moreover, if the effect occurs at different times and at different stages as the subjects age, the effects of history and maturation are probably not important.

Further refinements in this family of n = 1 (ie, single subject) designs are discussed by Hersen and Barlow.[16] They review tactics such as having multiple baselines (ie, establishing baselines for more than one variable with only some of the variables likely to respond to the treatment) and multiple treatments that might affect different variables. Despite these refinements, it is not possible to generalize from the case study because of individual variation, and there is no way of knowing whether the subject of the study is typical of those who have the condition. The case series is one attempt to improve generalizability.

Case-series analysis

Similar to the case report is the *case-series analysis*, a retrospective study of case records usually gathered in one institution or practice. Investigators then make some generalizations on the basis of their cases. The case-series analysis suffers from some of the same failings as the case report. In the first place, it is often difficult to ascertain how a patient came to be treated at a given institution or practice, but it is highly likely that the cases in the study are not selected randomly. Another problem is that with the passage of time, patients are exposed to many different treatments or conditions, and it can be difficult to determine which of the possible causes were related to the final effect. Mainland[17] lists two additional problems of retrospective studies: *(1)* records made for clinical purposes are seldom suitable for any profound analytic study, and *(2)* clinicians can lose touch with many patients over time. Despite these problems, a recent review found that the case series is a frequently adopted design and figured in some 30% of the Health Technology Assessments of the National Institute for Clinical Excellence

(UK).[18] Agnew and Pyke[19] have likened the retrospective analysis of cases to a murder investigation in which there are various suspects who are eliminated by different criteria, such as motive and opportunity, so that only the prime suspects are left. However, they stress that the after-the-fact method is used only when it is impossible, too difficult, or too late to experiment.

References

1. Einstein A. Cited in Brush SG. Should the history of science be rated X? Science 1974;183:1164.
2. Beveridge WIB. The Art of Scientific Investigation. New York: Random House Vintage Books, 1950:140.
3. Cawson RA. Stocker IP. The early history of fluorides as anti-caries agents. Br Dent J 1984;157:403.
4. Pennisi E. Audubon count now serves science too. Scientist 1989 Dec 11:1–4.
5. Robson C. Real World Research. Oxford: Blackwell, 1993.
6. Tuckman BW. Conducting Educational Research, ed 4. Fort Worth, TX: Harcourt Brace, 1994.
7. Trochim WMK. The Research Methods Knowledge Base, ed 2. Cincinnati: Atomic Dog, 2001.
8. Greenhalgh T, Taylor R. Papers that go beyond the numbers (qualitative research). BMJ 1997;315:740–743.
9. Paley J. Phenomenology as rhetoric. Nurs Inq 2005;12:106–116.
10. Sandelowski M, Davis DH, Harris BG. Artful design: Writing the proposal for research in the naturalist paradigm. Res Nurs Health 1989;12:77–84.
11. Gift HC. Values of selected qualitative methods for research, education, and policy. J Dent Educ 1996;60:703–708.
12. MacEntee MI, Hole R, Stolar E. The significance of the mouth in old age. Soc Sci Med 1997;45:1449–1458.
13. Moore R. Combining qualitative and quantitative research approaches in understanding pain. J Dent Educ 1996;60:709–715.
14. Streiner DC, Norman GR, Blum HM. PDQ Epidemiology. Toronto: Decker, 1989:viii.
15. Huth EJ. How to Write and Publish Papers in the Medical Sciences. Philadelphia: ISI Press, 1982:58.
16. Hersen M, Barlow DH. Single Case Experimental Designs: Strategies for Studying Behavior Change. New York: Pergamon, 1976.
17. Mainland D. Elementary Medical Statistics. Philadelphia: Saunders, 1963:25.
18. Dalziel K, Round A, Stein K, Garside R, Castelnuovo E, Payne L. Do the findings of case series studies vary significantly according to methodological characteristics? Health Technol Assess 2005;9:1–146.
19. Agnew NM, Pyke SW. The Science Game. Englewood Cliffs, NJ: Prentice Hall, 1978:69.

17 | Correlation

The scientific literature is a large graveyard for correlations that didn't "pan out" when more data became available.

—Peter A. Larkin[1]

The investigative strategies outlined in this chapter include: (1) cross-sectional survey; (2) ecologic study; (3) case-control design; and (4) follow-up (cohort) design.

Cross-sectional Survey

$$S \rightarrow OP_1 \rightarrow r$$
$$OP_2$$
$$OP_n$$

where S = pool of eligible subjects, OP_1 = observation of property 1, OP_2 = observation of property 2, OP_n = observation of property n, and r = calculation of correlation coefficient or other measure of association.

As an example of a *correlational cross-sectional study* in dental research, consider the data from Keene et al[1] in Table 17-1. The *correlational strategy* is used to relate two or more variables. Investigators classify the study subjects into groups and examine each subject indi-

vidually to measure the different variables. In this example, investigators measured three properties: the *Streptococcus mutans* biotype; decayed, missing, or filled teeth (DMFT); and caries-free status. Often in cross-sectional studies, one variable is concerned with exposure (S *mutans*), while the other variables relate to "caseness" (ie, presence of some conditions). Each group member is then assigned a value, depending on the particular variable measured. The degree of relationship between the variables is then assessed with statistical techniques. Notice that because the Keene et al[2] study is a correlational study, no attempt is made to manipulate the biotype of S *mutans* in the naval men. The biotype is simply measured. Hence, a correlational study is similar to the observation-description strategy and shares the same strengths and weaknesses. Two advantages of a simple correlational study (such as that of Keene et al[2]) are that (1) they are relatively inexpensive because no follow-up is required and (2) subjects are not exposed to potentially harmful agents or conditions.

Table 17-1 Correlation cross-sectional study measuring *Streptococcus mutans* biotype, DMFT, and caries prevalence*

S mutans biotype group	No. of subjects	DMFT Mean	SE	Caries-free subjects No.	%
c	64	3.16	0.37	17	26.6
d	22	2.36	0.39	5	22.7
e	14	3.93	0.88	1	7.1
Single (c or d or e)	100	3.09	0.28	23	23.0
Multiple (eg, cd, ce)	96	4.76	0.40	11	11.5
e-type carriers	56	4.91	0.48	4	7.1
Non-e-type carriers	140	3.51	0.28	30	21.4

*Data from Keene et al.[1]
SE = standard error.

Table 17-2 Odds for caries using data from Table 17-1

Factor	Caries present	Caries absent	Odds
e carriers [+]	52	4	13
Non–e carriers [–]	110	30	3.7

Statistical considerations and calculations

Correlational studies have statistical considerations. The groups formed from exposure and outcome (eg, caries-free individuals exposed to e-biotype *S mutans*) could end up with very different sample sizes, and statistical efficiency could be poor. Various calculations, such as the odds ratio, can demonstrate the presence or absence of a relationship between the two variables under study (in our example, caries and *S mutans* biotype). Some calculations may be better than others. The criticism of statistical tests used in correlation involves methods outside the scope of this book; detailed information is presented elsewhere.[3–6] However, two simple statistical approaches are given here: the odds ratio and the contingency table analysis using the Cohen Kappa.

Odds ratio

The *odds ratio* is a widely used means that can show the relationship between factors and disease. *Odds* are defined as the ratio that something is so, or will occur, to the probability that it is not so, or will not occur. In looking at the odds, we could express the data in Table 17-1 in a different way (Table 17-2). For e-type carriers, the odds of having caries are 52/4 = 13. For non-e-type carriers, the odds are 110/30 = 3.7. The *odds ratio*—the ratio of one odds to another—is 13/3.7. An odds ratio of 1 means there is no association between the factor and the disease. Here, the odds ratio is greater than 1, and there is an association between having *S mutans* e-type and the disease.

The Cohen Kappa

In the view of Norman and Streiner,[7] the best measure of association for a contingency table with an equal number of rows and columns is the *Cohen Kappa*. It is defined as:

$$K = \frac{\text{observed agreement} - \text{chance agreement}}{1 - \text{chance agreement}}$$

The data on caries presence or absence in relation to e-biotype can be extracted from Table 17-1 in the form of a *contingency table* (Table 17-3) (see also chapter 14).

The Cohen Kappa concentrates on the diagonal cells. That is, the upper left cell, *a* (positive for caries and positive for e-type), would be expected to have a high frequency if there were a strong association between e-type and caries, as would the lower right cell,

Table 17-3 Contingency table using data from Table 17-1

Factor	Caries present	Caries absent	Marginal row total
e carriers [+]	a 52	b 4	a + b 56
Non–e carriers [–]	c 110	d 30	c + d 140
Marginal column total	a + c 162	b + d 34	a + b + c + d 196

d (absence of e-type and absence of disease). If there were a perfect association, all the cases would be found only in those two quadrants. However, in Keene et al's data,[2] the sum of quadrant *a* (52) with quadrant *d* (30) divided by the grand total (196) is 0.42 of the sample; this is the *observed agreement* for the association. If there were no association between e-type and caries, the individuals would be distributed into the four cells by chance, and the number in each cell could be determined by using the marginal totals as follows:

Quadrant *a* would contain $\frac{(56 \times 162)}{196} = 46.3$ cases;

and quadrant *d* would contain $\frac{(140 \times 34)}{196} = 24.3$ cases.

The proportion of cases expected to be distributed into the *a* and *d* quadrants by chance is thus:

$$\frac{\text{No. expected in 2 cells by chance}}{\text{Total no. in samples}} = \frac{46.3 + 24.3}{196} = 0.36$$

Therefore, for these data:

$$K = \frac{0.42 - 0.36}{1 - 0.36} = 0.09$$

For a perfect association, K = 1, and for no association, K = 0. Thus, the association between e-type and the presence of caries is weak.

Interpretation of correlation

Authors can interpret correlation to predict future events. In our example, if the next Saudi naval recruit we saw was a carrier of the e-biotype *S mutans*, we might predict on the basis of the data in Table 17-1 that the recruit's DMFT index might be higher than that of a non–e carrier. This is a legitimate use of the data. A second, and less conservative, use of the data would be to assert that the e-biotype *S mutans* is more

effective than other serotypes in causing caries. The data are compatible with such a proposal, but the authors carefully avoid asserting it. Instead, they state, "it will be most interesting to determine whether these relationships can be demonstrated under carefully controlled laboratory conditions in the animal model."[2]

The reason for their caution is the *fallacy of concomitant variation,* which is the fallacy of assuming that Mill's principle of concomitant variation is necessarily true. While it is possible that two events showing a high incidence of correlation are causally connected, it is not always the case. For example, Huff[8] states that there is a close relationship between the salaries of Presbyterian ministers in Massachusetts and the price of rum in Havana. However, there is no reason to suspect that the one influences the other. Thus, when applying the principle of concomitant variation, we must remember Hume's second criterion for causation (see chapter 7): There must be some plausible reason explaining cause and effect.

Another problem with correlational studies is the *linked* or *confounding variable* (or *confounder*). Sometimes, when varying one condition, an investigator also varies another factor, either knowingly or unknowingly. The hoary example used to illustrate this problem relates the story of a philosopher who started out drinking scotch and soda at a party. When the host ran out of scotch, the philosopher switched to rye and soda, and finally to bourbon and soda. Carefully selecting the best correlation, the philosopher concluded that soda water was the cause of his intoxication. This example illustrates the common problem of a confounder producing an apparent association (drunkenness and soda) where none actually exists, but confounders can also diminish, reverse, or exaggerate an apparent association.

The effect of any confounder can be important only if its association with the effect of interest is strong. The most common strategy used by epidemiologists to eliminate confounders begins with consideration of possible confounding variables that might be associated with the independent variable of interest. A number of variables that are often relevant to epidemiologic studies would be investigated, including sex, parity, ethnic group, religion, marital status, social class, education, occupation, rural or urban residence, and geographic mobility. The investigator then regroups the data to see if the possible confounder has any effect on the association. A study on the prevalence of root caries for individuals living in an extended-care facility might show that caries was more prevalent in women than men. However, subsequent analysis might demonstrate that the association was modified by the sample containing more elderly women than men (because women live longer) and that prevalence of root caries was related to age, not sex.

Investigators generally accept that the best way to elucidate causation is to vary experiment factors separately, and scientists are skeptical when surveys are substituted for experiments. In a survey, investigators try to define their groups precisely, but it is always possible that two variables will be confounded and that an investigator will attribute the effect to the wrong cause. In the example of the drunken philosopher, the linked variables were alcohol (the hidden variable) and soda.

A second difficulty arises because all the data are collected at a single point in time. This leads to problems in interpreting cause-effect relationships, because—as David Hume[9] noted—one of the criteria often used for establishing cause-effect relationships is that the cause precedes the effect (see chapter 7). In cross-sectional studies, interpretation becomes a chicken-and-egg problem. Gehlbach[10] has used the example of findings from cross-sectional studies that demonstrate that children who are overweight are less active than their normal counterparts. The conclusion drawn from the studies is that children who have a low level of activity are more likely to become obese. However, it could be equally inferred that obese children have difficulty getting around and are inactive because they are obese rather than obese because they are inactive.

Gehlbach[10] notes that the cross-sectional design is efficient and flexible and has been increasingly used in medical research. A common problem is sample selection (eg, study populations drawn from hospitals sometimes bear little resemblance to the community at large).

In addition to the cross-sectional study, a number of study designs use the basic correlational strategy but differ in the way the data are collected over time or the way subjects are selected. A brief description of the merits and deficiencies of the more common designs is given here; the interested reader is referred to Gehlbach[10] for more detail.

Ecologic Study

$$P(1) \rightarrow \%E \text{ (and not E)} \quad \%OV \text{ (and not OV)}$$
$$P(2) \rightarrow \%E \text{ (and not E)} \quad \%OV \text{ (and not OV)}$$

where P(1) = population in a geographic or social unit (country, province, hospital) no. 1; P(2) = population in a geographic or social unit (country, province, hospital) no. 2; %E = percentage of subjects exposed (eg, to water fluoridation); and %OV = percentage having a given outcome variable (eg, dental caries).

Ecologic studies attempt to establish the relationship between exposure to a factor (eg, fluoride in the drinking water) and an outcome variable (eg, caries) by using aggregate data. The groups are often defined geographically (eg, Toronto, Vancouver), and the investigator does not know the relationship between exposure and outcome variable on an individual-by-individual basis. The major advantage of the ecologic study is that it is inexpensive; the data are usually available.[11]

A significant disadvantage is that, although we know how many people are exposed and how many have the outcome, we do not know how many of the exposed people have the outcome. It is possible that unexposed people exhibit the outcome—as is illustrated in Fig 17-1. The proportion of black cats and the proportion of hatted cats is the same in four populations (see Fig 17-1a); but blackness and hattedness are not necessarily linked in individuals. The ecologic design is very susceptible to the problem of the *hidden variable*. Correlations based on individuals are almost always lower than ecologic correlations. In our pictorial example of black and hatted cats, Cohen's Kappa equals 0.33, even though the correlation coefficient is a perfect 1.0 (see Fig 17-1b). Widely used in cancer research, ecologic studies can be constructive in forming hypotheses that could prove useful for directing future research.[13]

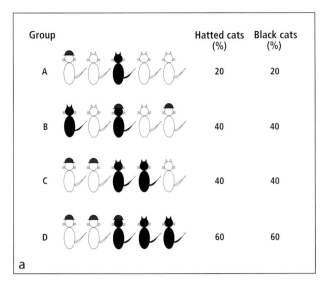

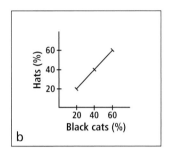

Fig 17-1 Example of an ecologic study showing that well-correlated variables are not necessarily linked. *(a)* Percentages of hatted cats and black cats in four groups. *(b)* Graphic representation of data showing a perfect correlation coefficient of 1. (Adapted from Rosen et al.[12])

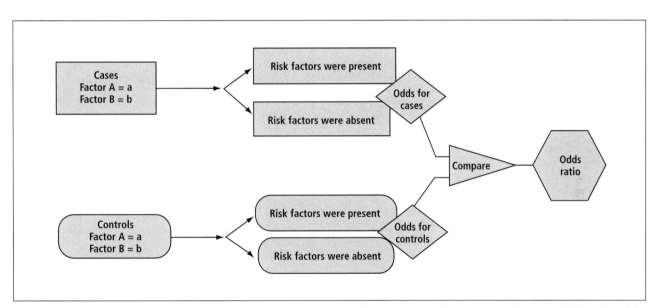

Fig 17-2 Case-control design. In this highly efficient design, the study begins after the event, ie the "causes" are known. The factors (A, B) for which the cases are matched may vary from the specific to the general, such as being treated in the same hospital. Many possible causal conditions (risk factors) can be assessed.

Case-Control Design

In the *case-control design* (Fig 17-2), investigators first examine people who already have a certain condition (the cases) and look for characteristics they share, such as exposure to an agent in the past. A valuable feature of the case-control approach is that investiga-tors can test a variety of possible causes that led to the disease or condition of interest. It is quite a flexible and inexpensive means of exploring possibilities and particularly powerful when searching for the causes of a new problem. Case-control design is also practical for studying conditions or diseases that take a long time to appear; lung cancer is a classic example. An investigator could compare lung cancer incidence in a group of nonsmokers with a group of smokers, but it would likely take a long time before any difference is evident.

Case-control–like approaches are informally used in problem-solving situations both in everyday life and in the laboratory. For a problem with contamination of cultures, an investigator might examine the history of the cultures to search for the factors that the contaminated ones held in common, such as batch of media, type of culture dish, source of antibiotic, technician who initiated the cultures, and other factors. In fact, the investigator would systematically go through all the components of the culture system.

The characteristics chosen for examination as possible causes for a disease or condition will probably be influenced by the theories currently being used to explain the condition. Patients with juvenile periodontitis would be examined for the presence of a particular type of bacteria or for unusual characteristics of their leuckocytes. If the cases share certain characteristics (eg, if the juvenile periodontitis patients have defective leukocytes), then an explanation of the condition is suggested. The problem is that many people who do not have the condition might also share the same characteristics; a *comparison group* is needed. In the case-control design, the comparison group (the controls) is often selected so that it resembles the cases as closely as is possible. When we consider the many ways that people can be matched—by age, sex, race, religion, dietary habits, human leukocyte antigen (HLA) type, and other traits—it becomes clear that it is difficult to get a perfect match. Without a perfect match, there is always an alternative explanation.

In Fig 17-2, the cases and controls have been matched for two factors, A and B. So, for example, A could be sex, and a in the diagram could stand for male. B could be age and the value b in the diagram could stand for age older than 60 but younger than 65. The controls would be 60- to 65-year-old males who were not poor. An investigator can overmatch. If the cases and controls are matched by age, sex, race, or any other factor, the matched factors can no longer be evaluated as etiologic agents, because they will be equalized in the cases and the controls. Sometimes case-control studies are not done with specific matching factors; there might be a sample selected from all the people who did not have the condition.

Two additional problems with the case-control design relate to *information bias*, that is, shortcomings in the way the information is obtained or processed. The ideal is for there to be no major differences in quality or availability of the data between the cases and the

controls. This is difficult because of *biased recall*. People who have unpleasant conditions may recall the past quite differently from nondiseased individuals; sick people have the tendency to think deeply about what caused their problem.[10]

Information bias is not necessarily detrimental to interpretation. Sometimes investigators can devise approaches that can—if not overcome it—possibly determine its relative unimportance. Elwood[14] examines an early and important study on the relationship of smoking and lung cancer[15] to illustrate how bias can be assessed. As the data indicated that smoking was related to lung cancer, the problem might be that the cancer patients (who may well have wondered what caused their condition) might overreport their smoking, or, alternatively, the controls might underreport their smoking. The investigators examined the records of subjects who were suspected of having lung cancer at the time of the interview, but whose final diagnosis was something else. These non-cancer patients, who at the time of interview thought they had cancer, reported smoking patterns similar to the non-cancer control patients, indicating that reporting bias may not have been an important issue. This example teaches us that while some investigative designs may be susceptible to certain problems, creative investigators can often find ways to assess just how much the problems are affecting their conclusions and can work out ways of minimizing them.

Second, case-control studies often utilize data that were collected in the past under uncertain conditions. It is difficult to get reliable bias-free information for such factors as exposure to asbestos, smoking habits, fluoride ingestion, and therapeutic drug usage. Moreover, in any given study, some of the most important data may not have been collected, because it would clearly be difficult to assess in advance what information will be of interest in the future. The collected information may be of questionable reliability, because standardized techniques for collecting the data may not have been practiced. This point is sometimes overlooked. Some years ago, our clinic director (at the time) asked the faculty council for permission to destroy some outdated records. In the ensuing debate, a number of faculty argued that this action would amount to destroying a potential treasure trove of data that could be used for research. However, considering how the data were obtained, it is improbable that much useful data would be lost. The students responsible for the treatments had different diagnostic, technical, and record-keeping skills. They had never been calibrated to any standard, and it is likely that

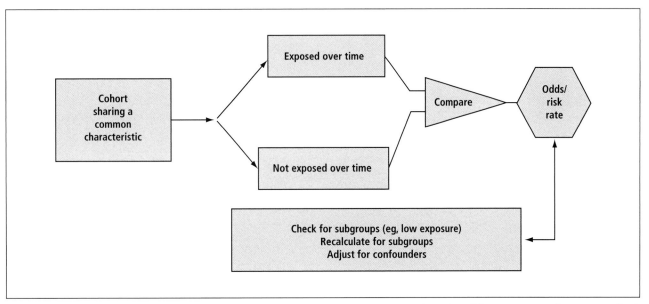

Fig 17-3 Follow-up (cohort) design used to study effects of a particular exposure. Members of a cohort differ in important characteristics (such as age). The date may be stratified into subgroups and analyzed separately or adjusted for confounding by methods such as Mantel-Haenszel.[17]

the standards changed, because there was considerable faculty turnover during the period. To date, those debated but probably useless records have not been used for research purposes.

Gehlbach[9] recommends that a reader ask three questions when considering the controls in a case-control study:

> 1. What sort of population do the control subjects represent (ie, do they behave like people in the general population)?
> 2. Are there likely to be relationships between the control population and the factors under study that would influence the results?
> 3. Was matching used appropriately?

As in the other correlational designs, there is still the problem of the hidden variable. For example, exposure to some agent may be correlated to some other factor that is correlated with the outcome (eg, socioeconomic status).

Despite these difficulties, there are merits in the case-control design. In comparison with other, more rigorous methods, case-control design is very efficient. For example, one way that a dentist could study juvenile periodontitis would be to characterize patients completely for a number of properties and follow these patients over time (ie, a follow-up design). The dentist could then compare the patients who developed juvenile periodontitis with those who did not.

There would be no problem with obtaining accurate data, because the data collection could be completely under the dentist's control. There would be little problem with selection of a control group, because it would comprise the patients who did not get the disease. However, there would be a problem in the number of cases of juvenile periodontitis; some dentists never encounter a single case. The dentist might end up with all controls and no cases. The follow-up design might be more rigorous than the case-control design but is much less practical. Gehlbach[10] believes that the case-control design is ideally suited for initial exploratory investigations. Analysis of case-control designs is best done by calculating the odds ratio. Simon[16] provides a detailed discussion of this point.

Follow-up (Cohort) Design

A *cohort* is a group of people who share a common characteristic (eg, year of birth, place of employment, or exposure to a risk factor such as radiation). Sometimes considered the crème de la crème of observational studies,[10] the *follow-up* or *cohort design* (Fig 17-3) begins with a study population free of the condition or outcome of interest. The population is then measured or classified on the basis of the characteristics of interest. At the start of the study, investigators can gather information that is as complete as they have resources or desire to acquire without the problems of accuracy in data gathering associated with the case-control study. The investigators then observe the subjects repeatedly over time and note when and if the outcome of interest occurs. In fact, they can measure multiple outcomes. Traditionally, *cohort design* has referred to groups formed on the basis of exposure to some agent, but the same principles are applied when the exposure is a treatment or other intervention. The outcome is correlated with the properties measured or recorded initially, as it may be necessary to adjust for confounders. In other words, the exposed and nonexposed groups might differ in important properties that may be relevant to the outcome. In particular, cohort studies are vulnerable to *selection bias*. Volunteers for the intervention would be expected to differ from non-volunteers in characteristics such as compliancy with treatment and education. Confounding would be expected in cohort design studies, because there is no randomization process that equalized the groups before treatment or exposure. Moreover, there may be some strata or gradient of exposure that might also require adjustment. Normand et al[18] provide a guide to analytical methods used to adjust for confounding, and new methods are available that attempt to adjust for unmeasured confounding—an impressive feat of statistical legerdemain.[19]

Cohort studies come in different flavors. Figure 17-3 illustrates a *prospective* cohort study, but cohort studies can also be done using data collected in the past (*retrospective*) or using a combination of data collected in the past as well as over time. The key feature is that the subjects are selected for the groups on the basis of exposure without knowing the outcome at the time. In other words, the subjects are free of the outcome at the time their exposure status is defined.

This approach obviously has more power than the cross-sectional design for elucidating cause-effect relationships, because the patients are classified before the outcome is observed. A thin child who became fat could be tested to see which changed first, the child's level of activity or the child's weight.[10] Follow-up studies are susceptible to selection bias, because various factors tend to select the subjects observed at the end of the study. Most studies will lose some subjects as people die, move, or simply quit the study. Investigators should compare the dropouts or other lost subjects to those who remain to determine whether they differ in such a way that the outcome could be affected. Another problem is that people can change their habits from the beginning to the end of the study, so

that smokers could become nonsmokers and drinkers could become teetotalers. Sometimes subjects may change their habits because they are in the study.

Technical problems of this design include the following: *(a)* it may be difficult to retain control of the therapy; *(b)* blindness among subjects (see chapter 18) and consensus may be difficult to achieve; *(c)* it may violate some statistical tests based on the assumption of randomization; *(d)* for some disorders, large sample sizes are required, and the study can be expensive.[9]

Scientific Standards in Correlational Experiments Involving Humans

Epidemiologic studies have led to splendid achievements, including demonstrations of a dietary deficiency leading to pellagra, the association between cigarette smoking and cancer, the protective dental effect of fluoridated water, and the role of thalidomide in phocomelia.[20] But epidemiology is also plagued with controversies. In one survey, 56 different postulated cause-effect relationships were found in which epidemiologic studies contradicted one another.[21] Perhaps because of this plethora of conflicting evidence, there is now widespread skepticism about the continuing stream of reports implicating such common items of daily life as eggs, coffee, or sugar as menaces to health. Feinstein[20] has argued that epidemiologic studies often lack the precautions, calibrations, and relative simplicity that are taken for granted in experimental science. To rectify this problem, he advocates the application of five scientific standards commonly assumed in experimental research to epidemiologic studies:

1. *High-quality data.* Persons should be directly examined with methods that can be carefully calibrated for their reproducibility and validity. Epidemiologic data are often not of high quality. The clinical diagnosis of the outcome disease in the cases is usually accepted as stated, although, on occasion, investigators may check for false-positive errors by reviewing the available diagnostic evidence. However, in the control group, which is chosen because the target disease was not diagnosed, evidence of the disease's absence is almost never verified, and members of the control group do not receive the appropriate di-

agnostic tests. Another problem is that exposure, caseness, or both depend on recall, which is fallible.[22]

2. *A stipulated research hypothesis.* Epidemiologic studies generate vast quantities of data. The advent of high-power computing enables these data to be dredged for numerous statistical associations. However, associations gleaned in this way do not have the acceptability associated with data that conform to a previously stipulated research hypothesis.

3. *A well-specified cohort.* Each person included in a study should be checked for suitable eligibility for the study, and each person should be accounted for thereafter.

4. *Avoidance of detection bias.* Disease should be sought with equally intense methods of surveillance and examination in the exposed and nonexposed groups.

5. *Analysis of attributable actions.* The complexity and erratic nature of human exposure to multiple agents makes it difficult for epidemiologists to define exposure to an agent as precisely as would be desired.

In the future, Feinstein concludes, investigators will have to focus more on the scientific quality of the evidence, and less on the statistical methods of analysis and adjustment.[20]

References

1. Larkin PA. Notes for Biology 300 (Biometrics). A Handbook of Elementary Statistical Tests. Vancouver, BC: University of British Columbia, 1978:131.
2. Keene HJ, Shklair IL, Anderson DM, Mickel GJ. Relationship of *Streptococcus mutans* biotypes to dental caries prevalence in Saudi Arabian naval men. J Dent Res 1977;56:356.
3. Abramson JH. Making Sense of Data. Oxford: Oxford Univ Press, 1988.
4. Gilbert N. Biometrical Interpretation. Oxford: Clarendon, 1973.
5. Streiner DS, Norman GR, Blum HM. PDQ Epidemiology. Toronto: Decker, 1989.
6. Willemsen EW. Understanding Statistical Reasoning. San Francisco: Freeman, 1974.
7. Norman GR, Streiner DL. PDQ Statistics. Toronto: Decker, 1986:96.
8. Huff D. How to Lie with Statistics. New York: Norton, 1954.
9. Hume DA. Treatise on Human Nature (1739–1740), ed 2, vol 1. Oxford: Clarendon Press, 1978:173–175.
10. Gehlbach SH. Interpreting the Medical Literature. Lexington, MA: Collamore, 1982:39–71.
11. Streiner DL, Norman GR, Blum HM. PDQ Epidemiology. Toronto: Decker, 1989:48.
12. Rosen M, Nystrom L, Wall S. Guidelines for regional mortality analysis: An epidemiological approach to health planning. Int J Epidemiol 1985;14:293–299.
13. Streiner DC, Norman GR, Blum HM. PDQ Epidemiology. Toronto: Decker, 1989:45–52.
14. Elwood JM. Critical Appraisal of Epidemiological Studies and Clinical Trials. Oxford: Oxford Univ Press, 1998:29–32.
15. Doll R, Hill AB. Smoking and carcinoma of the lung; A preliminary report. BMJ 1950;2:739–748.
16. Simon S. Odds ratio versus relative risk. StATS Web site. Available at http://www.childrens-mercy.org/stats/journal/oddsratio.asp. Accessed July 19, 2007.
17. Elmwood JM. Critical Appraisal of Epidemiological Studies and Clinical Trials. Oxford: Oxford Univ Press, 1998:116–160.
18. Normand SL, Sykora K, Li P, Mamdani M, Rochon PA, Anderson GM. Readers guide to critical appraisal of cohort studies: 3. Analytical strategies to reduce confounding. BMJ 2005;330:1021–1023.
19. Oakes JM, Church TR. Invited commentary: Advancing propensity score methods in epidemiology. Am J Epidemiol 2007;165:1119–1121.
20. Feinstein AR. Scientific standards in epidemiologic studies of the menace of daily life. Science 1988;242:1257.
21. Mayes LC, Horwitz RI, Feinstein AR. A collection of 56 topics with contradictory results in case-control research. Int J Epidemiol 1988;17:680.
22. Sackett DL. Evaluation: Requirements for a clinical application. In: Warren KS (ed). Coping with the Biomedical Literature. New York: Praeger, 1981:123.

18 | Experimentation

Argument is conclusive . . . but it . . . does not remove doubt, so that the mind may rest in the sure knowledge of the truth, unless it finds it by the method of experiment.

—Roger Bacon[1]

Independent and Dependent Variables

A shorthand model for a simple experiment design follows:

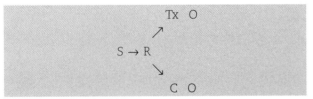

where S = selection of eligible subjects; R = randomization, an essential difference between experiment and quasi-experimental designs; Tx = treatment or manipulation of the independent variable; C = control; and O = observation of the dependent (or response) variable.

Ideally, an experiment is designed so that all properties, apart from those under investigation, are held constant. A property fixed in this way is commonly called a *parameter*. In *Great Scientific Experiments*, Harré[2] notes that many classic experiments depended on the skill of the experimenters in fixing parameters. For ex-

ample, caries incidence may be related to host factors, dietary factors, and microbiologic flora, and, to study any one of these factors, an investigator must consider the effect of the other variables. The variables under study are the dependent and independent variables. The factor, treatment, or variable manipulated by the experimenter is called the *independent variable*. The particular attribute measured in response to changes in the independent variable is called the *dependent variable*.

Consider the experiment[3] in Fig 18-1 in which the investigator applied a known load to a periodontal ligament and measured the amount it stretched (ie, the extension). The applied load is controlled by the experimenter and is, therefore, the independent variable. The extension of the ligament is the response to the load and is, therefore, the dependent variable. This figure is unusual, because the independent variable normally is plotted on the abscissa (x axis) with the dependent variable plotted on the ordinate (y axis). The dependent variable in one investigation may be the independent variable in another. Hence, in this example of periodontal ligament extension, it is possible that another investigator would stretch the ligament vari-

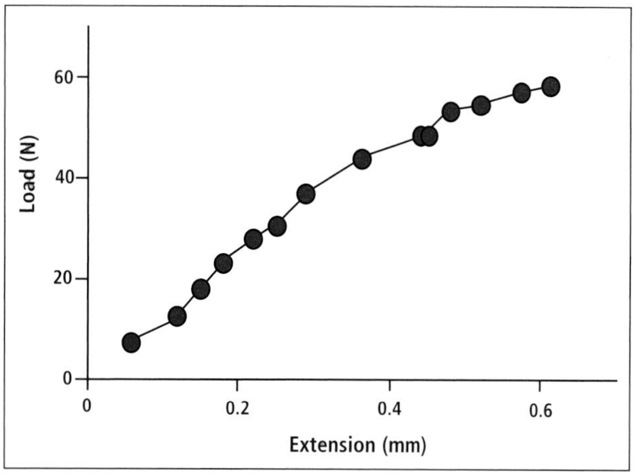

Fig 18-1 A known load (N) was applied to periodontal ligament and the extension (in millimeters) was measured. (Reprinted with permission from Atkinson and Ralph.[3])

ous distances and record some response (eg, the orientation of cells in the collagen fibers). The independent variable may be only one among many conditions that can affect the dependent variable.

Controlled vs uncontrolled or uncontrollable variables

In designing experiments, an investigator is often faced with an array of variables, some of which can be controlled and others of which cannot. The variable selected as an independent variable must be *controllable*. In a study on the effectiveness of dentifrices, it is fairly easy to control the type of toothpaste used by the subjects but difficult to control their diets. The golden rule in such situations appears to be to control what can be controlled and to measure (or observe) the rest. The measurements of the *uncontrolled variables* might prove useful in a retrospective analysis and help explain unexpected results.

Requirements for a Good Experiment

An experimenter must make decisions regarding factors such as definitions, sampling, experiment design,

measurement, statistics, and generalizing.[4] In a good experiment, these decisions are made satisfactorily. Some characteristics of a good experiment in biologic and clinical research follow.[5]

Adequate controls

The value of controls is that they eliminate plausible alternative hypotheses. A good experiment has *adequate controls*.

Difficulties

The most common method of induction is Mill's method of difference, which requires the experimental group to differ from the control group with respect to only one variable. However, obtaining a one-variable difference between groups is difficult to achieve. Consider the apparently simple problem, outlined by Heath,[6] of studying the effect of different concentrations of potassium ion (K^+) on cell cultures. For such an experiment, it is unfortunate that K^+ is only available in combination with an anion such as chloride (Cl^-). Thus, to change the K^+ concentration, an experimenter would also have to change the concentration of the anion. Second, in varying the K^+ concentration, the experimenter also varies the ratio of K^+ to all the other cations and anions in the culture medium. The effects of changes in these other variables are said to be *confounded* in this experiment; in other words, if an effect were found, it would be impossible to tell which of the changed variables (K^+, anion, ratios) caused the effect. Heath[6] has stated that "a treatment applied in an experiment is never simple in the sense that it alters only one factor," and, moreover:

> The limit to the number of such confounded effects for any experimental treatment is set only by our knowledge and powers of imagination. An experiment in which the application of treatments to the material under investigation has been properly randomized can yield an unbiased estimate of the effects of those treatments as applied; it gives no information as to which of the myriad components in any treatment comparison are responsible for the effects observed. That is a question of interpretation and is entirely a matter for the experimenter's judgment.

The reader of a scientific paper may not share the author's interpretation and may propose that the effect was really produced by one of the confounded variables.

Investigators have some options when confronted with confounded variables or concomitant effects. The first, and weaker, alternative is to quote the literature; in this example, investigators would need to reference papers stating that changes in Cl⁻ concentration had no effect on culture growth. However, relying on other work may be dubious, because there are inevitable differences between different experimental systems. These differences weaken the form of inductive argument used by the investigator in this situation (ie, argument by analogy). The better option is to design an experiment so that the particular variable causing concern is no longer confounded.

A significant difference between experiments in physics and chemistry and those in biology and medicine is that the variables that must be controlled in the physical sciences are often known and can be controlled. In studying chemical reaction rates, we know that we must control the temperature, but we do not have to worry about the phase of the moon. In contrast, in psychiatry, there are a vast number of factors that might influence behavior, including a subject's upbringing, genetic composition, biochemistry, and even—if apocryphal tales of correlation between criminal activity and a full moon are true—the phase of the moon. Moreover, in physics and chemistry, there are often laws that describe the relationship between variables so that an investigator can make valid comparisons between observations that were made under different conditions. In biology and medicine, no such precise laws are available. Thus, in physics and chemistry, although the equipment required must be precise and sophisticated, experiment designs are often, but not always, simple in comparison with the elaborate designs used in psychology and medicine.

Technical or conceptual sophistication does not cancel the need for controls. The challenge becomes devising appropriate controls when new investigational tools are developed. For example, antisense oligodeoxynucleotides (ODNs) can be used for the specific manipulation of gene expression. In theory, inhibition of gene expression is brought about when ODNs bind a complementary messenger RNA (mRNA) sequence and prevent translation of the mRNA. However, some early studies employing antisense ODNs gave erroneous results, because the investigators did not realize that there could be nonspecific effects of

ODNs and that ODNs did not necessarily enter the cell freely. The outcome was that additional controls were required to measure antisense effects and to differentiate them from nonspecific effects. Such controls included direct measurement of target RNA, careful choice of control sequences, and demonstration of cell permeability to the ODNs.[7] In summary, there was a development of knowledge about antisense ODN experiments that necessitated additional controls. These additional controls were recognized as being necessary only after the limitations and problems of the antisense ODN experiments were realized. This example shows that choosing appropriate controls requires a detailed and comprehensive knowledge of the biologic system under investigation.

It is difficult to have a well-controlled experiment in biology or medicine. It is a creative act to determine which of the many possible differences between the untreated control group and the treated (best thought of as the "treatment as applied") groups could be important and to devise appropriate control groups that eliminate plausible alternative hypotheses. Thus, it should be no surprise that many experiments published in the literature do not approach this standard.

Use and abuse of controls in the medical and dental literature

Studies on the use and abuse of controls have long appeared in the medical literature.[8] From such reviews, it is clear that:

1. *Controls are often absent in reports of clinical trials in the medical literature.* It seems that even the elementary principles of experimentation and the thoughts of J. S. Mill are not adequately appreciated by biomedical investigators.

2. *Experts vary in their estimate of the percentage of reports judged to be adequately controlled.* There could be many reasons for this variation, including the journal and time period studied, as well as the reviewer's standards. For example, Patterson[9] asserts that therapeutic regimens used in diseases whose known courses are quite constant require less rigid controls for evaluation, while Mahon and Daniel[10] believe that "probably the only clinical situation where no controls are necessary is the treatment of disease which is universally and rapidly fatal."

   Exactly what constitutes an adequate control is not a simple matter. A *true control* is one in which all the relevant variables (save the putative one being tested) are identical between the experimental and control groups. The number of relevant variables known depends on the state of knowledge of the particular area of science at a particular time. There is little investigators can do about this problem except to randomize their groups. In other cases, a relevant variable may be identified or known to be operative, and the problem becomes *how* investigators perform controlled experiments. This problem of experiment design will be discussed later (see chapter 19).

3. *Real controls are useful.* In a review comparing the results of controlled vs uncontrolled studies, Spilker[11] found that the success rate (ie, the proportion of papers that claimed that their therapy was useful) was much higher in uncontrolled than in controlled studies. In other words, authors whose studies lacked controls could not detect that other factors were at work that would explain their results. Spilker notes that his review supports "Muench's second law: Results can always be improved by omitting controls."[11]

Negative, positive, and active controls

In biologic experimentation, investigators examine the effects of biologic response modifiers (BRMs), which may be drugs, growth factors, changes in environmental conditions, genotype, or anything that might influence the components of a biologic system. However, biologic assay systems can exhibit day-to-day or batch-to-batch variation. In cell-culture experiments, experiments might not work on some days because some sort of contaminant, such as endotoxin, killed the cells or rendered them otherwise unresponsive. Such potential problems can be dealt with by incorporating positive and negative controls.

Negative controls

A *negative control,* is synonymous with most people's idea of a control and is easily understood. With the negative control, the biologic response is observed in an untreated group. The purpose of this control is to set up a direct comparison so that—as J. S. Mill would have liked—the experimental and control groups differ in only one important factor: the treatment.

Positive controls

Equally important, but less practiced, is the *positive control* that shows that the observed system is capable of response. In cell culture, a positive control for an experiment investigating a suspected growth factor would be to include a group in which the cells were exposed to a known growth factor. If the suspected growth factor did not produce any growth, but neither did the positive control, a technical problem would be suspected, and the effect of the suspected growth factor would be tested in another experiment. Without the positive control, the suspected growth factor might not be investigated further. Another value of positive controls is that they can identify an assay system in which no increased activity can be observed. The latter condition is sometimes called the *ceiling effect* (ie, when you are at the ceiling, there is no way to go higher). The frugal scientist might think that the effort placed in performing positive controls is wasted if the experimental treatment also produces a positive result. But such is not the case; even in the successful experiment, the positive control will enable the investigator to assess the potency of the BRM relative to that of the positive BRM in the control. Taken over time, positive controls also provide an estimate of assay variation by retrospective analysis. In short, positive controls are extremely useful and should be incorporated into more experiments.

Active controls

Sometimes it is not possible to perform a negative control in clinical studies. Suppose an investigator believes that a current therapy, while not optimal, does have some beneficial effect. Because there is a need to produce a better treatment, experimentation is required. Ethics dictate that the investigator could not withhold beneficial treatment to any patient, so there cannot be a group of untreated or placebo-treated controls. In such situations, it may be permissible to treat one group with the experimental BRM and the comparison group with the current best treatment. Those receiving the current best treatment are called the *active controls*; these subjects are really a type of positive control. The desired result is for the experimental BRM to outperform the active control. The other interpretable result is if the experimental BRM is less effective than the standard treatment. The problem occurs when there is no difference between the active control and the experimental BRM; then it is not clear whether either treatment was effective. In such a case, the standard problems in interpreting negative results occur, because there are many possible explanations for no effect. It is possible that the detection system was not sensitive enough, that the treatment was inadequate, that compliance with the treatment was inadequate, or that there was heterogeneity in those receiving treatment. If the population is heterogeneous with regard to response, the results will depend on the proportion of responders and nonresponders in the groups.

Adequate measurement and statistics

Absence of systematic error

For a clinical experiment, the absence of systematic error means that if the experiment were performed with a large number of subjects, it would give an accurate estimate of the treatment effects. In practice, this often means eliminating bias in the selection of the sample. In comparing Americans' heights with Canadians' heights, it clearly would be invalid to measure the heights of American men and compare them with the heights of Canadian women; the systematic difference (in this case sex) between the groups invalidates the comparison. In the parlance of experiment design, sex and nationality are confounded. If a significant difference occurred, the investigator would not know whether to attribute the difference to sex or nationality.

The second component of an experiment that must be free from systematic error is the scoring or measurement procedure. In the case of measurement, the instruments or techniques used must be accurate; that is, they must give a true indication of the value being measured. A third possible source of systematic error could occur if one group is examined more (or less) thoroughly than the other, as may happen when one group is hospitalized and the other is not.

Sufficient precision

If there is no systematic error, the estimate of the effect of treatment or variable will differ from the true value only by random error. A major challenge in designing experiments is to ensure that the random errors are not so large that they obscure the effects of the independent variable of interest. A number of techniques (see chapters 12, 14, and 20) are used to increase the precision of an experiment, such as refining methods or increasing the number of subjects.

Calculation of uncertainty

Every measurement is subject to variation caused by factors that cannot be controlled by the experimenter; this variation is called *random error*. Sensitive instruments can illuminate random error. The last digit on a digital pH meter will often change in the course of taking a measurement; one moment it will read 7.40; the next instant, 7.39; then, 7.41; and so on. Because it is known to exist in any experiment, the random error should be estimated. Otherwise, a critic could attribute the results to chance. To overcome such a criticism, investigators must have some estimate of the uncertainty in their results. When the random error is known, the investigators can assess the statistical significance of their data; that is, they can assess the probability that any difference between a treated and a control group was not just the result of chance.

A wide range of validity

As a general rule, the primary goal of experiments is to increase our understanding of nature and to improve our ability to control and predict events. But our ability to apply the knowledge gained from experiments to other situations is limited, because practical considerations dictate that only a small range of conditions can be examined. The more widely the experiment encompasses relevant variables, the greater the confidence we have in the extrapolation of the conclusions. Cox[4] believes that having a wide range of validity is particularly important in experiments performed to decide some practical course of action, and less important where the object is purely to gain insight into some phenomenon.

Case reports lack a wide range of validity. As a general rule, they are based on examination of a few individuals (perhaps even a single person) exhibiting unusual symptoms. The conclusions of case reports, if any, tend to have a very limited applicability. Case reports are seldom cited. Thus, if we accept the argument that citation frequency is a good indicator of the importance of a finding, the low citation frequency of case reports indicates that a wide range of validity is a condition for a significant result.

Simplicity

Simple experiments are preferred to complicated ones, because they are more likely to be executed correctly. Moreover, simple designs yield data that are easier to analyze. Nevertheless, complicated factorial designs can be more efficient when a wide range of conditions must be investigated. Hence, the investigator has to weigh the relative merits of simplicity, technical feasibility, cost, and range of validity.

Originality

Originality would appear to be a self-evident criterion, for the goal of all research is to make discoveries. Rewards in science are overwhelmingly allotted to scientists who demonstrate originality—that is, those who first arrive at a particular result.[12] At the simplest level, originality means that nobody has performed exactly the same experiment before. However, an investigator who only did experiments that met that simple requirement would not normally be classified as possessing an original mind. Original investigators have the ability to ask questions and perform experiments that add to our understanding. Such truly original work interests other investigators, who will subsequently cite it, because their own experiments will be based on it in some way.

Unfortunately, as Medawar[13] states, there is "no such thing as a calculus of discovery." Indeed, creativity has been analyzed from the perspectives of historians, biologists, psychologists, artists, and poets, but there is a continuing question of whether creativity can be learned. Root-Bernstein[14] has produced a book that exemplifies scientific discovery as it describes it. However, creativity can be abetted, Medawar[15] believes, "by reading and discussion and by acquiring the habit of reflection guided by the familiar principle that we are not likely to find answers to questions not yet formulated in the mind."

Types of Experiment Research

Beveridge[16] has discussed and classified types of experimentation in his book *The Art of Scientific Investigation:*

1. *Pure research* is done to gain knowledge for its own sake.
2. *Applied research* is a deliberate investigation of a problem of practical importance.
3. *Exploratory research* opens up new territory; however, some kinds of exploratory research are quasi-experimental. Anatomists are not *experimenting* in the strictest sense of the term when they dissect animals, but still they gather information by a manipulative act that would not normally take place in nature.
4. *Developmental research* consolidates the advances (also known as *pot-boiling*).
5. The *transfer method of research* applies an ordinary fact, principle, or technique from one branch of science to another, in which it may become novel. In Beveridge's opinion, this is the most fruitful and easiest method in research. From my experience on various granting committees, it seems also to be the most popular approach.

According to Harré,[17] the most common type of experiment is probably the measurement of some variable property under variable conditions. Robert Boyle's experiments on the relationship between pressure, volume, and temperature exemplify this kind of study to perfection.[18] They also illustrate—for Boyle had no effective way of controlling temperature—that in the real world, few processes are so simple that they comprise only a cause and effect, with no other variables entering the relationship.

The next most common experiments are those that attempt to link the structure of something found in an exploratory study to the processes going on in that structure.[17] Less common, but perhaps most important, are experiments that attempt to test a theory by proving the existence of something not previously identified in the real world. The search and isolation of cytokines and growth factors whose existence has been postulated but not verified exemplifies this type of study.

Both Beveridge[19] and Conant[20] have likened research to warfare against the unknown, and have outlined some useful tactics. On the psychology of discovery in biologic science, Beveridge advises use of the following tactics:

1. The investigator should follow up clues until the trail is exhausted; workers who change their problems repeatedly are usually ineffectual.

2. From time to time, the investigator should deliberately put the problem out of his or her mind for a while to get a fresh approach to the problem, a process Beveridge refers to as the *principle of temporary abandonment.*

3. The investigator should look for analogies between the problem presented and others that have been solved.

4. In publishing scientific papers, the investigator should present the results accurately, but should only cautiously suggest an interpretation, to distinguish clearly between facts and interpretation.

5. Discovery and proof are distinct processes. Discoveries are made by giving attention to small clues or discrepancies in data. Initially, a hypothesis formed on such a basis might not stand up to intense critical scrutiny. Such scrutiny should be reserved for later when the hypothesis is being proved.

Beveridge[19] recommends the following practical aspects of experimentation:

1. Test the whole before the parts. Before you can study anything, there must be some effect to study. Thus, it is often worthwhile to start with a complex system or extreme conditions of some kind, such as a massive dose of the compound of interest, to establish the effect.

2. After establishing the effect, the most important factors can be determined by systematic elimination.

3. Pilot or modest preliminary experiments are often useful in determining the types of problems that might be encountered and in identifying the approximate range of doses or other conditions that can be investigated in more detail later.

4. The investigator should understand the limitations and degree of accuracy of each technical method to obtain reliable results and to interpret them properly. The most common cause of error, according to Beveridge—and my own experience verifies his—is a mistake in technique.

Experiment Tactics

Experiment tactics can be thought of as the art of making experiments work. The general approach is to devise conditions so that the phenomenon of interest can be seen. The list of tactics used by investigators would

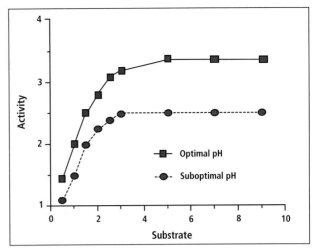

Fig 18-2 Relationship between velocity of an enzyme-catalyzed reaction and substrate concentration.

be almost endless, for any experiment involves tactical considerations. Three examples are presented here.

Assays and optimization

Many of the most-cited papers in biologic research deal with the development of methods to measure some biologic response. Indeed, much of the art of biologic and medical research consists of devising methods to quantify phenomena and to devise conditions where responses to various agents can be distinguished. Choosing the right conditions requires that decisions are made on how an experiment is to be done—a process that can be called *experiment tactics.* As an example of experiment tactics, we discuss *assays* here rather than in chapter 11 on measurement. Two general cases will be considered: *optimal* and *suboptimal conditions.*

To examine and better understand a complex process, it is often useful to isolate component phases and to consider each separately. Often, when biologic responses are depicted graphically, they take on a pattern where there is a linear (or nearly linear) portion of a curve and a plateau region. Consider the relationship between the velocity of an enzyme-catalyzed reaction and substrate concentration (Fig 18-2).

As the independent variable substrate concentration increases, the dependent variable reaction velocity increases almost proportionately. This is the *linear* (or, in this case, nearly linear) portion of the curve. At some point, there is a transitional zone, after which the reaction velocity remains constant despite the increase of the independent variable; this is the *plateau* portion of the curve. Depending on the nature of the problem, either portion of the curve may prove useful. If a biochemist were studying the effect of inhibitors on the reaction, it would be best to use the near linear portion of the curve, because it is the most sensitive portion for determining changes. However, if the goal of the experiment is to detect activity, it would be best to choose a substrate concentration on the plateau portion of the curve, as this is the area where optimal activity is found. Disturbances of the substrate (eg, by competitive inhibitors) would then be minimal. Note that, after determining the optimal substrate concentration, a biochemist might determine the optimum pH, ionic strength, or other factor. Thus, biochemists can control experimental variables reasonably well by breaking a complex problem (eg, enzyme activity) into parts (eg, substrate concentration, temperature, pH, etc).

This strategy works only after conditions have been established that allow the biochemist to see some activity. To arrive at this preliminary stage, tactics vary. Some investigators prefer the *synthetic approach* (adding factors one at a time until they see some response), while others prefer a *shotgun approach* (throwing everything conceivable into the mix or taking many precautions) and, if some response is seen, simplifying later.

For example, in developing his method for localized delivery of drugs, Max Goodson explained to me that he placed a periodontal pack on his patients, even though he did not think it was absolutely required. He simply wanted to take all possible steps to ensure that the released drug remained localized. This cautious type of approach is not unusual, but can result in needlessly complex procedures, if the subsequent step of simplification is not carried out.

Turning a problem into an asset

Another tactic—what might be called the "jujitsu method"—is to turn a problem into an asset. A common approach is the constructive use of variation. Variation is often viewed by investigators as a nuisance or problem to be overcome. Some experiment procedures, such as blocking (see chapter 19), are employed explicitly to reduce variation so that any experimental effects are more apparent. However, in some instances, variation can be employed productively, for it carries information about the experiment.

In 1943, Lüria and Delbruck[21] published a paper destined to become a classic of bacterial genetics. It had been discovered that resistant bacterial populations would emerge when exposed to a selective agent such as viruses (phages). The mechanism was not known. Do a few cells of the original population acquire resistance as a result of exposure to bacteriophage, or does the bacteriophage select for pre-existing resistant cells? Lüria and Delbruck devised an experimental test to answer the question (Fig 18-3). A broth culture of *Escherichia coli* was split into two; one half was cultured in a single culture (the mainline), whereas the other was further divided into multiple cultures (sublines). After growth, the cultures were tested for resistance to bacteriophage in replicate cultures. The replicate cultures from the mainline culture showed similar numbers of resistant colonies, while the sublines showed wide variation. This result could be explained by mutations conferring resistance that was random and spontaneous. If the mutation arose early in the subline culture, the subline would yield a large number of resistant cells, whereas if it arose later, only a few cells in the subline would be resistant. In contrast, the mainline culture would include some cells that mutated early and some late, giving rise to an intermediate number of resistant cells relative to the extremes found in the subline.

Note that in this assay Lüria and Delbruck were not interested in the absolute number of bacteria resistant to the bacteriophage, but rather in the variation between cultures. This experiment relied on recognizing the role of chance and using it constructively. In his autobiography,[22] Lüria, a Nobel laureate, recalled that he conceived the idea while watching a colleague play a slot machine at a faculty dance. The colleague hit a jackpot. The jackpot was analogous to the cultures that produce high numbers of resistant cells, and it dawned on Lüria that "slot machines and bacterial mutations have something to teach each other."

Use of inhibitors

A frequent approach in studying regulation of biologic processes such as cell proliferation is the use of *inhibitors*. Typically, inhibitors are used to identify a catalytic or regulatory activity that affects an end process. Many inhibitors are reversible and act conditionally, depending on the inhibitor's concentration and its duration of exposure to the biologic system. Inhibitor studies can be combined with biochemical and

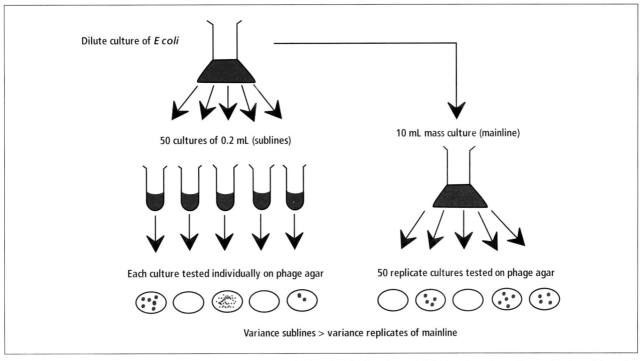

Fig 18-3 Culture of *Escherichia coli* split into single culture (mainline) and multiple cultures (subline) to investigate the mechanism of bacterio-phage resistance.

genetic approaches to determine the exact protein that interacts with the inhibitor and the contribution of the protein to the end process. A specific inhibitor should block the proposed process, but not other closely related reactions; for example, an inhibitor of DNA synthesis should not also block RNA synthesis. Failure of an inhibitor to affect a process suggests that the reaction normally modified by the inhibitor is not involved. A common problem in studies using inhibitors is the uncertain specificity or, worse, the known lack of specificity of some inhibitors. In some instances, the specificity is dose-dependent (ie, at low doses, the inhibitor might be specific and affect only one process, but, at higher doses, it might affect several). Thus, studies using inhibitors should use the lowest possible concentration.[23]

Tactical Considerations in Clinical Experiments

Clinical studies have a host of strategic and tactical considerations, many of which result from the interac-

tions of patients and investigators, and their state of knowledge and ethics. The investigator's intention also influences clinical research trial design; the investigator might strive to demonstrate *efficacy* (the ability of the intervention to produce effects in an ideal setting) or *effectiveness* (what the intervention accomplishes in actual practice). Spilker[24] has reviewed many of these studies in his *Guide to Clinical Studies and Developing Protocols*. Friedman et al[25] discuss the fundamentals of clinical trials, with an emphasis on trials demonstrating effectiveness. Some of the key considerations follow.

Outcome measures

In clinical studies, the selection of the *outcome measure* is a key decision. Ideally, it should be easy to ascertain or measure accurately. The outcome measure should be clinically relevant and, ideally, should avoid the problems associated with surrogate variables. The investigators should be able to observe or measure the outcome in all treatment groups. The measure should be chosen before the experiment begins, so that investigators may be spared the temptation of choosing the variable that best supports their hypothesis after data are collected. Moreover, the investigators have an ethical responsibility to monitor the safety and clinical benefit of an intervention during a trial, so that if the intervention was showing a clear benefit, the trial could be stopped so that subjects in the control group could benefit. Statisticians have devised *stopping rules* to determine the appropriate point at which a trial can be discontinued. These methods can entail repeated testing for significance that must adjust for the number of comparisons being made.[26,27] Similarly, a clinical trial may have to be discontinued if harmful effects are noted in those receiving treatment or the data are unlikely to show any significant effect.

The choice of outcome measure will influence the statistical test used to analyze the results—and thus the number of subjects required to obtain suitable power. The formula for determining the number of subjects for a *dichotomous response variable* (ie, success or failure) differs from one used for determining *continuous response variables* (eg, see Friedman et al[28]). The general rule is that a clinical trial should have sufficient statistical power to detect clinically interesting differences between groups.

Clinical therapies in dentistry are often evaluated in terms of technical performance, such as quality of margins. Technical performance is appropriate in evaluating quality only to the extent that the technical indicator is related to the clinical outcome. Bader and Shugars[29] state that the support for the relationship between some technical performance indicators (eg, amalgam polish) and adverse outcomes is often not well documented, for the outcomes of the treatments themselves are not well documented. The breadth and depth of knowledge vary across outcome categories, including such dimensions as physiologic (eg, pain, presence of pathologic states, assessment of function), psychological (eg, esthetics, satisfaction), economic (costs), and longevity/survival (eg, pulp death, tooth loss, time until repeat treatment). Bader and Shugars[29] conclude that dentistry is in an early period of the development of outcomes analysis and that most of dentistry's day-to-day procedures are rendered in the absence of comprehensive knowledge of their expected results.

Blinding

Research has repeatedly found that the clinician's or patient's faith in the treatment (or in the physician) can result in a considerable alleviation of symptoms, even when the treatment is a placebo with no active ingredient. The term *blind* refers to a lack of knowledge of the study treatment. Blinding the investigator and the patient to the treatment is done to prevent the placebo effect from interfering with a study. In an *open-blind* or *unmasked* study, both the clinician and the patient are aware of the treatment. In a *single-blind* treatment, one of them (usually the patient) does not know the treatment, but the other (usually the clinician) does. In a *double-blind* treatment, neither clinician nor patient knows which treatment the patient received. In some cases, it is difficult to disguise the treatment; for example, any treatment that stains teeth would be obvious to both the clinician and the patient. Spilker[30] cites instances where different results were obtained in single- and double-blind studies. For example, patients significantly improved their perceived taste acuity when treated with zinc sulfate in a single-blind study, but not in a double-blind, crossover study. One method of checking for the effectiveness of the blinding is to ask patients and investigators which treatment the patient received. Clinicians and patients can be quite perceptive in identifying treatments. In a supposed double-blind test of a betablocker in heart-attack patients, nearly 70% of physicians and more than 80% of patients correctly guessed whether the patients had received the drug or the placebo.[31]

Compliance

A *compliant* subject is one who is willing to carry out the procedures specified in the study protocol. Subjects may not wish to comply or may be incapable of complying for many reasons, including factors such as unpleasantness or complexity of the treatment, personality of the subject or the investigators, insufficient motivation, and lack of any discernible effect. Obviously, it is best to enroll only subjects who are likely to be compliant into an efficacy study. Compliance can be assessed by techniques such as counting pills, directly observing and questioning patients, obtaining biologic samples at spot checks, and examining patient diaries kept for this purpose. In our study of the effects of chlorhexidine-soaked dental floss, my graduate student checked compliance by both self-reports and measurements of the actual floss used. Compliance was important to assess in that study, because compliance is best obtained with simple interventions and using floss properly seems difficult for many people. Compliance can be improved by simplifying the demands, minimizing unpleasant events for the patients, allowing frequent contact between the patient and his or her family, and employing other motivational methods.[32]

Subject recruitment and loss

Clinical studies have eligibility criteria that define the type of subject that is required. Obtaining eligible subjects and retaining them is a major problem for investigators, for both these factors can introduce bias into the study. In setting the eligibility criteria, an investigator must strike a balance between obtaining a homogeneous population that will enhance the probability of seeing a result and a heterogeneous group that will better represent the general population. In general, ease of recruitment is inversely proportional to strictness of the eligibility criteria, but some criteria cannot be relaxed. Designing effective recruitment strategies requires some consideration of the target population's characteristics. Perri et al[33] found that the placement of advertisements in senior citizen newsletters was the most cost-effective method of recruiting for prosthodontic subjects from that group.

Ethics dictates that clinical studies should employ subjects who have the potential to benefit from the intervention; conversely, those who would be harmed by the treatment must be excluded. Patients who are assigned to a group by a randomization procedure but fail to complete the study because they are unwilling or unable to participate are called *dropouts*. *Withdrawals* are patients who have entered the study but have been excluded because there is an assignable cause for removing them, such as noncompliance. Spilker[34] has reviewed patient sources, factors that influence their recruitment, and techniques to increase recruitment. The most rigorous analysis, in which patients' results are analyzed in the groups to which they were assigned regardless of whether they complete treatment, is called *intention-to-treat analysis*. The intention-to-treat approach makes sense for effectiveness studies, because it estimates what happens when an intervention is prescribed for a patient. However, for efficacy studies, the goal is to evaluate under ideal conditions, a situation that would normally entail a subject's receiving the intervention.

Data quality

Much of the effort in performing clinical trials is spent ensuring that the data are collected in accordance with a protocol and are recorded accurately. Investigators must design data collection forms that collect standard information, such as the subject's name, schedule of treatments received, and values of measurements performed. In addition, the forms often allow for recording abnormal events or adverse reactions, as well as investigator comments. Any laboratory performing the measurement should have standard protocols and quality control measures to determine, for example, if values drift with time. Strategies to deal with unexpected values must be devised. Should measurements be repeated on samples that gave severely abnormal results? Should samples be tested at two separate laboratories and discrepant results checked? What standards should be used for the laboratory, and how frequently should instruments be calibrated? In addition, investigators must standardize procedures for clinical measurements; must prepare detailed instructions for subjects, clinicians, and support staff; and must follow protocols carefully.

Significant problems in data quality include (1) missing data, (2) inaccurate data, and (3) highly variable data. There are several ways of dealing with these problems; nevertheless, random external audits of clinical trial data[35] have found problems with data quality, such as failure of investigators to comply with recruitment criteria (6%), deviations from treatment protocol (11%), and recorded treatment responses (5%).[35] Altogether, problems with data quality seem to be sufficient to interfere with research efficiency.

Other strategic and tactical considerations for randomized controlled trials are discussed in chapter 19.

Typical Variables to Control or Consider in Biologic Research

Each scientific discipline has its own traditions about what variables must be closely controlled. For instance, even at the mundane level of washing glassware, differences exist. In general, chemists are meticulous in this regard, whereas microbiologists (at least before the advent of molecular biology) are typically more lax. Biologists might often be downright sloppy, unless performing cell culture, in which case they are ritualistic. These differences in standards of cleansing exist because the importance of clean glassware depends on the kind of experiment being done. Trace amounts of sulfur compounds could ruin an experiment on chemical catalysis but would likely have no effect on the growth of a hardy bacterium. Thus, for each type of study, there are variables that have been found to be important and that must be controlled. Knowing which variables are important is central to expertise in any discipline, and, given the diversity of biologic experimentation, no one could provide an exhaustive list of these variables. Nevertheless, Ingle[36] has outlined the major extrinsic and intrinsic variables that affect biologic and medical research; some of these are mentioned briefly here:

1. *Genetics.* Breeds and strains of animals differ in metabolic behavior in ways that can be crucial to investigators. In general, rodents seem to require the same vitamins as humans. But, unlike humans, rats synthesize their own vitamin C (do not attempt to make rats scorbutic by placing them on an ascorbic-acid–deficient diet). There is a whole industry developed for the production and distribution of inbred strains of animals with specialized features.
2. *Sex.* Sex differences have been found in metabolism, responsiveness to hormones and pharmacologic agents, susceptibility to pathologic changes, and longevity.
3. *Age.* The sensitivity of animals to hormones, food factors, and drugs varies with age.
4. *Activity.* The voluntary activity of laboratory animals and of humans varies greatly among individuals and may be cyclic in the same individual. Thus, it is said that civil servants do not look out the windows in the morning, because that is all they do in the afternoon. Muscular activity correlates with age up to sexual maturity and begins to decline when growth has stopped.
5. *Emotionality.* Ingle[36] states that in humans, correlations between emotional behavior and metabolic changes are abundant, but cause-effect relationships have been difficult to establish.
6. *Microbiologic pattern.* Dentists hardly need any reminder that the pathogenesis of periodontal disease and dental caries depends on the presence of certain microorganisms. Bacteria can also exist in a symbiotic relationship with animals—a relationship that might be adversely affected by antibiotics. There is growing evidence that latent viruses are involved in many diseases. These considerations complicate the interpretation of the responses observed to agents that might exert their influence indirectly by affecting the microbiologic pattern.
7. *Environment.* Environmental factors that must be controlled include light, temperature, ventilation, bedding materials, population density, juxtaposition of different species, and cage design. Like hospitals, animal-care facilities are now required to be accredited, a process that involves a site visit and a minute examination of conditions.
8. *Diet.* Navia[37] states that a common error in the design of experiments involving animals is the use of diets that are nutritionally and organoleptically inadequate. In such experiments, treatments are applied to animals that are not healthy; consequently, the results will be confounded by the presence of nutritional diseases, which may independently affect the parameters being measured.

References

1. Bacon R. Opus Maius. Part IV: Mathematics in the science of theology. 1267.
2. Harré R. Great Scientific Experiments. Oxford: Oxford Univ Press, 1983:16.
3. Atkinson HF, Ralph WJ. In vitro strength of the human periodontal ligament. J Dent Res 1977;56:48–52.
4. Plutchik R. Foundation of Experimental Research. New York: Harper and Row, 1974:33.
5. Cox DR. Planning of Experiments. New York: Wiley, 1958:10.
6. Heath OVS. Investigation by Experiment, No. 23, Institute of Biology's Studies in Biology Series. London: Edward Arnold, 1970:9–16.
7. Wagner RW. Gene inhibition using antisense oligodeoxynucleotides. Nature 1994;372:333.
8. Ross OB. Use of controls in medical research. JAMA 1951;145:72.
9. Patterson HR. Controls in clinical studies. Lancet 1962;1:90.
10. Mahon WA, Daniel EE. A method for the assessment of reports of drug trials. Can Med Assoc J 1964;90:565.
11. Spilker B. Guide to the Clinical Interpretation of Data. New York: Raven, 1986:340.
12. Meadows AJ. Communication in Science. Toronto: Butterworths, 1974:54.
13. Medawar PB. The Limits of Science. Oxford: Oxford Univ Press, 1984:16.
14. Root-Bernstein RS. Discovering: Inventing and Solving Problems at the Frontiers of Scientific Knowledge. Cambridge, MA: Harvard Univ Press, 1989.
15. Medawar PB. Induction and Intuition in Scientific Thought. London: Methuen, 1969:57.

16. Beveridge WIB. The Art of Scientific Investigation. New York: Vintage, 1950:171–175.

17. Harré R. Great Scientific Experiments. Oxford: Oxford Univ Press, 1983:17.

18. Conant JB. On Understanding Science. New York: Mentor, 1951:41–68.

19. Beveridge WIB. The Art of Scientific Investigation. New York: Vintage, 1950:20–35.

20. Conant JB. On Understanding Science. New York: Mentor, 1951:102–111.

21. Luria SE, Delbruck M. Mutations of bacteria from virus sensitivity to virus resistance. Genetics 1943;28:491–511.

22. Lüria SE. A Slot Machine, A Broken Test Tube. New York: Harper and Row, 1989:75.

23. Pardee AB, Keyomarsi K. Modification of cell proliferation with inhibitors. Curr Opin Cell Biol 1992;4:186.

24. Spilker B. Guide to Clinical Studies and Developing Protocols. New York: Raven, 1984.

25. Friedman LM, Furberg CD, DeMets DL. Fundamentals of Clinical Trials, ed 3. New York: Springer, 1998.

26. Friedman LM, Furberg CD, DeMets DL. Fundamentals of Clinical Trials, ed 3. New York: Springer, 1998:246–283.

27. Elwood JM. Critical Appraisal of Epidemiological Studies and Clinical Trials, ed 2. Oxford: Oxford Univ Press, 1998:182–185.

28. Friedman LM, Furberg CD, DeMets DL. Fundamentals of Clinical Trials, ed 3. New York: Springer, 1998:94.

29. Bader I, Shugars DA. Variation, treatment outcomes, and practice guidelines in dental practice. J Dent Educ 1995;59:61.

30. Spilker B. Guide to Clinical Studies and Developing Protocols. New York: Raven, 1984:16.

31. Byington RP, Curb JD, Mattson ME. Assessment of double-blindness at the conclusion of the beta-blocker heart attack trial. JAMA 1985;253:1733.

32. Spilker B. Guide to Clinical Studies and Developing Protocols. New York: Raven, 1984:133–139.

33. Perri R, Wollin S, Drolet N, Mai S, Awad M, Feine J. Monitoring recruitment success and cost in a randomized clinical trial. Eur J Prosthodontics Restorative Dent 2006;14: 126–130.

34. Spilker B. Guide to Clinical Studies and Developing Protocols. New York: Raven, 1984:236–240.

35. Friedman LM, Furberg CD, DeMets DL. Fundamentals of Clinical Trials, ed 3. New York: Springer, 1998:167.

36. Ingle DJ. Principles of Research in Biology and Medicine. Philadelphia: Lippincott, 1958:67–79.

37. Navia JM. Animal Models in Dental Research. Birmingham, AL: Univ of Alabama Press, 1977:51.

19 | Experiment Design

But for the moment, let us stop with the idea that the scientist cannot just go off and "experiment." It takes some long and careful thought—and often a strong dose of difficult mathematics.
—David Salsburg[1]

In designing experiments, investigators typically make decisions about five major components: *(1)* treatments or interventions, which are generally the research interests driving the experiment; *(2)* experimental units, which might be teeth, mouths, animals, or plots in a field; *(3)* population/sample, which defines the group about which the investigators want to generalize and from which they must sample; *(4)* allocation, which is the manner in which the treatments are allocated to experimental units (usually by a specified randomization procedure); and *(5)* outcome, which comprise the counts or measurements to be made on the experimental units.

The *precision* of an experiment, like the precision of a measurement, indicates the closeness with which the experiment estimates some quantity; it is measured as the reciprocal of the variance per observation.[2] If an experiment were changed so that the diet of the subjects was no longer controlled, the variance in the amount of bacterial plaque found in the subjects' mouths might increase twofold. In that event, twice as many subjects as were used in the experiment in which diet was controlled would be required to estimate the mean for the treatment with the same variance. The *efficiency* of experiment designs may be considered the number of experimental units required to gain a certain precision. The relative efficiencies of two experiment designs are given by the ratios between their precisions.[2] Because most investigations operate under financial constraints, efficiency is an important concept, since it relates directly to the cost of the experiment. The greater number of experimental units used in a less efficient design will add to the cost.

Experiment design is a complex subject that has received comprehensive treatment in numerous textbooks.[2–6] Only some of the simpler designs and more essential issues will be considered here.

Managing Error

A fundamental goal of experiment design is to minimize the effects of error. In dealing with error, the investigator has four basic options: avoid the error, distribute the error, measure the error, or make the error relatively small.

Avoiding sources of error

Avoiding the sources of error is the usual approach in the physical sciences and is most often accomplished by identifying relevant variables and improving methods to bring the variables under control.

Distributing error

If the source of error cannot be eliminated, it may still be possible to arrange the experiment so that the particular error is distributed equally among the groups in the experiment. This principle was first applied in agricultural science to divide fields and partition the treatments into different areas. Indeed, much of the terminology used in experiment design reflects this agricultural heritage (eg, experimental units are called *plots*). Several of the designs described in this chapter are effective because of the manner in which they distribute the error.

Measuring error

Some errors are unavoidable and cannot be distributed. In such cases, the investigator must measure the error and report it or correct for it.

Example 1: Measurement of absorbance

Among the first scientific laws formulated were the laws describing the absorption of light by solutions. Using a spectrophotometer to measure the amount of light a solution absorbs enables an experimenter to estimate the concentration of a chemical within that solution. This measurement is common in biologic and chemical laboratories, and the various problems associated with it are well recognized. In brief, the amount of light absorbed by a sample of solution contained in a cuvette is measured with a photocell, according to the Beer-Lambert law. This law states that absorbance $A = abc$; where a is a constant for the material in solution, b is the path length in the cuvette, and c is the concentration. The concentration c can be calculated after measuring A (since a and b are known).

One possible error is that some light could reflect off the walls of the cuvette and other interfaces and never reach the photocell. It is common practice to correct for this error by measuring it. In this case, the correction involves measuring the absorbance of a cuvette filled with water. This control is called a *blank*. The absorbance of the sample solution is then calculated as: A = A sample – A blank = abc. A second problem occurs when another molecule that interferes with the measurement is also in the cuvette. For example, in the Lowry method for measuring protein, the protein is reacted with Folin reagent in the presence of a buffer containing Cu^{2+} ions. However, the Folin reagent absorbs some light. In this instance, the blank is not distilled water but the reaction mixture without added protein to control for the absorption of the Folin reagent.

Another issue concerns the varying apparatuses used to measure absorbance; there are different kinds of spectrophotometers, which have different advantages. Dual-beam models are used to get around the problem of instability of the light source. Although such variability would not be a serious problem for routine measurements, it might be a significant source of error if very small differences were measured.

In any case, the purpose of this example is to show that measuring or correcting for the error is a common and useful procedure that can be applied at various levels of sophistication.

Example 2: Correction via internal controls or standards

In the previous example, adjustments were made to the system from the outside (ie, by using a blank or a dual-beam instrument that could be manipulated outside the solution itself). Sometimes this is not enough and an internal standard or control is used. One problem encountered in measuring radioactivity by liquid scintillation is *quenching*. When quenching occurs, some of the bursts of light that would normally be produced and counted are blocked by interfering substances or conditions. Ideally, the experimenter would remove the interference, but often this is not possible because the sample itself is responsible for the quenching. To circumvent this problem, a known amount of radioactivity is added to the sample. We can then calculate what the new (increased) count should be and compare it with what the count actually is. Suppose the observed counts per minute (cpm) of a sample were 200. One could add 100 cpm of a radioactive standard to the sample. The expected value would equal the sample plus the radioactive standard (ie, 200 + 100 = 300 cpm). If the new observed value = 250 cpm, 50 cpm were lost. Therefore 50 out of 100 means that 50% of the counts of the radioactive standard were lost. Thus, it seems likely that 50% of the counts in the sample were also lost when the original sample was counted. Furthermore, because one half of the counts was lost, the original value for the sample should be multiplied by 2. The corrected value would be 200 cpm × 2 = 400 cpm.

Example 3: The reconstruction experiment

Investigators often wish to demonstrate that the effect of a particular treatment or procedure is negligible. The lack of an effect can sometimes be demonstrated by means of a *reconstruction experiment*. To test various cavity cleansers, Vlietstra et al[7] devised a technique whereby a broth containing *Micrococcus luteus* was dripped into the cavity during preparation. The cavity was then treated (eg, with Cavilax), and the investigators attempted to recover *M luteus* from the cavity. However, they discovered a potential problem. During the cavity preparation, an aerosol was created that could recontaminate cavities to give false-positive results on their test. To estimate the magnitude of this potential problem, they did a reconstruction experiment whereby they prepared cavities without dripping the *M luteus* into them during preparation. These cavities were exposed to the atmosphere in the same manner as the treated groups. Because none of these controls was found to be contaminated, this reconstruction experiment was able to rule out the possibility that those treated cavities that contained *M luteus* were contaminated after treatment. Reconstruction experiments of this type are extremely useful in dealing with unavoidable errors due to observation or treatment.

Making error relatively small

Error can be made relatively small in two ways.

1. Increasing the potential difference between treated and control groups

When this strategy is adopted, the investigator tries to perform the experiment under conditions that are maximally favorable for demonstrating a given effect. It is one of the oldest and most effective techniques in the experimenter's arsenal. To take a historical example, one reason advanced for Lavoisier's success in 1775 in discovering the role of oxygen in combustion was that he used materials (sulfur and phosphorus) that demonstrated a *prodigious* (to use Lavoisier's

term) increase in weight on burning. Other investigators used metals, such as tin, which increased only by about 25%. With the crude instruments available at the time, Lavoisier could detect the large difference in weight after burning phosphorus, whereas others could not detect the increase in weight of the metals clearly enough to discount the phlogiston theory.[8] In biologic research, the potential difference between treated and control groups can often be increased by using a high-risk population. This stratagem ensures that something will likely happen.

In testing the effectiveness of oral hygiene procedures on gingival indices, the population under study is often ordered not to brush their teeth for some period of time prior to and/or during the experiment. This stratagem ensures that the subjects will have plaque on which the test procedure can work. If a study tested a mouthrinse on dental students (who often volunteer for experiments of this type) but gave no instructions to avoid teeth brushing, the chances of seeing any effect would be small, because the students' oral hygiene would inhibit plaque formation. The same principle applies to other instances in which investigators select a population that is likely not only to respond to whatever treatment is applied but to respond maximally. The idea behind such a strategy is to increase the signal-to-noise ratio. Thus, if the error remains the same, it is easier to distinguish the effect of a treatment from the error by using a high-risk population that increases the size of the response.

Chilton[5] notes that, because dental caries formation is most active during childhood and adolescence, the best trial would be run in a group in which these ages are well represented, rather than in an older population in which the caries process is no longer as active. However, the lowest age group studied should be one in which a sufficient number of permanent teeth are present to give a large enough susceptible tooth population. Too many primary teeth in the population makes for added difficulty because of the variability associated with the exfoliation of teeth.

In an experiment on the effect of diet on rat caries, the investigator feeds the animals some agent with potential anti-cariogenic activity, such as xylitol, and measures the number of caries lesions over time. The problem is that with a normal diet, few caries lesions might develop. Thus, the rats are fed a diet containing 20% sucrose and are inoculated with the caries-producing *S mutans*. In this way, an investigator can induce the caries process in 15 of the 16 fissures at risk, and the effectiveness of any treatment can be more readily demonstrated.

2. Making the error smaller

The error can be made smaller in several ways. For example, the method can be improved (precise and accurate methods of measurement produce smaller errors and increase the power of an experiment), and the homogeneity of the population can be increased. Homogeneity might be achieved by using experimental units of the same age, sex, genetic background, subculture, state of oral hygiene, or other factors. This will eliminate variability in the observations that arise because of systematic differences in the sample attributable to these factors. However, this method limits the generality of the conclusions.

Increasing the sample size reduces the *standard error* (SE). The decrease in the SE is proportional to the square root of the sample size. Thus, to reduce the SE by a factor of three, we have to increase the sample size nine times.

Increasing homogeneity and sample size are simple means to make the error smaller, but sometimes more complex methods are needed to measure and/or distribute the error.

Some Common Experiment Designs

Randomized controlled trial

The *randomized controlled trial* (RCT) is based on Mill's method of difference and is recognized as a strong research design. In an RCT, a group of experimental units (patients, animals, or cultures) are randomly allocated into two or more groups. The experimental groups receive treatment, while the control group gets nothing (negative control), conventional treatment (active control), or a placebo. In a parallel trial, the groups are treated separately but concurrently as part of the same study. Sometimes, an attempt is made to minimize biases by having neither the subject nor the investigator know which group received experimental treatment until the trial is over (a *double-blind* trial).

Randomization

Randomization is the control technique whereby each subject or object to be measured has an equal probability of being included in a given treatment group.

Therefore, the groups to be compared should, on a statistical basis, be the same at the beginning of the experiment, so that any differences observed at the end of the experiment are the result of some treatment. A second reason for randomization is that it removes investigator bias in assigning participants to groups. Randomization is not necessarily easy and is not synonymous with *haphazard selection* for several reasons outlined by Mainland,[6] including the possibility of the purposeful, although well-intentioned, steering of patients to a favored treatment. Nor is it synonymous with *alternated assignment* (ie, Patient 1 gets treatment; Patient 2 is a control; Patient 3 gets treatment, etc). In general, the use of an alternate subject method of assignment risks confounding sequence and treatment.[6] It has been said that nearly every human being has a tendency away from true randomness when making choices. Moreover, such procedures as the "every nth name technique," which appear to produce random samples, are not reliable, because alphabetical lists contain clusters from racial origins, blood relationships, and even marriage. Current standards of experiment design demand that the method used for randomization be reported.

Once the sample groups have been chosen, some characteristic is measured. Because (at least theoretically) the groups are identical in every other variable prior to treatment, it is concluded that any difference in the treated group is caused by the treatment. Randomization commonly occurs in two basic forms.

Stratified randomization entails classifying the subjects on some variable and dividing the subjects into strata (eg, high, medium, and low values for the measurement). Then, for each level, subjects are randomly allocated into the treated and control groups. For many purposes, this is the equivalent of *blocking* (discussed later in this chapter). Another form of randomized sample selection is *adaptive sampling,* which can take several forms and can introduce other considerations, such as balancing the numbers in the groups, baseline characteristics, or participant response to a given intervention. However, for all of these considerations, it remains true that a randomizing procedure will be involved in selecting which subjects go to which groups.

Along with its virtues, randomization has its problems as a guarantor of making comparisons free of systematic error, which might result because the groups are not equivalent in some important property that helps determine outcome. Chalmers et al[9] studied how such determinants are partitioned between groups and concluded that at least one determinant was significantly maldistributed in 14% of trials. The possibility of such maldistribution is highest when selections are made from small heterogeneous groups. Blair[10] discusses several ways to deal with this issue; in particular, *minimization* is an allocation strategy that seeks to minimize differences in the distributions of outcome determinants between groups.

Bivalent vs functional experiments

In a *bivalent* experiment, only two conditions are used. The *t* test is the usual statistical test employed in comparing the two groups. The main danger is *overgeneralization*, because bivalent experiments test a treatment under only very limited conditions. It is possible for the treatment to be ineffective at the particular level or time chosen but effective at higher (or lower) concentrations or at other times. Bivalent experiments do not demonstrate a pattern in the results, nor do they necessarily test the treatment under optimal conditions.

In *functional experiments,* one variable (the independent variable) is given three or more values, and the characteristic of interest (dependent variable) is measured at each level on randomly selected groups. The results of the measurement vs the value of the independent variable are plotted. Functional experiments have several advantages:

1. They test for the effect of the independent variable over a wider range of values.
2. They enable relationships between the variables to be seen. This is particularly important if there is a theory that explains the relationship. In those cases where a hypothesis predicts a certain mathematical relationship between the variables, it is important to remember that, simply because a group of data points fits a certain curve, this curve is not necessarily the only one that suits the data. There are probably other mathematical formulae that would also give a good fit. Gilbert[11] notes,

> There are no rules for choosing curves. Choice of an appropriate formula is largely a matter of experience. Where the data show a steady (even though nonlinear) progression, it is usually quite easy to find several different curves and different mathematicians tend to favor different types of curve. Provided there is no theoretical reason to prefer one over another and provided we do not want to extrapolate along the curve beyond the range of operations, any one of these curves may be adopted.

Thus, before accepting a well-fitted curve as evidence for a particular hypothesis, we must be sure (as always) that an alternative hypothesis does not predict a formula that also fits the data.

3. They enable *interpolation* (ie, estimation of the values of the dependent variable) between values of the independent variable. *Extrapolation* (ie, estimation beyond the range of the independent variable) is also more accurate than a bivalent experiment, but this procedure is obviously subject to more error than interpolation.
4. I believe that, like a house of cards—in which the group is more solid than any individual card—several data points demonstrating a pattern of response are much more believable than the evidence afforded by a single point. However, the appropriate statistical tests of the data must be made before the relationship can be deemed significant.
5. There is a problem when the points on the curve are sampled from a potentially heterogeneous population. In one part of my thesis research, I examined the effect of an inhibitor on an enzyme found in tissue-culture cells. I found a maximum of 80% inhibition and concluded that this was the most that this enzyme could be inhibited. To my embarrassment, it was pointed out at my oral examination that it was possible that the cells were heterogeneous. Thus, my data could be explained by supposing that in 80% of the cells, the enzyme was completely inhibited and in the other 20% of the cells, completely uninhibited. The points on many published curves are, in reality, the averages of samples taken from populations that may be heterogeneous. For example, a problem in measuring the growth of children is that there is a change in the rate of change (an acceleration or a deceleration), because different individuals spurt or slow down at different distances from the starting point. The method of averaging can create false estimates of the time and size of growth spurts in children.[12]

A major practical limitation with functional experiments is that often only one variable can be changed at a time. This, it shall be seen, can be a very inefficient way of finding information. The data are generally analyzed with regression analysis, using the least squares method.

Matched-group designs: Overcoming differences in relevant variables

Matching

When the number of subjects is small and the variation of the characteristic under consideration is large, randomization may not yield truly equivalent groups. *Matching* techniques perform a dual function of reducing the error and, at the same time, controlling the variable on which the subjects or objects are matched.

One problem with the random-groups design is that it is possible, because of random sampling fluctuations, that the two groups are not identical or even similar. One way to avoid this problem is to match the groups. For example, if we were testing the effect of some agent on bone growth in rat calvaria in organ culture, we would cut the calvarium in two, and one half would serve as a control while the other half would be treated. This procedure would be repeated for each of the rat embryos. In this way, one variable (size of a half calvarium, which exhibits much less variability within a rat than within a litter) could be controlled. Matching enables the experimenter to reliably detect differences between groups with a smaller number in the experimental groups than would be needed in the random-groups designs. Unfortunately, the matched-group design is more sensitive to the detection of small effects at the expense of the generality of the conclusions; one can only guess whether the effect is large enough to be observed in randomly selected heterogeneous populations.

Pairing

The power of *pairing* is evident from an example, cited by Beveridge,[13] in which growth rates of calves were studied; identical twins were about 25 times more useful than ordinary calves. Pairing is not always useful; one of van Belle's[14] statistical rules of thumb is that one should not pair data unless the correlation between the pairs is greater than 0.05.

Blocking: Building the extraneous variable into research design

Blocking is the practice whereby groups of experimental units that have some property (such as males, females, samples obtained from one patient, litter-mates) are made up in advance, and members of the block are assigned randomly to the treatments.

Blocking might be efficiently used in a test of a drug that was applied to both males and females (Fig 19-1). The block test population would be divided into male and female blocks, and members of each block would be randomly assigned to the treated and control groups. In this way you could control the variation (because for many kinds of measurements, there would be large differences between males and females), but you could also find whether there was a difference in male and female response to the drug. Blocking makes the experiment more efficient because the effects of variation are reduced. In studies on rat caries, Marthaler[15] found that a significant litter effect was found in 13 of 16 experiments. In other words, some litters were more or less caries-prone than others. To avoid this source of variation, we could arrange matters so that each treatment is applied to one member of each of a number of litters. By blocking the litters in this way, the investigators found that the efficiency of the blocked experiment was 143% relative to 100% for a completely randomized design.

Yoked controls

Another way of managing an extraneous variable is to incorporate a suitable control into the experiment design. Consider Fig 19-2, which shows the influence of ascorbic acid on weight gain in guinea pigs. Since vitamin C would usually be in the diet of these animals, the group having the diet with vitamin C would be considered the control. The experimental group would be vitamin C deficient, and these animals would not gain weight in the same manner as the controls.

However, most nutrient deficiencies cause a state of inanition, and the animal in the experimental group progressively restricts its intake of the deficient diet. Therefore, the experimental animals would be deficient not only in vitamin C but also in other nutrients. As explained by Alfano,[16] this problem may be solved by including a pair-fed control—that is, animals receiving the vitamin C diet would be allowed to eat only the amounts consumed by their counterparts on the deficient diet. The result is shown in Fig 19-3. Although vitamin C still has an effect, it is not as large as would be inferred from Fig 19-2. The pair-fed control is an example of a *yoked control*. In this example, a relevant variable (total food consumption) on weight gain has been controlled.

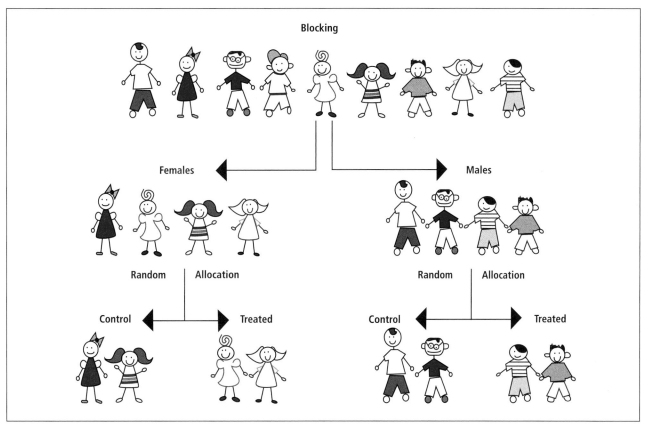

Fig 19-1 Illustration of blocking technique to reduce variation and determine if a drug affects males and females differently.

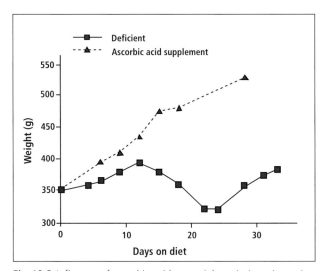

Fig 19-2 Influence of ascorbic acid on weight gain in guinea pigs. (Reprinted from Alfano[15] with permission.)

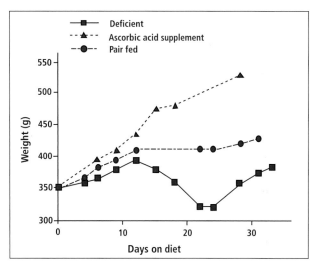

Fig 19-3 Addition of pair-fed control to study in Fig 19-2. (Reprinted from Alfano[15] with permission.)

Factorial design

A dogma for some scientists is that the only legitimate way of doing experiments is to vary one factor at a time. This dogma has proved to be false. According to Fisher,[17]

No aphorism is more frequently repeated in connection with field trials than that we must ask Nature few questions or ideally one question at a time. The writer is convinced that this view is

Table 19-1 Ulcerogenicity scores, varying one factor at a time*

Group	Aspirin dose (mg/kg)	Indomethacin dose (mg/kg)	Ulcerogenicity score
A	0	0	0
B	250	0	6
C	0	10	23
D	250	10	71

*Data from Shaw and Wischmeier.[19]

Table 19-2 Ulcerogenicity scores, varying one factor at a time*

		Indomethacin dose (mg/kg)	
		0	10
Aspirin dose (mg/kg)	0	0(A)	23(C)
	250	6(B)	71(D)

*Data from Shaw and Wischmeier.[19]

wholly mistaken. Nature, he suggests, will best respond to a logical and carefully thought-out questionnaire. Indeed, if we ask her a single question she will often refuse to answer until some other topic has been discussed.

The need to vary several factors at a time is particularly important in areas of research where time is an important factor, such as agriculture, where there may be only one growing season per year. Accordingly, Fisher designed experiments that resembled carefully thought-out questionnaires. These *factorial designs* have the following advantages:

1. It is possible to obtain information on the average effects of all of the factors economically in a single experiment of moderate size.
2. It broadens the basis of inference on one factor by testing it under varied conditions of others.
3. It is possible to study the interactions of the factors.[18]

Suppose we were investigating the production of gastric mucosal damage in rats that were being given aspirin and indomethacin, separately and in combination. The data given here (adapted from Shaw and Wischmeier[19]) were expressed as ulcerogenicity scores (Table 19-1). The data could also be arranged as shown in Table 19-2. First we will consider the effect of aspirin. Two comparisons can be made: the effect of aspirin by itself (ie, at 0 dose of indomethacin), which involves comparing groups B and A (ie, 6 vs 0), and the effect of aspirin at 10 mg/kg, which involves comparing groups D and C (ie, 71 vs 23). Note that in each of these two comparisons the only variable that differs between the groups is the presence of aspirin. The average effect for aspirin can be calculated as follows:

$$\text{Aspirin effect} = \frac{1}{2}[(B - A) + (D - C)]$$
$$= \frac{1}{2}[(6 - 0) + (71 - 23)]$$
$$= 27$$

Similarly, the effect of indomethacin can be calculated as follows:

$$\text{Indomethacin effect} = \frac{1}{2}[(C - A) + (D - B)]$$
$$= \frac{1}{2}[(23 - 0) + (71 - 6)]$$
$$= 44$$

The two effects calculated above are the so-called primary effects. If there were no interaction (discussed later) between the variables, a model of the data could be developed in which each observed data point could be constructed as follows:

$$Y \text{ (data point)} = M \text{ (mean)} + \text{effect of aspirin} + \text{effect of indomethacin} + \text{error}$$

The idea behind the model is that aspirin and indomethacin contribute to changing the observed data from the overall mean value.

For group C:

$Y_C = 23 =$

+25	The mean for all 4 data points equals 25
+ (−13.5)	The effect of aspirin was 27; this is partitioned as −13.5 to those groups that do not get aspirin, such as group C, and +13.5 to those that do
+ (+22)	The effect of indomethacin partitioned as −22 to those that do not receive indomethacin, and +22 to those that do receive indomethacin, such as group C
+ [error]	

Table 19-3 Interaction effect of aspirin and indomethacin on ulcerogenicity

Data		Mean		Aspirin		Indomethacin		Interaction	
0	23	25	25	−13.5	−13.5	−22	22	10.5	−10.5
6	71	25	25	13.5	13.5	−22	22	−10.5	10.5

From this we can calculate that the error term equals −10.5.

However, our model did not consider that there might be an interaction between the variables. The *interaction effect* can be considered the question of whether the increase in ulcers in rats treated with indomethacin depended on the presence of aspirin.

The interaction is calculated as follows:

$$\frac{1}{2}[(D - B) - (C - A)]$$
$$= \frac{1}{2}[(71 - 6) - (23 - 0)]$$
$$= 21$$

The interaction effect would be equally partitioned among all four points. To incorporate this idea, the model would be revised as follows:

$$Y_C = 23 = (\text{mean} + \text{aspirin effect} +$$
$$\text{indomethacin effect} +$$
$$\text{interaction}) + \text{error}$$
$$= 25 - 13.5 + 22 - 10.5$$
$$= 23$$

Thus, after considering the interaction, the error term equals 0. (Note that because there are no replications in this data set, error cannot be estimated.)

Overall, the model for this experiment can be represented as shown in Table 19-3. This model indicates how the data were produced (ie, why the data points are what they are). Next we must ask: How are the data analyzed? Is the effect of aspirin or indomethacin significant? The latter question cannot be answered for the example data set because there are no replications. If there were replications—ie, more than one data point per cell—the analysis would be accom-

plished by *analysis of variance* (ANOVA). For factorial designs, this can be quite complex; however, most statistics packages for microcomputers are able to perform such analyses.

Note that, generally, when we include the interaction term, the value estimated for the error drops. In ANOVA, the reduction of the error has an important consequence—it becomes easier to demonstrate a significant effect (because the mean square of the error is reduced). Because most research workers are interested in obtaining significant effects, this technique appears to be the royal road to happiness, but, like many good things, there is a catch. If an interaction proves significant, one must modify the conclusion concerning the two primary effects. It is possible that these primary effects are significant only because of the contribution of the data points where the interaction occurred (ie, the primary effects are only effective when they are applied together). This can be tested by another experiment—or in some cases by a reevaluation of the data, if they can be combined so that the points where the interaction occurred are not considered. In summary, the conclusions regarding the main effects have to be modified in such a way as to make them less general either by stating that there exists some subgroup within the experiment where the primary effect was greater than other subgroups, or by stating that the primary effect was not found at all in some subgroups.

Complex factorial designs are being used in biomedical research, but comparatively rarely. This is unfortunate given the method's power.

When we plot the data from a factorial design (Figs 19-4 and 19-5), we can get an indication of whether an interaction occurs. If no interaction occurs (see Fig 19-5),

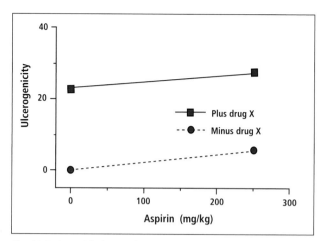

Fig 19-4 Data from factorial design, indicating an interaction between indomethacin and aspirin.

Fig 19-5 Factorial design data, indicating no interaction between drug X and aspirin. Lines are parallel.

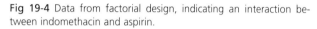

	Group 1 (G₁) Proxygel then placebo	Group 2 (G₂) Placebo then Proxygel	Difference Proxygel and placebo
Measured at end of period 1 (P₁)	2.44 ($Y_{P_1G_1}$)	3.17 ($Y_{P_1G_2}$)	–0.73
Measured at end of period 2 (P₂)	2.45 ($Y_{P_2G_1}$)	1.86 ($Y_{P_2G_2}$)	–0.59
Difference P₁ – P₂	–0.01	+1.31	

Table 19-4 Example of crossover design*

*Adapted from Zinner et al[20] with permission.

the lines are parallel. But in the paper by Shaw and Wischmeier,[19] there does seem to be some interaction between indomethacin and aspirin, because there is a marked difference in slope (see Fig 19-4). There is much more ulcerogenicity in the presence of aspirin than in its absence. Thus, the authors concluded that "the combined use of these nonsteroidal anti-inflammatory agents has high ulcerogenic potential at doses of each not heretofore considered as such."

Counterbalanced designs to reduce problems of individual variations

In *counterbalanced designs* each subject receives each treatment, but one subject or group is tested in one sequence of conditions, while another subject or group is tested in a different sequence. These are also called *crossover designs*, because the groups exchange treatments. Crossover designs have been used frequently in dental research studies using a placebo and an active compound. For example, Zinner et al[20] tested the

effects of Proxygel (Reed and Carnnick) and a placebo on the oral hygiene index (OHI).

An abridged version of the data is given in Table 19-4. At the end of the first period, the mean OHI value for Group 1 (which received the Proxygel first) is designated ($Y_{P_1G_1}$); the value for the same group at the end of the second period is ($Y_{P_2G_1}$). For the group that received the placebo first (Group 2), the values are labeled ($Y_{P_1G_2}$) and ($Y_{P_2G_2}$), respectively. We can see that the Proxygel apparently caused a decrease in the OHI, because:

1. At the end of the first period, the OHI value fell for the Proxygel group, and their score was less than the score for the placebo group:

$$(Y_{P_1G_1}) < (Y_{P_1G_2})$$

2. When, during period 2, the group that received the placebo first was given the Proxygel treatment, their OHI values declined:

$$(Y_{P_1G_2}) > (Y_{P_2G_2})$$

When the data from this experiment were treated as a simple bivalent random-groups design (ie, the groups were compared at the end of period 1 using the Student t test), a t value of 2.92 was obtained. However, the t value calculated using the differences between the periods for each group yielded the much higher t value of 5.91. (You will recall that the higher the value of t, the less likely the result can be explained by chance.) Thus, the use of a crossover design produced a more sensitive test. It is clear that the design could be improved by taking readings before any treatments were started because this would enable additional comparisons to be made. However, this level of complexity is beyond the scope of this book, and the interested reader is referred to Varma and Chilton's[21] article or Jones and Kenward's[22] book, both devoted to crossover designs, for more details.

The advantage of counterbalanced designs is that each subject serves as its own control. Because, as a general rule, there is less variation in a property of the same individual measured at different times than there is variation among different individuals at different times, it is easier to detect small differences. Another advantage of the design is that statistical analysis may show that effects of order are important. Weaknesses of the counterbalanced design surface when there is an interaction between the groups and variables being tested. In that event, the simple comparison of the means of the two tests would be valueless.

With regard to this problem, Schor[23] has suggested that some clinical investigators of new drugs seem to have contracted a contagious disease called *crossover-itis*. The symptoms of the disease include an investigator's belief that two drugs can be tested properly only by testing them on the same people (as occurs in a crossover design). As noted previously, if there is an interaction, or—in the case of drugs—if the effect of one treatment is so great that it does not disappear when the treatment is discontinued, then the results are not trustworthy. In crossover experiments, a key goal is to allow a sufficient period of time (called a *washout period*) between treatments, so that there are no residual effects from the first treatment. Sometimes this is difficult or impossible to arrange.

Split-mouth design

The *split-mouth design* used in dentistry subdivides the mouth into experimental units of halves, quadrants,

or sextants, and different treatments are applied to these experimental units. Because comparisons are made *within the patient*, variability is expected to be less than that in studies (with patients as the experimental unit) in which comparisons are made *between patients*. A potential disadvantage is that treatments performed in one part of the mouth can affect treatment in other parts of the mouth—a phenomenon that has been called the *carry-across effect*.[24] If carry-across effects exist, then treatment effects cannot be measured directly because they include the sum of all carry-across effects.[22] A study of the efficiency of split-mouth designs found that this design produces moderate to large gains in efficiency when disease characteristics are symmetrically distributed over the experimental units and a sufficient number of sites is available, but that, in the absence of a symmetric disease distribution, *whole-mouth clinical trials* may be preferable.[25]

Other possible relationships among time, testing, and treatment

Counterbalanced designs are only one option for the arrangement of time, testing, and treatment. Campbell and Stanley[26] developed a classification scheme that has become a standard for behavioral science and educational research. Appendix 5 lists these designs and their sources of invalidity in terms of the major relevant variables discussed earlier: history, maturation, testing, instrumentation, regression, selection, mortality, and their interactions. In experiment design, investigators consider internal and external validity.

Another way of thinking about *internal validity* (discussed in chapter 15) is that it refers to the degree to which the independent variable brings about change in the dependent variable. Extraneous factors that are not controlled decrease the internal validity because you cannot be sure that changes in the independent variable account for the results. When a study is said to not be internally valid, it means that plausible rival hypotheses could explain the results. Internal validity is of prime importance when the experiment is testing a hypothesis or establishing a mechanism. An experiment with poor internal validity will not add to our understanding of the processes under consideration.

As noted earlier, *external validity* refers to the degree to which a study reflects events that occur in the real world. Threats to external validity include failure (or inability) to select a random sample, or interactions between a treatment and the particular subjects studied. External validity is of prime importance when an experiment's purpose is related to an application. An experiment with poor external validity will not allow us to predict what will happen when a treatment is applied in the real world.

Campbell and Stanley[26] categorized experiment designs as *pre-experimental, quasi-experimental,* and *true experimental*. A brief summary of this classification system—some components of which were discussed earlier— follows.

Pre-experimental designs include the *one-shot case study* and the *one-group pretest/post-test design*. According to Campbell and Stanley, a design such as the one-shot case study has such an absence of control as to be of almost no scientific value.

Quasi-experimental designs include *time series, equivalent time series, equivalent material samples, nonequivalent control group, separate sample pretest/posttest, separate sample pretest/posttest control group, multiple item series, institutional cycle,* and *regression discontinuity designs*. The quasi-experimental designs resemble true experimental designs in that some manipulation is done to look for an effect on the dependent variable but differ from true experiments in that either a control or randomization is lacking. Campbell and Stanley[27] deem these quasi-experimental designs worthy of use where better designs are not feasible (see below).

In *true experimental designs,* the investigator is able to manipulate a variable (for example, apply a treatment), randomize the groups (so that experimental and control groups are, in theory, similar), and control (or eliminate) interfering and irrelevant influences from the study. True experimental designs include the *pretest/posttest control group, Solomon four-group,* and *posttest only control group* designs, as well as other more complex elaborations such as *factorial design*.

Quasi-experimental design

In several circumstances it is not possible to use randomization or to manipulate the introduction or withholding of treatment. Two main types of quasi-experimental design are the *nonequivalent control group* and the previously described *interrupted time series*. The nonequivalent control design entails using groups in which the subjects have not been assigned randomly. Lack of randomization raises the possibility that there may be preexisting differences between the groups that could explain differences in outcome between the treated and control groups. In particular, there is the possibility of

"confounding by indication." For example, in the evaluation of vaccine effectiveness, patients with poor prognoses are more likely to be immunized. Thus, selection for vaccination is confounded by patient factors that are likely related to clinical end points.[28] Similarly, the time series designs are subject to temporal confounders and maturation, as well as regression to the mean. Despite these drawbacks, necessity sometimes dictates the use of quasi-experimental designs, such as in the study of infection control and antibiotic resistance. For example, an outbreak of resistant organisms in a hospital might leave little time to implement all of the procedures used in an RCT, since it must be dealt with immediately. Harris et al[29] have systematically reviewed reports using quasi-experimental designs in infection control and antibiotic resistance and have concluded that the conduct and presentation of such studies needs to be improved so that interventions are evaluated more rigorously. For example, *segmented regression analysis* is a powerful tool for evaluating longitudinal effects of interventions that has considerable potential to improve conclusions from interrupted time series studies.[30] Although quasi-experimental designs lack the formal rigor of true experimental designs, they still can be informative; the challenge is for the investigators to consider—and, ideally, rule out—alternative explanations of their results so that their interpretations are sound.

Some issues related to RCTs

The dominance of the RCT in epidemiological thinking leads some to conclude that it is the only reliable way of seeking knowledge, but this is obviously not true. For example, Grossman and Mackenzie[31] relate a case where an evidence-based working group discounted the contribution of 13 observational studies that all agreed in favor of the single RCT with an opposing conclusion. Moreover, RCTs often use patients with less severe disease and can thus mislead one's understanding of a treatment's usefulness. RCTs also use patients who are relatively young, yet the results are extrapolated inappropriately to older patients; in fact, some generalizations are made to patients who have been excluded from the study.[32] In essence, the problem is that, to increase internal validity and maximize the size of effect, investigators typically choose relatively homogeneous groups of patients, usually those who have a strong potential to benefit from the treatment. In my own studies on agents that reduce oral malodor, for example, my colleagues and I selected individuals who had considerable oral malodor. This strategy was necessary to increase our chances of seeing a significant effect. But it came at a price, because it was no longer clear what benefit those with less extreme mouth odor would receive. In other words, as is often the case, we increased internal validity at the expense of external validity.

One approach to this problem is to widen the spectrum of subjects included in the trial. However, if people who can benefit only minimally from a treatment are included, the average effect size will be reduced. Moreover, interpretations normally made from homogeneous groups where everyone received a benefit cannot be made from heterogeneous groups where the benefit may have depended on a patient's particular characteristics. *Heterogeneity of treatment effects* is the term used to describe the differential response to the same treatment by different patients with different characteristics (such as severity of disease, age, sex, genetic makeup, and so forth). In the chlorhexidine-soaked dental floss trial, my graduate student Pauline Imai and I found that the treatment worked better for sites in which the pocket depth was less than 4 mm. The probable reason was that floss likely goes down into the pockets only about 2 to 3 mm, so the treatment was not being delivered to the bottom of the deeper pockets. The consequence was that our interpretation had to be modified to restrict the range of sites where this modality might be effective. One can imagine extreme instances where a treatment is superbly effective for some patients and ineffective, or even damaging, for others, yet the average effect would work out to be positive. Such a situation could result in a treatment being recommended on the basis of average effects to patients who would not benefit or who would even suffer from it.

Other challenges include problems of blinding and randomization availability of a suitable placebo, inaccurate statistical analysis, inappropriate surrogate outcome measures, and false negatives. Although the RCT is a powerful design, its interpretation and clinical application are not necessarily straightforward. In a review of 39 RCTs published in major general clinical journals, Ioannidis[33] found that 9 of the 39 studies had been contradicted or demonstrated to have stronger effects by other studies. A significant problem has been the tendency to view one well-controlled trial that achieved statistical significance to be definitive. As Fisher[3] always emphasized, the test of a firm conclusion is repeated studies, each of which demonstrates statistical significance.

References

1. Salsburg D. The Lady is Tasting Tea: How Statistics Revolutionized Science in the Twentieth Century. New York: Henry Holt, 2001:8.
2. Finney DJ. Experimental Design and Its Statistical Basis. Chicago: Univ of Chicago Press, 1955:43.
3. Fisher RA. The Design of Experiments, ed 8. New York: Hafner, 1965.
4. Fleiss JL. The Design and Analysis of Clinical Experiments. New York: Wiley, 1986.
5. Chilton NW. Design and Analysis in Dental and Oral Research. New York: Praeger, 1982:291.
6. Mainland D. Elementary Medical Statistics. Philadelphia: Saunders, 1963:75–78.
7. Vlietstra JR, Sidaway DA, Plant CG. Cavity cleansers. A simple in vitro test. Br Dent J 1980;149:293.
8. Conant JB. On Understanding Science. New York: Mentor, 1951:96–98.
9. Chalmers TC, Celano P, Sacks HS, Smith H Jr. Bias in treatment assignment in controlled clinical trials. N Engl J Med 1983;309:1358–1361.
10. Blair E. Gold is not always good enough: The shortcomings of randomization when evaluating interventions in small heterogeneous samples. J Clin Epidemiol 2004;57:1219–1222.
11. Gilbert N. Biometrical Interpretation. Oxford: Clarendon, 1973:104–105.
12. Mainland D. Elementary Medical Statistics. Philadelphia: Saunders, 1963:171–172.
13. Beveridge WIB. The Art of Scientific Investigation. New York: Vintage, 1950:29.
14. van Belle G. Statistical Rules of Thumb. New York: Wiley, 2002:61–63.
15. Cited in Konig KG. Design of animal experiments in caries research. In: Harris RS, Caldwell RC (eds). Art and Science of Dental Caries Research. New York: Academic, 1968.
16. Alfano MC. Controversies, perspectives, and clinical implications of nutrition in periodontal disease. Dent Clin North Am 1976;20:519.
17. Fisher RA. The arrangement of field experiments. J Minist Agric 1926;33:503.
18. Finney DJ. Experimental Design and Its Statistical Basis. Chicago: Univ of Chicago Press, 1955:83.
19. Shaw DH, Wischmeier C. Combined ulcerogenicity of aspirin and indomethacin in the rat. J Dent Res 1976;55:1133.
20. Zinner DD, Duany LF, Chilton NW. Controlled study of the clinical effectiveness of a new oxygen gel on plaque oral debris and gingival inflammation. Pharmacol Ther Dent 1970;1:7–15.
21. Varma AO, Chilton NW. Crossover designs involving two treatments. J Periodontal Res 1974;9(suppl 14):160.
22. Jones B, Kenward MG. Design and Analysis of Cross-over Trials. London: Chapman & Hall, 1989.
23. Schor SS. How to evaluate medical research reports. Hosp Physician 1969;5:95.
24. Hujoel PP, DeRouen TA. Validity issues in split-mouth trials. J Clin Periodontol 1992;19:625.
25. Hujoel PP, Loesche WJ. Efficiency of split-mouth designs. J Clin Periodontol 1990;17:722.

26. Campbell DT, Stanley JC. Experimental and Quasi-experimental Designs for Research. Chicago: Rand McNally, 1966:6.

27. Campbell DT, Stanley JC. Experimental and Quasi-experimental Designs for Research. Chicago: Rand McNally, 1966:34.

28. Hak E, Verheij TJ, Grobbee DE, Nichol KL, Hoes AW. Confounding by indication in non-experimental evaluation of vaccine effectiveness: The example of prevention of influenza complications. J Epidemiol Commun Health 2002;56:951–955.

29. Harris AD, Lautenbach E, Perencevich E. A systematic review of quasi-experimental study designs in the fields of infection control and antibiotic resistance. Clin Infect Dis 2005;41:77–82.

30. Wagner AK, Soumerai SB, Zhang F, Ross-Degnan D. Segmented regression analysis of interrupted time series studies in medication use research. J Clin Pharm Ther 2002;27:299–309.

31. Grossman J, Mackenzie FJ. The randomized controlled trial: Gold standard, or merely standard? Perspect Biol Med 2005;48:516–534.

32. Greenfield S, Kravitz R, Duan N, Kaplan SH. Heterogeneity of treatment effects: Implications for guidelines, payment, and quality assessment. Am J Med 2007;120(4 suppl 1):S3–S9.

33. Ioannidis JP. Contradicted and initially stronger effects in highly cited clinical research. JAMA 2005;294:218–228.

20 | Statistics As an Inductive Argument
and Other Statistical Concepts

A judicious man looks at statistics not to get knowledge, but to save himself from having ignorance foisted upon him.

—Thomas Carlyle[1]

Statistics ≠ Scientific Method

Scientific method does not necessarily require the use of statistics. Indeed, papers published in areas such as molecular biology and biochemistry rarely use sophisticated statistics; the power of their experiment systems is so great that differences between the items being compared are evident enough not to require statistical tests. These differences may be observed directly (eg, the appearance or disappearance of a particular molecule that can be identified by its location on a polyacrylamide gel). This disclaimer notwithstanding, it should be noted that most clinical dental research *does benefit* from a statistical approach, because the size of the effects being observed is often small, and it is difficult to distinguish the effects from natural variation. The number of articles in the dental literature that employ statistics has risen rapidly, and instruction in statistics is now common—though not necessarily effective[1]—in dental schools.

The statistics used in most research papers are different from the statistics of everyday usage, such as reported census data or baseball batting averages that provide comprehensive information about the population involved. For example, in calculating a batting average, we know every time a player went to bat, and we know the player's exact number of hits, so the batting average completely and accurately represents the player's performance.

Statistical Inference Considered As an Inductive Argument

Prior prediction

To be testable by standard statistical procedures, a hypothesis must predict some particular distribution of a measured value. The hypothesis is best made in advance of the experiment. This point can be illustrated by looking at a table of random numbers. The frequencies of certain numerals will be higher in some sequences than would be predicted by chance alone. A statistical test would judge the departures from predicted values to be significant. Could we then say that the tables of random numbers are not random? We could not, because such a test—constructed after the data had been collected—would not be valid. Any sample of random numbers can be expected to exhibit some unusual sequences, but if they are truly random numbers, we cannot predict what those sequences will be.

As noted in our discussion of evaluation of hypotheses (chapter 7), successful prediction is considered stronger support for a hypothesis than an equal amount of data known when the hypothesis was put forward. The same arguments hold true for statistical analysis of research data. If a set of data shows some effect that was not suspected prior to the experiment, the conservative strategy is to test for the effect in a subsequent experiment. An alternative is to use special statistical tests that have been developed for after-the-fact (a posteriori) analysis. In the example of hypothesis testing in chapter 9, prior prediction was assumed.

Golden rule of sample statistics

A number of features of statistical reasoning about samples were not illustrated in the previous chapters. Some of these may be summed up in what I will call the *golden rule*: Any sample should be evaluated with respect to size, diversity, and randomness.[2] The statistics in research reports are based on samples. The obvious questions to ask are: *(1)* How representative of the target population are the samples? Was the sample selected randomly, or were there factors present that could lead to biased selection? *(2)* How large is the sample? *(3)* How much diversity exists in the sample? Does it cover all of the groups that make up the population? Fallacies, as well as acceptable arguments, can arise from statistical inference.

Induction by enumeration

Induction by enumeration is commonly used in scientific thinking. In this form of reasoning, a conclusion about all of the members of a class is drawn from premises referring to observed members of that class.

premise   Four of the 20 patients experienced a problem after endodontic treatment.

conclusion   Twenty percent of all patients experience problems after endodontic treatment (inductive generalization).

Induction by enumeration, also called *statistical generalization*, can yield false conclusions from true premises. For example, there was no estimate of the error in the previous value. It is unlikely that a second sampling of 20 patients would also yield a value of exactly 20% failures. We could try to reduce the chances of being accused of a false conclusion by *hedging* the conclusion. For example, we could write "about 20% experience problems." Hedging does not solve the problem.

A more precise solution would be to use probability theory to calculate your confidence in the statement. Because this example is based on the binomial theorem with two mutually exclusive outcomes (success or failure) with a fixed probability, we could use the table in appendix 2. Using the example of University of Bristish Columbia (UBC) dental graduates in chapter 9, consider Dentist B, who had 16 successes and 4 failures. According to the table in appendix 2, this result indicates that Dentist B is 95% confident that his percentage of failures lies between 5.8% and 44%. We can see that precisely stating the confidence interval gives a rather different perspective on the data. There is no reason for Dentist B to be overconfident; a failure rate as high as 44% is included in this interval.

Fallacy of insufficient statistics (or hasty generalization)

In the *fallacy of insufficient statistics,* an inductive generalization is made based on a small sample.

premise   My mother and my wife smoke.
conclusion   All women smoke (fallacy of insufficient statistics).

If this argument were used as sole evidence for the conclusion that all women smoke, the argument would be classified as *proof by selected instances*.

Associated with this fallacy is the problem of how many is enough. The answer depends on how large, how varied, and how much at risk is the population being studied. Numbers that appear quite large can still be inadequate. Huff[3] recounts a test of a polio vaccine in which 450 children in the community were vaccinated, while 680 were left unvaccinated as controls. Although the community was the locale of a polio epidemic, neither the vaccinated children nor the controls contracted the disease. Paralytic polio had such a low incidence—even in the late 1940s—that only two cases would have been expected from the sample size used. Thus, the test was doomed from the start.

What is a reasonable sample size?

There is no simple answer to this question, but two general considerations appear to be relevant: tradition and statistics.

Tradition

In some research areas, experience shows that consistent and reliable results require a certain number of subjects or patients; for example, Beecher[4] recommends at least 25 patients for studies on pain. These *traditions* probably develop because of practical considerations such as patient availability, as well as inherent statistical considerations such as subject variability. The underlying philosophy in this approach is that the replication of results is a more convincing sign of reliability than a low P value obtained in a single experiment. If a number of investigators find the same result, we can have reasonable confidence in the findings. Means of combining and reviewing studies are given in *Summing Up* by Light and Pillemer.[5]

There are problems with the traditional method of choosing an arbitrary and convenient number of subjects. If the sample is too large, the investigator wastes effort and the subjects are unnecessarily exposed to treatments that may not be optimal. However, most often the number of subjects is too small; the size of the sample is usually limited by subject availability. Thus, studies that use low numbers of subjects and report no treatment effect should be considered with skepticism. In fact, some journals have a policy of rejecting papers that accept null hypotheses. Such *negative results papers* end up in a file drawer. They neither contribute to scientific knowledge nor enhance the careers of their authors. These "file-drawer papers" emphasize the need to understand the relationship between sample size and the establishment of statistically significant differences. Failure to use an appropriate sample size leads to much wasted effort.

Role of the sample size and variance in establishing statistically significant differences between means in the t test

The size of an adequate sample is a complex question that will not be addressed in great detail here. However, some insight into the problem can be gained by examining the formula for the t test, which is perhaps the most common statistical test used in biologic research. It should be used when comparing the means of only two groups. The t test exists in several forms that depend on whether the samples are related (eg, the paired t test) or independent. Below is the formula used for a two-sided comparison when comparing the means of the measured values from two independent samples with roughly equal variances of unpaired subjects:

$$t = \frac{\text{difference in means}}{\text{SE of the difference between means}}$$

$$t = \frac{\bar{X}_A - \bar{X}_B}{s_{\bar{X}_A - \bar{X}_B}}$$

$$s_{\bar{X}_A - \bar{X}_B} = \sqrt{\frac{(n_A - 1)s_A^2 + (n_B - 1)s_B^2}{n_A + n_B - 2}} \times \sqrt{\frac{1}{n_A} + \frac{1}{n_B}}$$

where n_A, n_B = number in samples A and B, respectively; $\bar{X}_A$, $\bar{X}_B$ = means of samples A and B, respectively; s_A^2, s_B^2 = variance of groups A and B, respectively; $s_{\bar{X}_A} \times s_{\bar{X}_B}$ = standard error (SE) of the difference between means; and $n_A + n_B - 2$ = degrees of freedom.

A high observed t value indicates the unlikeliness that the two samples are drawn from a population with the same mean. Having selected a significance level and calculated a quantity called *degrees of freedom* (*df*) (in this case $df = n_A + n_B - 2$), we can consult a table of published t values such as can be found in appendix 3. If the observed t value is higher than the critical level, we reject the null hypothesis. For example, consider once again the study by Keene et al,[6] who reported the decayed, missing, or filled teeth (DMFT) data found in Table 20-1:

$$t = \left[\frac{\bar{X}_e - \bar{X}_{non-e}}{\sqrt{\frac{55(3.59^2) + 139(3.31)^2}{194}}}\right] \times \left[\frac{1}{\sqrt{\frac{1}{56} + \frac{1}{140}}}\right] = \frac{1.40}{.54} = 2.59$$

$$df = 140 + 56 - 2 = 194.0$$

Table 20-1 Relationship of *Streptococcus mutans* biotype to DMFT*				
Biotype	**Mean**	**SE**	**SD**	**n**
e carriers [+]	4.91	.48	3.59	56
Non–e carriers [–]	3.51	.28	3.31	140

*Data from Keene et al.[6]

The critical value of t for 194 df at an α level of .05 ≈ 1.96.

Since the calculated value of $t = 2.59 > 1.96$, we can reject the null hypothesis and conclude that there is a significant difference in DMFT between the e and non–e carriers.

From the formula for the statistic, we realize the following:

1. A large difference between means will increase the t value. This makes sense. Large effects should be easier to see. If the effect is large, the sample size required to distinguish the groups will be smaller.
2. The t value is decreased when the variance is large. (Remember that variance is related to the spread of measured values around the mean.) A large variance tends to produce a small t value, making it harder to detect differences between groups.
3. The t value is increased when the number in the sample is large. From the formula, it can be calculated that the decrease in the SE value is proportional to the square root of the sample number. Thus, if you increase the sample size by a factor of 10, you only decrease the SE by 3.16. This may be an inefficient way of reducing the error, but it works. Bakan[7] notes that increasing the sample size (n) almost inevitably guarantees a significant result. Even very small alterations in experiment conditions might produce minute differences that will be detected by a statistical test made very sensitive by a large sample size.

In the dental sciences, the reverse is the more common problem; that is, frequently there is only a small number in the sample. Combined with a large variability in the subjects, this small sample often means that no difference is detected, even when it is likely that a real difference exists.

Effect-size approach

Choosing the optimal sample size is a complex business that depends on the difference between groups, the variability of the groups, the experiment design, and the confidence level. A rough-and-ready way to estimate an appropriate sample size using the *effect-size approach*[8] for a simple experiment with a treated and a control group follows:

1. Estimate what you think is an important (or important to detect) difference in means between the treated and control groups.
2. Use the results of a pilot study or previously published information on the measurement to estimate the expected pooled standard deviation (SD) of a reasonably sized sample.
3. Using the values found in *(1)* and *(2)* above, calculate the d statistic (formula given on page 252).
4. Choose your level of confidence (5% or 1%).
5. Look up the number of subjects needed in appendix 6.

Using the same approach, we can also work backward to decide if a paper's authors used a reasonable sample size. This is particularly important if no effect was seen, because the sample may have been too small to produce a sensitive experiment. To check this possibility:

1. Use the authors' data to estimate the d statistic.
2. Look up the table in appendix 6 to determine the number of subjects that should have been used.
3. Compare the number from the table with the actual number used. Effect- and sample-size tables for more sophisticated designs can be found in Cohen's[8] book *Statistical Power Analysis for the Behavioral Sciences*.

Dao et al[9] examined the choice of measures in myofacial pain studies. Based on the characteristics of the measurements, they calculated how many subjects would be required to observe significant groups differing from each other by specified amounts. Their technique was based on the *statistical power analysis* developed by Cohen[8] and is similar to the effect-size calculation given above. Their values for within- and between-subject variance were obtained from a population referred to as *University Research Clinic*. The technique used to measure pain was a *visual analogue scale* (VAS), shown to be a rapid, easy, and valid method that provides a more sensitive and accurate representation of pain intensity than the *descriptive scales*.

They found that detecting a 15% difference in pain intensity between treatment and control groups in an experiment with 3 groups would require 242 subjects per group. However, to detect an 80% difference in pain intensity, only 8 subjects per group would be needed, and the total study size would be 24 subjects. Even with the sensitive VAS method to measure pain, the traditional approach of using 25 subjects and descriptive scales could probably distinguish only very large differences between groups (ie, ≈ 80% differences, if three groups were used).

A handy rule for the effect of sample size on confidence intervals

Van Belle's *Statistical Rules of Thumb*[10] includes a chapter on calculating sample sizes and provides a number of other "rules of thumb" useful in performing practical statistical analysis. Figure 20-1, taken from van Belle,[10] shows the half-width of confidence intervals with sample size. One can see that the width of the confidence interval decreases rapidly until 12 observations are reached and then decreases more slowly.

The Fallacy of Biased Statistics

To review briefly, *descriptive statistics* are simply efficient ways of describing populations. For our purposes, a *population* is a collection of all objects or events of a certain kind that—at least theoretically—could be observed. The specific group of objects (events, subjects) observed is the *sample*. *Inferential statistics* are concerned with the use of samples to make estimates and inferences about the larger population. This larger population from which the sample is selected is also called the *parent population, or*, perhaps

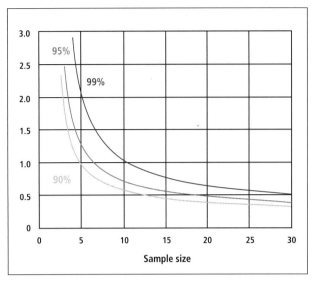

Fig 20-1 Half-width confidence interval assuming a *t* statistic with n − 1 *df* and sample size n. Confidence level curves are shown for confidence levels of 90%, 95%, and 99%. (Reprinted from van Belle[9] with permission.)

more accurately, the *target population*. This is the population that we hope the sample represents, so that we can generalize our findings.

The *fallacy of biased statistics* occurs when an inductive generalization is based on a sample that is known to be—or is strongly suspected to be—nonrepresentative of the parent population. This problem of *nonrepresentative samples* is associated with the randomness of sample selection and the spread of the sample. Gathering numbers to obtain information may be likened to an archer shooting at a target. The bull's-eye represents the *true value* of the population in question. The place where the arrow hits represents one value from the sample. *Bias* is the consistent repeated divergence of the shots from the bull's-eye. For an archer, this bias may be caused by a factor such as a wind blowing from one direction that causes the arrows to hit predominantly on one side of the target. In research experiments, bias may be caused by factors leading to nonrandom sampling. There are many examples of biased polls giving erroneous results. Perhaps the most famous is the *Literary Digest* poll that predicted, on the basis of a telephone survey and a survey of its subscribers, that a Republican victory was assured in the 1936 election.[3] The number of people polled was huge—over two million—but the prediction was wrong because the people polled were not representative of the voting public. In fact, they were wealthier than average because, at that time, telephones were found mainly in the homes of the wealthy. Thus, the *Literary Digest* poll selected relatively wealthy people, who stated that they would vote Republican. Today, the public opinion polls conducted by the Gallup and Harris organizations interview only about 1,800 persons weekly to estimate the opinions of US residents age 18 and over, but these polls are reasonably accurate because the sample is chosen by a *stratified random sampling* method that is not biased.

Bias can appear in many different ways, as denoted by Murphy's[11] definition:

> Bias is any trend in the choice of a sample, the making of measurements on it, the analysis or publication of findings, that tends to give or communicate an answer that differs systematically (nonrandomly) from the true answer.

Much of epidemiology is concerned with searching out various kinds of bias. An entertaining guide to this topic is the *Biomedical Bestiary* by Michael et al.[12] The topic also is discussed comprehensively by Sackett,[13] who catalogued no fewer than 56 types of bias. Only a brief overview is presented here.

Who is studied (selection bias)

Persons being studied may differ in important ways from the larger population they are supposed to represent; this is known as *selection bias*. Selection bias was exemplified in the case of the *Literary Digest* poll. Persons who seek medical attention for a disease are likely to be those who are the sickest—sometime leading physicians to conclude that the disease is more debilitating than it really is. Selection bias in clinical studies can arise in different ways; following are two types that particularly affect dental research.

> 1. *Volunteer bias* can occur if a significant number of eligible subjects do not agree to participate. Participants tend to be more motivated, more compliant, and, in clinical studies, destined for better outcomes than those who decline to participate. Compliant volunteers likely practice oral hygiene more rigorously than the general population; treatments that require strict plaque control would be expected to be more effective on volunteers. Dental research often uses dental students as volunteers, but this group obviously differs from the general

> population in their attitude about oral hygiene.
> 2. *Withdrawal bias.* Patients who are withdrawn from a study or refuse treatment may differ systematically from those who remain or accept treatment. This bias probably explains the results of a review of a periodontal practice that found those who elected surgical treatment had better periodontal health than those who refused treatment and left the practice.

In a trial of a beta-adrenergic blocking agent on patients recovering from heart attack, 13.9% of patients in the placebo (control) group died suddenly, whereas only 7.7% of the drug-treated patients suffered the same fate.[14] The data were statistically significant, and it appeared that the drug produced a potentially clinically important reduction. However, because of the side effects of the drug (such as bradycardia and hypotension), drug-treated subjects withdrew from the study more frequently than the placebo-treated subjects. It is possible that patients who are sensitive to drug side effects are also susceptible to arrhythmias and sudden death. The observed *selective withdrawal* raises the possibility that the difference in outcomes may be caused by the high-risk people removing themselves from the treated group, and that the drug itself has no effect. Therefore, at least three alternatives could explain differences found between treated and control groups: *(1)* chance fluctuations—but these can be shown to be unlikely by statistical techniques; *(2)* a real effect—ie, the drug does prevent sudden deaths; or *(3)* the withdrawal of high-risk patients from the treated group.

Because a plausible alternative hypothesis exists, a critic would be on solid ground in refusing to believe that the drug had an effect. The investigators would have to defend their hypothesis from such a criticism by gathering more data, referring to other data, or—as was done in this study—analyzing the data in a different manner so that the criticism could be met.

How the sample is studied

Detection biases

For various reasons, such as knowledge of exposure to a putative cause (*diagnostic suspicion bias*), some patients (cases) may receive more intensive or prolonged examination than the controls. Cases may be examined many times on each recall visit, whereas the controls are examined only once (*recall bias*).

Observational error biases

Certain measures may differ systematically from their usual level because of the procedures or conditions used to make the measurement—eg, blood pressure during medical interviews. Measurements that hurt, embarrass, or invade privacy may be systematically refused or avoided. Instruments or techniques may be inaccurate or insensitive.

Response bias

This *systematic error* results when subjects respond inaccurately to an investigator's questions. For instance, dental floss sales do not correspond to the number of people who report using dental floss in surveys. Presumably, the subjects lie about their oral flossing practices to give a more positive impression of their personal hygiene to interviewers. A subset of the response bias is the *obsequience bias*, in which subjects systematically alter their responses in the direction they perceive desired by the investigator. For this reason, reviews of teaching effectiveness are best done with the students remaining anonymous.

Sampling and treatment allocation bias

Bias can also occur in sampling or allocation of treatments within an individual. For example, in a study on the effect of an antibiotic on periodontal disease, the authors proceeded as follows: *(1)* microbiologic samples were obtained from the most severely periodontally involved site and were therefore not representative of all sites; *(2)* the most severely involved quadrant was treated with root planing; another quadrant served as the control. Thus, there was a systematic difference between the control and treated quadrants.

Other Statistical Concepts

When the null hypothesis is rejected

There are at least five possible explanations for the deviation of a sample from the real value or the value proposed by a hypothesis.

Sometimes there are more than two alternatives

Statistical methods are useful when random errors are the primary source of variation, but there are other types of error. As outlined previously, when testing a hypothesis it is assumed that there are two mutually exclusive alternatives. One is that the two samples differ only as a result of chance fluctuation. When this alternative is rejected, it is surmised that the reason the samples differ is the reason put forward by the investigator (ie, that the difference is caused by the difference in, for example, treatments between the treated and control groups). It is assumed that all other relevant variables have been held constant. This is not always true. There may be more than one difference between the groups. This is a variant of the *UFO fallacy;* the statistical test assumes there are only two possibilities that are mutually exclusive and exhaustive. In reality, there may be other possibilities.

Sample vs target populations

In evaluating research reports, one must always bear in mind that there are two distinct populations: the target population, about which the investigator wishes to draw a conclusion; and the sampled population, from which the sample was actually taken. The possibility of bias is such an important consideration that it bears repetition. When clinicians report the results of various therapeutic procedures, a question that immediately comes to mind is: How representative of the general population (or, even more cynically, of all of the patients treated by the clinician) are these particular patients? Selective factors may operate to cause the two populations being compared to be different.

Unreliability of observation

Some techniques do not measure what they claim. Other techniques are inherently unreliable. Some investigators are habitually incompetent. All of these factors can produce unreliable results. For this reason, if you are suspicious of or unfamiliar with a particular technique on which a scientific paper depends, it is worthwhile to talk with someone who has used it. It might also be helpful to conduct a citation analysis of the publication in which the technique was originally described.

Sampling fluctuations (type I error): Real difference between the populations and hypothesis

In this event, a number of other questions arise that are related to the importance of the findings or the size of the effect. The importance of the findings is best assessed by an expert or by citation analysis. The size of the effect can be calculated using several indicators; one is the d statistic. When the null hypothesis is rejected, it is often of interest to calculate the effect size. Cohen[8] has devised methods for evaluating the size of an experiment effect for a number of different experiment designs. The effect-size index d for a comparison between means of two groups is calculated as follows:

$$d_s = \frac{\bar{X}_a - \bar{X}_b}{S_p} \qquad s_p = \sqrt{\frac{(n_a - 1)s_a^2 + (n_b - 1)s_b^2}{n_a + n_b - 2}}$$

where d_s = effect-size index for means in a standard unit

n_a = number in sample of Group A
s_a = SD of sample of Group A
n_b = number in sample of Group B
s_b = SD of sample of Group B
$\bar{X}_a$ = mean for Group A
$\bar{X}_b$ = mean for Group B

Note that the d statistic is related to the t statistic simply by the formula:

$$d = \sqrt{\frac{n_a + n_b}{n_a \times n_b}} \times t$$

A convenient way of thinking of these values is in terms of *population overlap* (see appendix 7), which is given here as the percentage of the area covered by both populations that is not overlapped.
When:

d = 0	0% not overlapped; either population is perfectly superimposed on the other
d = 0.1	7.7% not overlapped

d = 0.2	14.7%; eg, height differences between 15- and 16-year-old girls
d = 0.5	33%; eg, height differences between 14- and 18-year-old girls
d = 0.8	47.4%; eg, height differences between 13- and 18-year-old girls, or mean IQ difference between PhDs and typical college freshmen
d = 1.0	58.9%
d = 2.0	81.1%
d = 3.0	92.8%
d = 4.0	97.7%

Cohen[7] has calculated effect-size indicators for other statistical tests.

Finally, truly large differences do not require statistical tests. Most people will believe that a difference in size exists between apples and pumpkins without the calculation of the d statistic. Indeed, it has been argued that any effect so small that it requires statistics for its demonstration is not important. A quote attributed to Lord Rutherford states, "If your experiment needs statistics, you ought to have done a better experiment. . . ." There is an element of truth in such an argument—particularly in laboratory studies in which investigators can manipulate several factors to demonstrate an effect or reduce the variability in the groups. Nevertheless, most dental research requires appropriate statistical analysis.

What is regarded as an acceptable size of an experimental effect differs according to field. In behavioral science, Cohen[8] has defined d values of 0.8 as being large differences. Such a difference would probably not be regarded as large in biologic studies. Nevertheless, small effects can be important, particularly in situations where large numbers of people or large amounts of money are involved.

When the null hypothesis is accepted

As noted earlier, it is relatively rare to see H_0 accepted; a negative result may mean only that the techniques used to demonstrate the effect were not sensitive enough. One should note that the test does not say H_0 is true. It merely says there is no significant difference, or, expressed alternatively, either H_0 is true, or there is not enough information to prove it false.

In an assessment of 71 negative randomized control trials (RCTs), 50 of the trials used a sample size so small that the trials could have missed a 50% improvement. Many of the therapies labeled as *no different from control* had not received a fair test.[15] A quality assessment of RCTs in dental research found that none of the 17 studies reporting no significant differences calculated a type II error to ensure that a sufficient sample size had been used.[16]

In a study of psychological journals, Sterling[17] found that investigators generally do not publish experiments that do not show significant differences at the 5% level or better. This is not surprising, because negative results—ie, reporting that the experimental conditions had no effect—could always be interpreted as meaning that the methods used were not sensitive enough to detect any effect. Such studies do not often end up in good journals. (In Sterling's report, about 3% of the articles did not reject the null hypothesis, while 97% did at the 5% level.) Although I have no precise data on the dental literature, my impression is that acceptance of the null hypothesis is not rare. Nevertheless, suppose that an idea for a given treatment occurred to 40 investigators. Next, suppose that the treatment, in reality, did not have any effect. It is likely that 2 of the 40 would get significant results at the 5% level. The first would publish the result, and the second would confirm it. A nonexistent effect could become enshrined in the literature without being refuted because of the other 38 authors' reluctance to publish negative results.[7] The 38 investigators who do not publish their results exemplify what has been called the *file-drawer problem*. Studies that do not show a statistically significant effect are not published, but rather placed in a file drawer. In trying to interpret the generality of results—for example, of the effectiveness of some form of therapy—reviewers have to guess at how many file-drawer manuscripts exist.

In summary, H_0 (ie, the *no-difference hypothesis*) can never be proven because subsequent experiments with more replicates or more accurate measurements might show that a treatment does have an effect and so disprove the hypothesis. This reasoning leads to the statistician's common caveat against interpreting a lack of statistical significance as counterevidence. This "weakness" in statistical reasoning—ie, that statistics can *disprove* H_0 (by showing that it is highly improbable that H_0 is true), but that it cannot *prove* H_0—has been discussed in detail by Bakan.[7]

Sometimes it is to the investigator's advantage to accept the null hypothesis for at least a part of a study. For example, if an experiment design requires two or more clinicians to make observations, it is common to compare them to determine if they differ significantly in their assessments. In such cases, it simplifies the analysis and interpretation of the data if it can be assumed that the clinicians do not differ significantly. In such papers, authors are glad to accept the null hypothesis.

Choice of computational unit

Experimental units can be considered at various levels, such as sites, half mouths, or patients. Blomqvist[18] has recommended that the highest-level unit should be used because, in statistical inference, use of a lower-level unit will underestimate the SE and level of significance. This was evident to Mainland,[19] who used a dental example in his classic text as follows:

> Let us suppose that a dentist, having attended to the teeth of two boys, instructs one of them to use Toothpaste A and the other to use Toothpaste B, and ensures by parental cooperation that his instructions are carried out. After a certain length of time the dentist finds that the boy who used Toothpaste A has eight carious teeth, whereas the other boy has no caries. In terms of numbers of teeth, this looks like an impressive difference, but we need no profound knowledge of dentistry or of statistics to realize that it provides no adequate evidence that the difference in toothpaste was responsible. Persons differ in their tendency to develop caries; therefore the individual teeth in any mouth do not provide independent pieces of information about the effect of a toothpaste. It is boys, not teeth, that are the sampling units, and there is only one sampling unit in each of the A and B samples and no true replicates, that is, sampling units that receive the same test treatment but are otherwise independent.
>
> In this simple case, the point is obvious, but it was not obvious to a distinguished worker in nutrition and dentistry who reported on the caries in 36,196 teeth in the mouths of 1,870 children. By examining about 20 teeth per child, the investigator has measured over and over again the same tendency (or resistance) to caries, but in the analysis each tooth was counted as if it gave an independent piece of information. The error—the error of wrong sampling units—can also be called spurious enlargement of samples, spurious

replication, or counting the same thing over again.

In the large dental caries study, the proper sampling units were children, and one way to express the information would be by the numbers of children with, and without, caries (and this was done in another part of the report). A finer measure would be the number of carious teeth per child, with some form of adjustment for the number of filled and missing teeth.

This issue of sampling units has caused hot debate in dental science. At the 1983 Gordon Conference on periodontal disease, some clinicians argued that, because periodontal disease was a localized lesion, each site could be treated as though it were independent. The statisticians echoed the arguments made by Mainland—namely, that the sites were not independent and that the statistical methods should be modified. The debate continues, but it appears that the statisticians are winning. Fleiss and Kingman[20] state, "Theory and data both indicate that it is a mistake to employ statistical procedures that take individual sites as the unit of analysis; it is the patient who must be the unit of analysis." Sophisticated methods have now been developed for determining and selecting the optimum number of sites and patients for clinical studies in dentistry.[21]

A related problem that is a frequent source of error is the choice of a unit that solves a problem related to, but different from, the one under investigation. Schor[22] points out that in contraception research, a reduction in sperm count does not necessarily mean a reduction in fertility. If you were interested in the effects of a drug on fertility, the appropriate unit would not be the number of sperm in a sample of semen, but the percentage of men whose sperm count was reduced to subfertile range.

Violation of assumptions

The debate about independent sampling units illustrates that many assumptions underlie statistical tests. Studies of the medical research literature have found that statistical tests have been applied inappropriately to data because the assumptions underlying the tests were probably false.

Errors in analysis and spotting faked data

This group of problems is concerned with errors in the statistical analysis of data. A large number of these, including mistakes in computation, would be expected to be hidden from the reader because the raw data often are not reported. However, sometimes errors in analysis are evident even at the level of simple arithmetic computation. An example is furnished by a paper submitted to the *Journal of Experimental Medicine* by Summerlin, who later admitted to falsifying data.[23] Summerlin performed transplants on six groups of animals; each group had 20 animals. Summerlin reported the percentage that were not rejected in each group. Because any nonrejection is a discrete event, the percentage had to be a multiple of five: $\frac{1}{20}$ = 5%, $\frac{2}{20}$ = 10%, etc. The percentages Summerlin recorded were 53, 58, 63, 48, and 67. An alert referee should have noticed that something was wrong with Summerlin's data.

In 1881, astronomer Simon Newcomb observed that the earlier pages of logarithm tables showed more wear than the later pages in the books, and concluded that, for natural observations, the first significant number is more often the number 1 than it is 2; the number 2 is more frequent than 3; and so forth.[24] This pattern was later confirmed by Benford, a physicist at General Electric, who analyzed some 20,229 observations; the first significant digit rule eventually became known as *Benford's Law*, given by the following: The probability P that the first significant digit (D_1) equals a particular value d (where d = 1, 2, 3, . . . 9).

$$P(D_1 = d) = \log_{10}(1 + 1/d)$$

Benford's Law was an empirical affair until 1991, when it was given a rigorous mathematical foundation by Georgia Tech mathematics professor Theodore Hill. Today it is widely used to identify fraudulent data (or unintentional errors) not only in naturally occurring data but also in financial data. Frey[24] provides a history of Benford's Law, some applications, and even references where one can find Mathlab code to do calculations on Benford's Law.

A Final Warning and a Set of Rules

Statistics are powerful tools for estimating the effects of random error. However, conclusions based on statistical inference should not always be accepted at face value but, like any other technique, should be viewed critically. Statistical analysis is not sacred but based on empirical findings (such as distributions of data) and assumptions that are sometimes dubious. To quote Epstein: "The field of statistics bows to no master for ability to furnish subterfuge, confusion, and obscuration."[25] The foregoing principles refer to only a small fraction of the possible problems that can be considered in statistical analysis. Indeed, despite the highly sophisticated types of statistical analysis that are now performed, there is ongoing debate on the foundations of statistical inference.[26] It is not uncommon for statisticians to disagree. There are journals that deal solely with biostatistics, suggesting that many problems related to analyzing biologic data remain.

Despite the sophistication found in some studies in dental research, there are numerous articles that use inappropriate or less-than-optimal statistical methods.[27] Because it is not conceivable that every student will become an expert in biometrics, I offer the following rules:

1. Always apply the golden rule: Examine every sample for size, diversity, and randomness.
2. Ask if the data should be evaluated with statistical techniques. Statistical testing is sometimes absent when it should be present. Dental journals still publish papers that claim differences in treatments or effectiveness of treatments in the absence of statistical testing. Readers can either perform the statistical test themselves or simply disregard the paper because nothing has been proved. A brief, excellent guide to the selection of statistical tests and a readable, nontechnical explanation of the most common techniques has been published by Norman and Streiner.[28]
3. If a simple statistical test was used, determine whether it was applied appropriately.
4. If unusual statistical tests were applied, there are two choices:
   a. If the paper is important to you, look up the test in a statistics textbook. Textbooks such as Norman and Streiner[28] and Zar[29] give straightforward explanations of the conditions under which particular tests are applicable. This may give you more insight into the reliability of the data, or perhaps the authors' desperation to get a significant result.
   b. Assume that the authors chose the right test for the application, and accept the result of the test as given.
5. For all papers, try to formulate alternative hypotheses that can also explain the results.

Now, Something Completely Different: The Bayesian Approach to Induction

The logic of statistical inference presented previously is called the *Neyman-Pearson approach,* but it also might be termed *classical* or *standard statistics.* This standard approach has several logical problems.[30,31] First, the standard approach evaluates evidence according to the intentions of the investigator. Investigators have to decide in advance what comparisons they are going to make, and whether they will be testing for greater-than or less-than differences (ie, a *one-tailed test*), or any differences at all (ie, a *two-tailed test*). Intuitively, it is difficult to understand how the intentions of the investigators bear on the assessment of the actual evidence, but the standard approach decrees that the investigator's intentions matter. Thus, one could argue that the standard approach is not truly objective because it incorporates not only the objective data but also the subjective intentions of the investigator.

A second problem is that the theory considers evidence that was not actually obtained. As illustrated in the example from chapter 9, in computing the probability of obtaining a certain number of successes for UBC dental graduates, we added the probabilities of the more extreme values as well. For example, for Dentist C, who had 13 successes, we added the probabilities for 1, 2, 3, 4, . . . 12, 13 successes. But these events—eg, 12 successes—were never observed for C; they just had a possibility of being observed. Some statisticians argue that the probability of data that have not been observed is irrelevant in making inferences from an experiment based on actual observations.

255

Table 20-2 Probabilities of rain with pain		
	Actual state	
Condition and prediction	Rain (R_1)	No rain (R_2)
Pain (P_1) → rain	.80	.30
No pain (P_2) → no rain	.20	.70

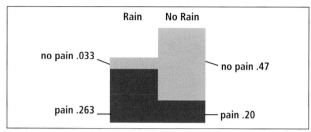

Fig 20-2 Probabilities of rain with pain.

A third problem is that researchers utilizing the standard approach end up testing the most untenable and outlandish null hypotheses. Researchers who are aware of differential effects have hopelessly inappropriate means of quantifying them; thus, they are reduced to implying that a result giving P < .000001 is more important than one for which P < .01.[32]

A fourth problem is that science should be *cumulative*. It would be an unproductive strategy to ignore the huge amount of available data and design experiments in which the null hypothesis is likely to be true. Instead, scientists try to perform experiments with high probabilities of revealing new information. As noted by Ross,[33] the *hypothesis of no effect* commonly used in hypothesis testing is correct for improbable claims; however, it is not correct when investigators have a body of knowledge to draw from and a theory designed to predict not just that something will happen but *what* and *how much*.

The *Bayesian approach* to statistics is named after the Reverend Thomas Bayes, a nonconformist clergyman who proposed the basic ideas in 1763. In Bayes' method, we start with a subjectively determined *prior probability* for a hypothesis. After obtaining evidence that bears on the hypothesis, we calculate the likelihood of obtaining the observations if the hypothesis is true. Then we combine the subjective prior probability with the likelihood to obtain a *posterior probability* of the hypothesis being true. The net effect of the calculations is that the evidence alters your assessment of the probability of the hypothesis being true. This posterior probability could be used as the starting prior probability for a second experiment. After successive iterations, one would expect the posterior probability to approach the truth. Thus, the Bayesian approach is cumulative and reflects the real world of science more accurately than the standard method of hypothesis testing. The main criticism of the Bayesian approach is that the best assessment of the first prior probability is *subjective,* while science is an *objective* business. However, recent theoretical work has shown that prior probabilities normally have relatively little influence on the corresponding posterior probabilities, and what influence they do have diminishes rapidly as evidence accumulates.

We will consider the Bayesian approach to decision making with the example of someone visiting Vancouver in the month of June.[34] The probability of rain on a day in June in Vancouver is .33, and the probability of no rain is 1 − .33 = .67. Suppose that the visitor has an arthritic joint that he uses to predict rain. He has documented the following data (Table 20-2) when experiencing pain on days when it did or did not rain. That is, on 80% of the days that it did rain, he experienced pain and rightly predicted that it would rain. But on 30% of the days that it did not rain, he also experienced pain. Thus, pain is an imperfect predictor of rain but clearly has some predictive value.

Suppose that the visitor travels to Vancouver and, on awakening, feels pain in the joint. How can he use the information about rainfall in Vancouver in June, as well as his pain, to assess the chances of rain?

Application of Bayes' theorem to this problem yields the following:

$$p(R_1, P_1) = p(R_1) \times p(P_1/R_1)$$

Or, in words: The combined probability of rain (R_1) and pain (P_1) equals the probability of rain $p(R_1)$ times the probability of pain given rain [($p(P_1/R_1)$]. In this example:

$$p(R_1, P_1) = .33 \times .80 = .263$$

Similarly, the combined probability of no rain and pain is:

$$p(R_2, P_1) = p(R_2) \times p(P_1/R_2) = 0.67 \times 0.3 = .20$$

Diagrammatically, we can look at the problem as creation of a new sample space, as shown in Fig 20-2.

Before pain was observed, the sample space was the total area of the diagram in which all days were either rain (.33) or no rain (.67). After pain was observed, the sample space became constricted to the hatched area—ie, the instances where pain occurs, which is found in an area of .263 in the rain column and .20 in the no-rain column. Note that these two probabilities no longer sum to 1 because we are no longer considering some of the previous possibilities—ie, the no-pain areas. To make this into a true probability distribution (which must sum to 1.0), we have to inflate the probability of the values by dividing by the total probability of pain (.463). Thus, the probability of rain given pain becomes:

$$p(R_1/P_1) = \frac{p(R_1/P_1)}{p(P_1)} = \frac{.263}{.463} = .57$$

The probability of no rain given pain is:

$$p(R_2/P_1) = \frac{p(R_2/P_1)}{p(P_1)} = \frac{.20}{.463} = .43$$

In summary, on the visitor's arrival in Vancouver and without considering pain, the proper betting odds for rain were 2:1: Rain was less likely than no rain. But after pain was observed, the betting odds became 43:57 (ie, rain was slightly favored).

In clinical medicine, the most widespread application of Bayes' theorem is in the adjustment of probabilities of a disorder being present after the results of a diagnostic test are known.[35] The form of Bayes' theorem that is commonly used in such an instance follows:

$$\begin{array}{ccc} \text{Pretest odds} & \text{likelihood} & \text{posttest odds} \\ \text{for the disorder} \times & \text{ratio (LR)} = & \text{for the disorder} \\ & \text{for the test} & \end{array}$$

The LR is calculated as:

$$LR+ = \frac{\text{true-positive rate}}{\text{false-positive rate}} = \frac{a/(a+c)}{b/(b+d)}$$

$$LR- = \frac{\text{false-negative rate}}{\text{true-negative rate}} = \frac{c/(a+c)}{d/(b+d)}$$

where a, b, c, and d refer to the four outcomes of a diagnostic test described in chapter 14, on sensitivity of clinical tests.

Like sensitivity and specificity, LRs do not change with prevalence of the disorder. Suppose that a patient with pretest odds of having periodontal disease of 1.0 (ie, even money) tested positive for bleeding on a probing test, which was a LR+ of 3. When we apply Bayes' theorem, the posttest odds of the disease would be $1 \times 3 = 3$. The relationship between probability and odds is given by: odds = probability / (1 − probability). If we rearrange the terms, the posttest probability of the disor-

der can be calculated for this bleeding-on-probing example as follows:

$$\begin{aligned} \text{posttest probability} &= \text{posttest odds/(posttest odds + 1)} \\ &= 3/(3 + 1) = .75. \end{aligned}$$

With pretest odds of 1, the pretest probability equaled $1/(1 + 1) = .5$ (ie, a 50/50 chance of the disorder). Thus, the results of the test have made the presence of the disorder more probable, and the probability can be calculated.

References

1. Carlyle T. Statistics. In: Carlyle T. Chartism Past and Present. London: Chapman Hill, 1858. Available at http://www.stat.ucla.edu/history/chartism.pdf. Accessed August 20, 2007.
2. Scheutz F, Andersen B, Wulff HR. What do dentists know about statistics? Scand J Dent Res 1988;96:281.
3. Huff D. How to Lie with Statistics. New York: Norton, 1954:40.
4. Beecher HK. Pain, placebos and physicians. Practitioner 1962;189:141.
5. Light RJ, Pillemer DB. Summing Up: The Science of Reviewing Research. Cambridge, MA: Harvard Univ Press, 1984.
6. Keene HJ, Shklair IL, Anderson DM, Mickel GJ. Relationship of Streptococcus mutans biotypes to dental caries in Saudi Arabian naval men. J Dent Res 1977;56:356–361.
7. Bakan D. On Method. San Francisco: Jossey-Bass, 1967:8.
8. Cohen J. Statistical Power Analysis for the Behavioral Sciences. New York: Academic, 1977.
9. Dao TT, Lavigne GJ, Feine JS, Tanguay R, Lund JP. Power and sample size calculations for clinical trials of myofacial pain of jaw muscles. J Dent Res 1991;70:118.
10. van Belle G. Sample size. In: Statistical Rules of Thumb. New York: Wiley, 2002:19; 29–51.
11. Murphy EA. A Companion to Medical Statistics. Baltimore: Johns Hopkins Univ Press, 1985:40.
12. Michael M, Boyce WT, Wilcox AJ. Biomedical Bestiary. Boston: Little Brown, 1984.
13. Sackett DL. Bias in analytic research. J Chronic Dis 1979; 32:51.
14. Norwegian Multicenter Study Group. Timolol-induced reduction in mortality and reinfarction in patients surviving acute myocardial infarction. N Engl J Med 1981;304:801.
15. Freiman JA, Chalmers TC, Smith H Jr, Kuebler RR. The importance of beta, the type II error and sample size in the design and interpretation of the randomized control trial. Survey of 71 "negative" trials. N Engl J Med 1978;299:690.
16. Antczack AA, Tang J, Chalmers TC. Quality assessment of randomized control trials in dental research. II. Results: periodontal research. J Periodontal Res 1986;21:315.

17. Sterling TD. Publication decisions and their possible effects on inferences drawn from tests of significance—Or vice versa. J Am Stat Assoc 1959;54:30–34.

18. Blomqvist N. On the choice of computational unit in statistical analysis. J Clin Periodontol 1985;12:873.

19. Mainland D. Elementary Medical Statistics. Philadelphia: Saunders, 1963:59.

20. Fleiss JL, Kingman A. Statistical management of data in clinical research. Crit Rev Oral Biol Med 1990;1:55.

21. Hujoel PP, DeRouen TA. Determination and selection of the optimum number of sites and patients for clinical studies. J Dent Res 1992;71:1516.

22. Schor SS. How to evaluate medical research reports. Hosp Physician 1969;5:95–99.

23. Moore DS, Notz WI, Nester DK. Do the numbers make sense? In: Moore DS, Notz WI, Nester DK. Satistical Concepts and Controversies, ed 6. New York: Freeman, 2006: 154–162.

24. Frey B. Statistics Hacks. Sebastopol, CA: O'Reilly, 2006: 268–278.

25. Epstein RA. The Theory of Gambling and Statistical Logic. New York: Academic, 1967:415.

26. Godambe VP, Sprott DA (eds). Foundations of Statistical Inference. Toronto: Holt, Rienhart and Winston, 1971.

27. Emrich LJ. Common problems with statistical aspects of periodontal research papers. J Periodontol 1990;61:206.

28. Norman GR, Streiner DL. PDQ Statistics. Toronto: Decker, 1986.

29. Zar JH. Biostatistical Analysis, ed 2. Englewood Cliffs, NJ: Prentice Hall, 1984.

30. Urbach P. Clinical trial and random error. New Sci 1987;116:52–55.

31. Berger JO, Berry DA. Statistical analysis and the illusion of objectivity. Am Sci 1988;76:159.

32. O'Quigley J, Baudoin CE. Null hypotheses and the misuse of statistics. Nature 1985;316:582.

33. Ross J. Misuse of statistics in the social sciences. Nature 1985;318:514.

34. Wonnacott TH, Wonnacott RJ. Introductory Statistics. New York: Wiley, 1969:312–314.

35. Sackett DC, Haynes RB, Tugwell P. The interpretation of diagnostic data, including likelihood ratios. In: Sackett DL, Haynes RB, Tugwell P. Clinical Epidemiology: A Basic Science for Clinical Medicine. Boston: Little Brown, 1985: 59–138.

21 | Judgment

> *Systemic decisions based on a few explicable and defensible principles are superior to intuitive decisions—because they work better because they are not subject to conscious or unconscious biases on the part of the decision maker, because they can be explicated and debated, and because their basis can be understood by those most affected by them.*
>
> —Robyn M. Dawes[1]

Critical Thinking As Applied to Scientific Publications

A number of common standards are used to evaluate critical thinking, including the assessment of scientific publications.

Clarity: Authors must make their points understandable to the reader. A good way to do this is to present the material so that it matches reader expectations; Gopen and Swan[2] provide an excellent introduction to this topic for writers of science in their article "The Science of Scientific Writing."

Accuracy: The criterion of accuracy applies not only to measurements but also to references to the literature. For example, have the cited authors' views been accurately portrayed in the discussion section, or have they been subtly shifted so as to align with the views of the writers?

Precision: Scientific writing should be precise with no ambiguity and little wiggle room. The *fallacy of equivocation* should be avoided. Scientific writers should not emulate the famous oracles at Delphi, whose predictions were worded so that they could be construed to be true no matter what events came to pass. Similarly, scientific measurements should be sufficiently precise so they can be used to distinguish between hypotheses.

Relevance: Both the introduction to and the discussion of scientific papers should include only materials relevant to the conclusions. Mere parading of knowledge by incorporating extensive references irrelevant to the problem under investigation wastes readers' time and tests their patience.

Depth: Scientific papers should explore the topic to a depth appropriate to the standards of the field in which they are published. Thus, a clinical study on the effects of chlorhexidine published in a dental journal would include discussion of the clinical measurements but would not include molecular orbital calculations on the molecule. The article's depth will be determined largely by the standards of the journal in which it is published.

Breadth: The authors should consider the points of view of other investigators in the topic area, as well as relevant insights from related areas.

Logic: Readers who labored through the early chapters of this book need no more preaching on the importance of logic. Here, I will merely mention that writers on critical thinking find logic indispensable.

Significance: Because readers invest their time in understanding a scientific publication, it is only fair that they receive something of value in exchange. Thus, papers should present meaningful information that can impact the research, understanding, or clinical practice of the reader. Assessing significance is a difficult task, particularly soon after publication; however, over time, impact can be assessed by tools such as citation analysis.

Putting It All Together: Argumentation Maps

At the end of the day, investigators have to consolidate their diverse set of observations, literature references, and arguments into cogent conclusions. Often, more than one set of observations contribute to the conclusion. This situation is exemplified in Fig 21-1, which shows an *argumentation map* that my former postdoctoral fellow Douglas Hamilton and I constructed in preparation for writing a paper subsequently published in *Biomaterials*.[3] The paper concerned the response of osteoblasts to the specific topographic features of the surface on which they were cultured. Among the responses examined were cell signaling cascades—inherently complex pathways, whereby cells transmit signals received from the environment into appropriate actions (such as activating specific genes). The experiments tend to be similarly complex, involving multiple procedures such as immunostaining, Western blots, and inhibitors of various pathways. Despite the complexity, the results must be clear to referees and editors. An argumentation map provides a way of clarifying matters for the authors, but it may also be used to understand the arguments of others.

Argumentation maps were developed by Horn[4] as an aid in teaching philosophy and resolving or clarifying real world debates. Related approaches are *mind mapping* and *concept mapping,* which is part of a learning movement called *constructivism.* Developed by Novak and Gowin[5] in the 1970s, concept mapping visualizes relationships between different concepts. Not all of the features of argumentation maps are used in Fig 21-1, but the main feature employed is that a claim (ie, a conclusion) is placed in what is called a *focus box.* In this case, the focus box is the paper's conclusion: "Substratum-induced topographic activation is mediated by the FAK-ERK complex." Surrounding the focus box are the results of specific experiments (eg, "P-ERK levels increased on grooves & DES"), which I will call *data boxes.* The finding in the "P-ERK" data box supports the conclusion by providing evidence for the involvement of ERK. That support is indicated by a *link* (in effect, an arrow connecting the boxes, which includes the relationship between them). In this case, the link is labeled "Evidence for role of ERK." (In fact, more than one link is labeled this way, as is not uncommon in science, because there are multiple ways of demonstrating a relationship.)

A second group of links are labeled *caveats,* or warnings of possible problems with the link. The box connected to the "P-ERK data box" by the caveat link is inscribed "True for all times?" This box told Hamilton and me that a referee might want more data at different times. If that request had been made, we would have had little choice but to comply. Another caveat-linked box, inscribed "Possibility that as . . . ," is linked to the data box "Inhibitor studies," by a link labeled *rebuttal.* In other words, we thought the inhibitor studies refuted the possible criticism made in the "Possibility . . . " box. The rebuttal-linked box "SOF" constitutes another means of rebuttal, invoking the current *standards of the field* (SOF). In other words, were a referee to criticize on the basis of the "Not quantified" box, we could argue that most investigators do not quantify immunostaining (in terms of intensity of the fluorescence). The SOF argument is one that might or might not work. You will recall from chapter 1 that the philosopher Fisher advocated the importance of having realistic standards. Normally referees are realistic because, like others, they do not want to face unreasonable standards when they submit their own papers for publication. Indeed, one sign of personal hostility to which scientists are acutely sensitive is unrealistic demands made by a referee or editor. Observing the influence principle of *liking* (discussed in chapter 3), alert scientists will go to some trouble to avoid having their work evaluated by a hostile person. Thus, scientists often try to surmise who is the source of the comments on their reviewed papers and grants.

Another kind of box, not shown in the diagram, is an "information missing" box, indicating that some information normally vital to establishing a conclusion is not currently available. How do you know what you do not know? The key to answering that question is to examine publications on similar topics in the same journal and determine what is normally required, although it must be conceded that identifying such requirements is not always easy.

Preparation of an argumentation map simplifies the writing of a paper. For this particular map, we could write, "there are several lines of evidence supporting the view that substratum-induced . . . ," then go around the supporting evidence boxes sequentially. We would still have decisions to make; should we discuss possible weaknesses in advance, or let the referees find them out for themselves? An author has an obligation to provide a balanced discussion; for example, the author would have to cite and explain any evidence in the literature contradicting the conclusion.

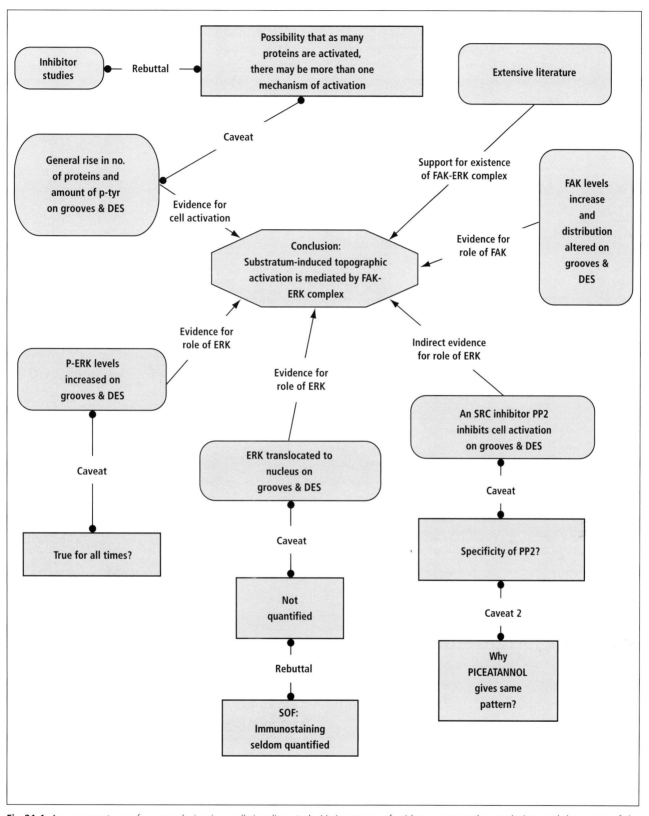

Fig 21-1 An argument map for a conclusion in a cell-signaling study. Various types of evidence support the conclusion, and the nature of the support is indicated on the linking arrows. Caveats to the conclusion and possible rebuttals may also be mapped.

The author also has an obligation to be reasonably concise—no one wants a discussion that examines minor points in mind-numbing detail.

Another use of argumentation maps is to assess the evidence for a conclusion in the paper. Sometimes in the dental literature one will find a conclusion supported by no evidence whatsoever in the paper. Some of these phantom conclusions may be platitudes relating to proper technique or widely accepted views. Other conclusions might be poorly supported. These are perhaps the most worrying because if the paper is accepted, they may undergo what I call "conclusion creep" in the author's subsequent papers, in which the weak sister conclusion transforms itself into a Goliath (albeit one ably brought down by the single stone of Fisher's assertability question, discussed in chapter 1).

By constructing an argumentation map that makes the support for a conclusion explicit, the reader is also able to consider the links more closely, look for missing information boxes, and think of other interpretations of the data.

Because of the difficulty of making complex arguments understandable to readers, authors should consider hiring professional editors or medical writers to help them present their arguments in a convincing fashion. After all, the hiring of statisticians to deal with data analysis is commonly accepted, yet statistical considerations are only one part of the total argument. The success of a study in terms of its eventual publication and impact might be well served by investing resources in rhetorical presentation, for readers will be hesitant to cite what they do not understand.

Balanced Judgments

A study that contains errors of logic, method, or design is not necessarily useless or unimportant. James Lind studied a group of 12 British sailors with scurvy and divided them into subgroups of 2 that received the following dietary supplements: cider, elixir vitriol, vinegar, sea water, two oranges and one lemon, or bigness of nutmeg.[6] By current standards of experiment design, Lind's findings would be considered rubbish. There was no random allocation of subjects; the treatments were not applied blind; there was no placebo; only one dose of each agent was used; and there was no statistical analysis. Yet, Lind's findings revealed a

way to prevent scurvy. In June 1854, Pasteur's anti-rabies vaccine was investigated by a committee of scientists appointed by the French government. For Pasteur's definitive test, he had used only two vaccinated dogs, two untreated dogs, and two rabbits.

Consider Ninio's analysis[7] of how a strict reviewer might evaluate the signal papers of molecular biology:

The double helix? Our reviewer has found two major faults: The authors wrongly assume the bases to be in the keto form and they conveniently ignore the fact that the A/T and G/C ratios differ significantly from unity by at least 10%. Furthermore, the authors have no original data to present that would substantiate their speculations. The genetic code? Dr Mathaei and Nirenberg's work will not be credible as long as the authors persist in using nonbiological templates, at nonphysiological Mg^{2+} concentration in a system that is five orders of magnitude slower than the cell's apparatus. . . . Had all the referees done the kind of job they are asked to do, molecular biology would hardly exist."

These examples illustrate the principle that assessing scientific papers is not a black or white proposition; defects in one aspect can sometimes be compensated by strengths in another. Thus, while Watson and Crick may not have presented much original data in their *Nature* article, the overall brilliance of their proposal won them a Nobel Prize.[8] Even a humble case report can contain the germ of an observation that could prove valuable for future study. The existence of errors or weaknesses in a study does not mean that the conclusions are necessarily wrong. We should not make the judgment error humorously known as "throwing out the baby with the bathwater." The problem of assessing a paper, then, is a balancing act in which the relative merits of originality and execution are considered.

Judgments Under Uncertainty

In some instances, sound judgments about the scientific merits of a proposal might be of practical importance. For example, the field of resin composites is changing rapidly, and there is believed to be a growth market for esthetic dentistry that uses these formulations. When new formulations become available, dentists must decide whether to adopt them. If a dentist adopts a new product and it fails, he or she may be stuck with the responsibility of replacing a lot of failed restorations. If the dentist does not change to a newer formulation that subsequently performs better than others, the dentist may lose patients to another practitioner who offers this better service. A dentist does not necessarily have the luxury of waiting; at a recent conference, it was stated that improved composite formulations are being prepared every 6 months. In short, dentists, like other clinicians, are forced to make judgments about the quality of scientific information under uncertain conditions.

While the preceding chapters of this book provide a guide to evaluating scientific information, there is still the mental act of forming a final judgment, which involves balancing the various components of the evaluation process. The process whereby people form judgments under uncertain conditions has been a topic of considerable investigation by psychologists.[9] Several principles have been developed that explain how people make judgments and errors in judgment. Following are some of the characteristics of human judgment that are particularly applicable in evaluating scientific work.

Belief in the law of small numbers

Experimental evidence shows that even scientists are rather insensitive to sample size and are willing to draw recklessly strong inferences about populations from knowledge about even a small number of cases.[10] Clinical seminars exemplify this principle when clinicians propose treatments based on their experience with few patients.

Greater impact of concrete vs abstract information

People are not very good at handling probabilistic data. Information on things such as prevalence of a disease will not have the same impact as one good illustrated example. This has long been recognized as the case; in 1927 Bertrand Russell wrote, "popular induction depends upon the emotional interest of the instances, not upon their number."[11] In experimental tests, where sheer number of instances is pitted against emotional interest, emotional interest has in every case carried the day.[10] I have noticed that when clinical scientists give lectures to dental students, the students remember the clinical slides illustrating a single patient at one point of time who had received a particular treatment, but have little ability to recall statistical data that represent many patients and better indicate treatment effectiveness.

Problems of causal reasoning

There is an irresistible tendency to perceive sequences of events in terms of causal relations, even when the perceiver is fully aware that the relation between the events is incidental and that imputed causality is illusory.[12] This statement merely affirms that the post hoc fallacy is common, as manufacturers of over-the-counter medicines are profitably aware.

In attributing causes to certain events, people usually assess the degree to which observed behaviors or outcomes occur in the presence of, but fail to occur in the absence of, each causal candidate under consideration.[13] Thus, they seem to apply Mill's canons of induction—particularly the method of agreement. Moreover, in the case of single observations, the assessment strategy involves a discounting principle whereby the observer discounts the role of any causal candidate in explaining an event, so that other plausible causes or determinants can be identified.[13] Thus, people adopt the inductively correct policy of considering plausible alternatives. However, in applying these rules, they may make certain errors. For example, there is some evidence to suggest that when people are called on to assess their role in a given sequence of events, they may give themselves more credit for success and less blame for failure than do independent observers.[10] This concept would seem intuitively obvious to anyone who has worked in large institutions or who has seen case presentations.

Model building and revision

Most inferences in everyday life rely on models that are imprecise, incomplete, or incorrect.

1. People commonly overpredict from highly uncertain models.[12] This could be called the *horse-race fallacy*.
2. It appears easier to assimilate a new fact within an existing causal model than to revise the model in light of this fact. In experiment studies, subjects are

reluctant to revise a rich and coherent model, even if the model is very uncertain; instead, they easily use an existing model to explain new facts, however unexpected.[12] Thus, theories—like the *focal infection hypothesis* from dentistry—can linger on even when they are highly improbable.

Use of heuristics

In assessing probabilities, people typically use certain *heuristics*—that is, exploratory problem-solving techniques—to reduce complex tasks to simpler operations.[9] Three examples are:

1. *Representativeness heuristic*. An object is assigned to one category rather than to another, insofar as its principle features resemble the category.

   Example: Two professors of chemistry have a friend who also is a professor and is shy, small in stature, and likes to write poetry. What is this friend's area of study—Asian studies or chemistry? Most people answer Asian studies, even though at the university there are four times as many professors of chemistry as there are professors of Asian studies, and two chemistry professors are much more likely to know another chemist than a member of any other department. People ignore these probabilities, because the description would appear to match a preconception of an Asian studies professor. They assign too much weight to the representativeness heuristic.

2. *Availability heuristic*. Objects or events are judged as frequent or probable, or infrequent or improbable, depending on the readiness with which they come to mind.

   Example: Is it more likely that a word selected at random from an English text starts with *r* (eg, *rich*) or that *r* is the third letter (eg, *car*)? People approach this problem by recalling words that begin with *r* and then recalling words that have *r* in the third position. Because it is much easier to search for words by their first letter than their third letter, most people judge words that begin with a given consonant to be more numerous than words in which the same consonant appears in the third position. They do this even for consonants such as *r* or *k*, which are more frequent in the third position than in the first.[7]

3. *Adjustment and anchoring*. In many instances people make estimates by starting from an initial value that is adjusted to yield the final answer. Typically, adjustments made to the initial value are insufficient. Thus, to get a good price on the sale of a house, it might be best to price it significantly higher than the market value. This will anchor the value in buyers' minds, and typically buyers will not adjust sufficiently when they make their offers.

Belief perseverance in the face of empirical challenges

Beliefs from narrow personal impressions to broader social theories seem remarkably resilient in the face of empirical challenges that seem logically devastating.[13] To some extent, this may be the result of the ability of the human mind to accommodate new data into an existing accepted model. Ross and Anderson[13] state that professional scientists are not immune to this offense:

> Again and again one sees contending factions that are involved in scholarly disputes whether they involve the origins of the universe, the line of hominid ascent, or the existence of ego-defensive attribution biases, draw support for their divergent views from the same corpus of findings.

Therefore, we can expect that authors of scientific articles will resort to mental gymnastics to justify their findings and to defend their theories.

Clinical vs Scientific Judgment

Clinical judgment can be thought of as a combination of knowledge, skills, and abilities based on personal experience and reading that allows a clinician to make correct diagnostic and therapeutic decisions based on information that is incomplete and uncertain. Clinical judgment requires the ability to choose relevant data from a larger set; formulate an overall view of the clinical problem; develop a plan to evaluate the clinical problem; monitor and modify the plan as needed; and determine what additional resources are needed.[14]

In medicine, clinical judgment is developed by exposure to many patients with a wide variety of diseases and presentations; experience in treating patients and following their courses; reading the literature; evaluating the validity of decisions by trial and error; and interactions with peers and superiors by discussion as well as by attendance at lectures, seminars, and professional meetings.[14]

One problem with the acquisition of clinical judgment is that clinical experience is often gained in a haphazard manner, because it depends on the problems of the patients that show up for treatment. Moreover, typically, a clinician must make judgments rapidly.

On the other hand, scientists are concerned with exact and systematic investigation. *Academic science* is a social institution devoted to the construction of a rational consensus of opinion over the widest possible field[15]—a time-consuming process. Thus, scientists can keep their minds open if the information is not definitive, whereas clinicians have to act. However, both groups face some common problems in forming their judgments.

Problems with clinical judgment

An understanding of clinical judgment is sometimes required in the evaluation of clinical research. Arkes[16] described four impediments to accurate clinical judgment in medicine:

1. Inability to assess covariation accurately. Many people overemphasize the percentage of cases in which both symptom and outcome are present. The cases in which the symptom is absent and the outcome is present are not accorded their full importance.
2. Preconceived notions or expectancies.
3. Lack of awareness of factors that influence judgment.
4 Overconfidence by physicians about the accuracy of their judgment, a condition brought about by:
   a. Placebo or *Hawthorne effect*. Receiving any treatment or attention is often beneficial.
   b. Gathering of selective information that tends to support the favored hypothesis.
   c. Selectively disregarding evidence that contradicts the present judgment.
   d. Hindsight bias. Many data sets contain observations that may be used to support many different interpretations. When a physician knows that a specific outcome has occurred, the data are observed and put together to support that outcome.

In reviewing behavioral decision theory and clinical information processing, Dowie and Elstein[17] emphasize the following problems:

1. Failure to retrieve correct hypothesis from memory.
2. Pursuit of exotic categories at the expense of more probable diseases.
3. Misinterpretation of data, whereby the data best remembered are those that fit the hypotheses generated.
4. Poor use of probabilistic information, such as the neglect of Bayes' theorem in revising probabilities, and confusion of the diagnostic value of a test with its predictive value. Base rates are often neglected in favor of individualizing information. This is an example of what has been called the *vividness problem*.[18] In solving problems or making decisions, people are most likely to employ the most readily accessible facts. One factor that strongly affects accessibility is the vividness of the information—and individual cases abound with vivid, concrete information.

From the preceding lists, we can conclude that clinicians have many of the same problems and tendencies with judgment as the general population.

A formal approach to clinical judgment: Decision theory

Formal decision analysis is an approach that enables decision makers, such as clinicians, to carry out a comprehensive and logical evaluation of alternative strategies and to choose the best decision, using rational criteria. The topic has been the focus of an issue of the *Journal of Dental Education,* and there is continued interest within the field of dentistry.[19]

The following example, supplied by Fung et al,[20] is based on a computer program for instruction in periodontal diagnosis. Application of decision analysis comprises the following steps:

1. The first step in clinical decision analysis is to identify and structure the problem. For example, a patient may have bleeding gums, and the decision problem may be deciding on the appropriate treatment (Fig 21-2).
2. The second step is to assign probabilities to each of the possible outcomes for each course of action. In this example, the two possibilities are the desirable

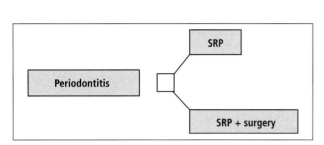

Fig 21-2 Application of decision analysis: A patient with periodontitis may be treated with scaling and root planing (SRP) or SRP plus surgery. □ = decision node.

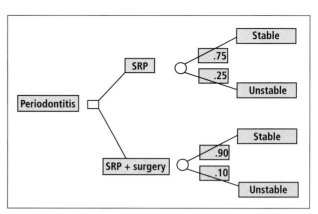

Fig 21-3 Assignment of probabilities to each outcome of treatment. ○ = chance node that the outcome is described in terms of probabilities and decision maker has no influence on outcome.

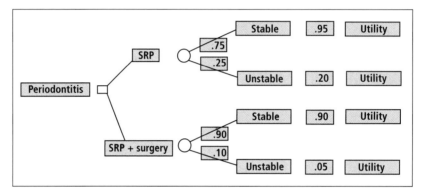

Fig 21-4 Decision tree based on utility of outcome.

outcome of *stable attachment* or the undesirable outcome of *continuing deterioration*. For illustrative purposes, suppose that the probabilities are as shown in Fig 21-3. That is, for this class of patient, SRP plus surgery has an increased probability of producing the desirable outcome (.90) relative to SRP alone (.75).

3. In formal decision theory, an additional piece of information is required—the *utility of the outcomes*. The stable outcome obtained by SRP alone might be assigned a value of .95, whereas the stable result obtained by SRP plus surgery might be assigned a value of only .80, because there would be additional costs to the patient in time, money, and pain. Here the utility values are chosen arbitrarily, but they could be measured, at least in theory. For example, for adults, it has been found that, in general, if a normal day of health is assigned a value of 1, a day feeling ill has a value of .80, and a day sick at home

or in the hospital has a value of .40. An unstable result obtained by SRP would have a higher utility than the same outcome with SRP plus surgery because of these additional costs of the surgical treatment. With this information, a decision tree can be generated that looks like Fig 21-4.

4. The fourth step is to combine the utilities and probabilities. Typically, this is done by multiplication, but there conceivably might be different weights assigned to the two informational components. For example, one might have a much more precise estimate of the probability than the utility and might want to weigh the less certain information less heavily. In this example, we will simply combine the values by multiplication to calculate the expected utility, as in Fig 21-5.

5. In the last step of decision making, the clinician chooses the path that leads to the highest expected

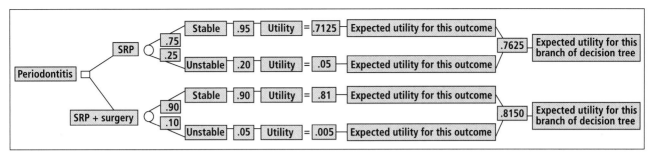

Fig 21-5 Decision tree based on utility and probability of outcome.

utility. In this case, SRP plus surgery would be chosen because the expected utility of this form of treatment is .815, whereas that of SRP is only .7625.

6. The last step in decision analysis is *sensitivity analysis*, whereby the decision maker judges the sensitivity of the solution to inputs—in our example, the probabilities and utilities.

The probabilities and utilities will differ, depending on the particular case in question. The probabilities of success of the SRP treatment for a patient with localized juvenile aggressive periodontitis might be less than those for a patient with generalized chronic periodontitis. They might also be expected to differ between geriatric and young patients. Thus, the probabilities used in the decision analysis would have to be adjusted to be appropriate for the case in question.

A major problem in applying decision analysis is that uncertainty in the probabilities or utilities may make the analysis useless. There are few precise data on the probabilities of success for different treatments, particularly when it is necessary to consider the precise attributes of the patient, such as age, sex, oral hygiene habits, and other factors. Only a limited number of large-scale unbiased medical databases exist that are suitable for the probabilities required for decision analysis. Subjective probabilities would be useful if they corresponded to the truth, but subjective determinants of probabilities by people in general and by physicians in particular are poor and show a strong tendency to overestimate the likelihood of an event occurring.[21]

In clinical dentistry, the first question about utilities is: utility to whom? The problem is that the measurement of the utility function of an individual or group of individuals is not easy.[22] The utility to the dental practitioner for providing additional therapies is usually high because the service is delivered on a fee-for-service basis. Calculating the utilities for the patients is difficult and almost inevitably involves subjective judgments. In prosthodontics, for example, some patients are perfectly happy with removable partial dentures, whereas others demand expensive crown and bridge restoration. Researchers have undertaken promising work on meaningful measuring utilities in clinical research and have identified a number of the problems.[23,24] Nevertheless, it is probably fair to say that relatively little information is available on this topic for dental decision making.

There are several advantages to a formal approach to decision making. First, it forces the clinician to identify all of the possible choices and to separate and consider the probabilities of success for the treatments and utilities for the outcomes. This is undoubtedly done informally and less rigorously in ordinary clinical decision making. Another advantage is that decision analysis will improve as clinicians obtain better data and means of assessing probabilities and utilities. It seems likely that formal decision analysis will occupy a greater role in dentistry and dental research in the future.[25,26] By 2000 some 67 papers had already appeared using this approach.[27]

Forming Scientific Judgments: The Problem of Contradictory Evidence

Differences among studies

The science of reviewing research and combining the results of various studies, a procedure termed *meta-analysis*, has been summarized by Light and Pillemer.[28] Some of the topics in this book give at least a partial explanation for the disagreements in the findings of

Table 21-1 Review of the use of dentifrices to control dental caries*

Agent	No. of negative findings	No. of positive findings	Range of caries reduction reported (%)
Urea and ammonium dentifrices	4	7	25–90
Enzymatic dentifrices	3	3	43–53
Antibiotic dentifrices	4	2	26–56

*Data from DePaola.[29]

different studies. Table 21-1, adapted from DePaola,[29] summarizes review findings on the results of dentifrice use to control dental caries. All of the agents tested produced conspicuous effects in some trials but little or no effect in others. At first glance, this is depressing; scientific findings should be reproducible, as noted earlier. There are many reasons why exact replication of results does not occur.

Random fluctuations

In a single trial consisting of the five flips of a coin, the odds of getting five heads in a row with a fair coin are $(\frac{1}{2})^5$ or 1 chance in 32. This is less than the commonly used choice of 1 = 5% or 1 in 20. If the trial flips were done 100 times, it is likely that five heads would occur at least once. This unlikely event of five consecutive heads could appear on the first trial. If we only did a single trial and obtained these results, we might conclude erroneously that the coin was not fair. A similar effect could have occurred in some of the caries studies. Because DePaola reviewed 45 studies, it is likely that in some of the experiments, contrary to the findings, the treatments did not really have any effect, but instead a statistical type I error occurred.

Differences in test conditions

A more common problem is that all of the studies would vary somewhat in the method of treatment or the population studied. For studies in dental caries, relevant differences might include location, age range, oral hygiene habits, diet, previous exposure to fluoride, and diagnostic criteria used by the examiners. In

illustrating this point, DePaola[29] used data to show that two nonfluoridated communities 12 miles apart varied greatly in their dental characteristics. Moreover, he points out that if independent tests of the same agent were performed in each of these locales, it would be hard to imagine that the strikingly different dental characteristics of the subjects in each study would not cause the clinical results to vary. Similarly, the age distribution of the subjects would also be important. For example, unlike in 8- to 10-year-old subjects, the measurement of caries activity in 6- to 7-year-old subjects is dominated by the first permanent molar—a tooth that is notoriously difficult to protect. The size of effect of a protective agent would be expected to change depending on the relative numbers of children in each age group. However, despite these explanations, the discrepancies between various studies are disturbing.

The fallibility of a single study demonstrating statistical significance has been emphasized by prominent pioneers in the field of statistics. Tukey[30] stated:

The modern test of significance before which so many editors of psychological journals are reported to bow down owes more to R. A. Fisher than to any other man. Yet Sir Ronald's standard of firm knowledge was not one very extremely significant result but rather to repeatedly get results significant at 5%.

Fisher[31] phrased his criterion for belief as follows:

In order to assert that a natural phenomenon is experimentally demonstrable we need, not an isolated record, but a reliable method of procedure. In relation to the test of significance we may say that a phenomenon is experimentally demonstrable when we know how to conduct an experiment which will rarely fail to give us a statistically significant result.

Readers of clinical journals need to keep these thoughts in mind because, not uncommonly results of a single trial are often reported, perhaps because of the expense in clinical trials.

Yet even some of the most widely accepted dogmas of dentistry fall short of Fisher's standard. It becomes obvious that continuing work is required to put dentistry on a sound scientific footing. The reproducibility (or lack thereof) of various dental measurements and diagnostic tests is part of the problem. Differences in test conditions and methods of measurement are more likely causes of discrepancies between studies than is type I error.

Discrepancies: Opportunities for research

There is a long-standing tradition of discrepancies between observations providing opportunities for research. For example, the inert gases (argon, xenon, etc) were discovered after it was noted that the molecular weight of nitrogen prepared from air (which contained inert gases) differed from that found for nitrogen prepared from ammonia. To return to the example of the efficacy of dentifrices, the discrepancies between studies present opportunities for research. One might want to investigate the possibility that positive or negative findings for enzymatic dentifrices correlate with fluoridation in the test community—or other characteristics, such as age of subjects, or some attributes not presently known to affect dental caries.

Problems with meta-analysis

Despite the difficulties outlined in the previous sections, it is useful in some instances to rigorously combine the results of different studies to incorporate all of the available information. Clearly, this approach of meta-analysis is most feasible when investigators use similar techniques on similar populations and look at similar outcomes. However, a major problem is that research studies on the same topic can vary in many ways, and the reporting of data can be incomplete. For example, Creugers and Van 't Hof[32] examined 60 pub-

lications presenting clinical data. Their aims were to assess an overall survival ratio of three- and four-unit resin-bonded partial dentures and to explore relationships between success factors, including type of retention, cementation material, preparation of the abutment teeth, and location of denture. However, many of the publications did not give sufficient information to address these questions, so that only 14 of the studies were selected for further analysis. It transpired that sufficient information was available to perform analysis on type of retention and location of denture, of which weighted multiple-regression analysis did not reveal a significant effect. This may not indicate that the factors were unimportant but may simply reflect the high variability in patient selection, tooth preparation, luting resin cements, and operator experience. The most useful information that came out of the study was that the overall survival curve showed an almost linear slope.

Using Others' Judgments: Citation Analysis As a Means of Literature Evaluation

No one can be an expert on everything; few people are experts on even one topic. Thus, to some extent, everyone must rely on other people's opinions. Opinions are not facts but judgments or beliefs based on grounds short of proof, and therefore they can be biased. It is possible that experts with different biases will disagree. A traditional approach to this problem is to collect informed opinions from as many experts as possible. The primary source that enables us to collect scientific opinion on published papers is the *Science Citation Index* (SCI). The fundamental question we can answer quickly with the SCI is where and by whom a particular paper has been cited. For example, if we were interested in the model system for studying gingivitis introduced by Löe et al[33] in the *Journal of Periodontology* 1965;36:177, we could find, by means of the SCI, that it had been cited 1,282 times as of July 2007. We would also discover who had cited this paper and where they had cited it. There are two ways to use this information:

1. First, we could read these papers and see exactly what the authors said about Löe et al's paper. Thus, we would be canvassing 1,282 papers for an opinion. For a highly cited paper like Löe et al's, this ap-

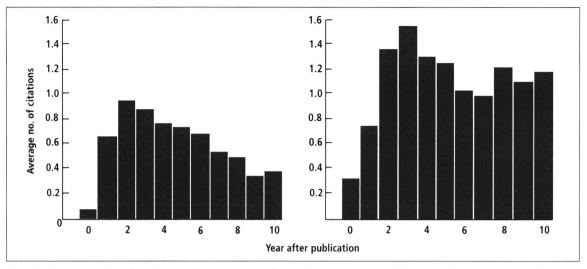

Fig 21-6 Average number of citations to all papers vs time after publication in *Journal of Periodontology* and *Journal of Periodontal Research*. (Reprinted from Brunette DM et al[37] with permission.)

proach would be thorough, but it would require an inordinate amount of work.

2. A second use of the SCI would be to simply count the number of authors who cited Löe et al. This can be instructive because most authors cite publications in a positive sense. Thus, the very fact that a paper (such as Löe et al's) has been cited frequently probably indicates that the paper has received wide acceptance.

However, most papers do not acquire such a large number of citations, and to interpret the numbers at all requires some background information.

Number of references per paper

Garfield[34] has stated that the number of references per paper is an important factor in *citation impact* (defined as the number of citations per paper). Papers published in math journals cite an average of eight references, whereas papers published in biochemistry journals have more. For example, the *Journal of Molecular Biology* cites around 29 references per paper. Clearly, this gives the biochemists an edge in collecting citations simply by virtue of the habits of their field. Studies published in the *Journal of Periodontology* and the *Journal of Periodontal Research* have around 20 references per article, which is close to what Price[35] defines as the normal range of references per paper. On average, papers in science journals cite about 15 refer-

ences, of which about 12 refer to other journals rather than to books.[34] The core dentistry journals (see Table 4-2) average 17 references per article, which is slightly higher than the average for all scientific journals (which is at 14.5).

Age distributions of references

Calculation of Price's index (PI) proportion of references dated in the past 5 years offers another insight into research. The benchmarks for such a study are provided by the data of Price,[36] who examined 162 journals from various subjects and dates and found that the median PI is 32, with a lower quartile of 21 and an upper quartile of 42. Hard sciences are found in the upper quartile and are called *research front areas*. Physics and biochemistry are two examples of this group, and it is thought that such fields are undergoing rapid progress. Does dental research go quickly or slowly? The PI of research in periodontology varies. In some years it is found in the rapid progress group, but in other years it is found in the range occupied by the normal group of sciences—that is, those that move at a somewhat slower pace.

Another way of looking at this aspect of literature usage is to calculate the average number of citations to all papers as a function of time after publication. Figure 21-6 presents this information for the *Journal of Periodontology* and the *Journal of Periodontal Research* between the years of 1966 and 1971.[37] It is evident that, as for

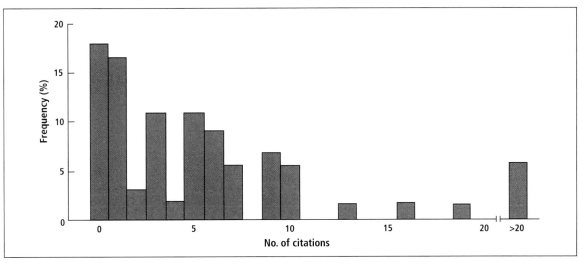

Fig 21-7 Distribution of the percentage of articles having a given number of citations in the first 5 years after publication in the *Journal of Periodontology* from 1966 to 1971.

other biomedical literature, the maximum frequency of citation of papers in both journals occurred 2 to 3 years after publication. This finding has a practical consequence; it means that our chances of locating citations to an article of interest are small in the first year after its publication. This is not surprising when we consider the mechanics of publication. Even if the reader of an article were writing a paper and decided to incorporate a reference to the newly published paper in his or her manuscript, a considerable delay in the appearance of the citation to the first article would be required as a result of the time necessary for the second article to be published. The length of that delay depends on factors such as the promptness of the referees, the diligence of the editorial staff, and the amount of revision required. For example, in 1989 it typically took about 8 to 9 months after submission for a paper to be published in the *Journal of Dental Research*. The processing of papers has been speeded up in recent years because most refereeing is now done over the Internet. Nevertheless, these delays conspire to reduce the effectiveness of citation analysis in the evaluation of an article in the first year after publication.

Distribution of citations among individual papers

All papers are not created equal. The number of times individual papers are cited varies widely. Data from an early study that I conducted with Simon and Reimers

(Fig 21-7) shows the distribution of articles that appeared in the *Journal of Periodontology* from 1966 to 1971 in the first 5 years after their publication.[37] This figure shows that there is a wide variation in the number of times articles published in the same journal are cited. The distributions are highly asymmetric, and the majority have low citation counts. The shape of Fig 21-7 is roughly what would be expected from earlier work on the distribution of citations among individual papers. Price[36] found that the percentage of papers cited a given number of times was proportional to $n^{-(2.5 \text{ to } 3)}$, where n is the number of citations. *Power-law distributions* of this type imply that a small proportion of the items under examination are responsible for a large proportion of the desired products. Figure 21-7 demonstrates that different papers in the *Journal of Periodontology* have a widely varying impact on subsequent research. The majority of papers have very little impact, and a significant proportion (18%) were never cited in the journals covered by the SCI (which includes most of the major journals of dental research) in the 15 years following publication. There may be other nonresearch uses of this material; hence, it is not fair to say that those articles not cited are useless. Nonetheless, it cannot be denied that their influence on subsequent research appears to be small.

One can only speculate on the reasons so many papers are ineffective in stimulating further research. First, on the whole, many authors seem to choose topics that are inherently uninteresting both to other research workers and, after publication, to the authors themselves. Second, many scientific publications appear to contain weaknesses. For the present purpose, it should be noted that the citation record of a paper can be used as a screen to sort papers of varying impact.

Role of citation analysis in the evaluation of individual scientific papers

Acceptability and reproducibility of published results

Many scientific articles undergo some sort of refereeing process. In theory, at least, the referee may be held responsible for checking on matters such as the validity of the stated conclusions, the clarity of presentation, and the suitability for publication of an article in a particular journal. However, he or she cannot be expected to reproduce the data that constitute the results section of a scientific paper. Consequently, the publication of such results represents an act of faith in the authors, in that the editors accept that the given results were obtained under the given conditions. However, subsequent workers may be unable to reproduce those results, for a number of reasons. In addition, others may be reluctant to accept the authors' interpretation of the results. Such differences in either fact or opinion can often be discerned with *citation analysis* (CA), by which we look up the authors who have cited a particular paper to see if they have done so in an affirmative or negative manner. Therefore, CA can serve as an instrument (albeit not a very sensitive one) for checking on the reproducibility and acceptability of published results.

Collective judgment

One strong argument for the use of CA in the evaluation of scientific work is the collective nature of the citation index. Because it covers the vast majority of the significant journals of science, the SCI in effect canvasses the writings—and thus the judgments—of the majority of scientific investigators. This large number of judges means that CA may be the fairest means of evaluating a paper, because the effect of individual biases becomes less pronounced. As noted earlier, *academic science* has been defined as the social institution devoted to the construction of a rational, consensual opinion over the widest possible field.[14] CA provides science with the most efficient means of demonstrat-

ing that a given piece of work has been absorbed into the scientific framework of a given subject.

Relationship of CA to peer judgment

A common means of evaluating scientific work is through the peer-review mechanism. In this system, a committee of experts (typically, investigators in the given subject) review and assess the quality of an investigator's work in that subject. A major problem of the peer-review system is that it has the appearance of a "buddy system" (ie, you approve my work and I will approve yours).[38]

Citation frequency (the number of times a given article has been cited) is objective and is therefore an improvement on review by only a few peers. Nevertheless, a number of objections to the method have been raised. Overall, it appears that ratings made by CA corroborate the decisions made by other methods, including peer review.[39] Perhaps the ultimate accolade awarded by peer judgment is the Nobel Prize.

Sher and Garfield[40] found that there are 30 times as many citations per average Nobel Prize winner as there are per average cited author. In a sample of 13 Nobel Prize winners, 11 were in the top 0.185% of the citation frequency file. Although part of the high citation rate was because the Nobel Prize winners produced more papers than the average scientist, still, the average number of citations per cited paper was roughly two times that of the average scientist.

Objections to CA

The objections to CA are largely based on the uncertainty about the reasons people cite papers. The role and significance of citations in scientific communication have been reviewed by Cronin.[41] Perhaps the most frequent objection is that papers that have been proved wrong might be quoted frequently. However, this is not the case; negative citations are rare.

Another objection is that scientists could inflate the value of their work by citing themselves frequently. Because this strategy is exceedingly obvious, it would likely be self-defeating. In any case, in periodontal literature self-citation comprises a significantly greater proportion of the citations of infrequently cited papers than frequently cited papers. It is hard to pull yourself up by the bootstraps.

A third objection—that citation frequency is dependent on the popularity of the specialty—has been answered by the observation that, though more papers are published in popular fields, there are also many more papers available to quote. Thus, the chance of a particular paper being quoted will be about the same in a popular field as in any other, providing other factors such as number of references per article remain constant.

Nevertheless, it is true that there are differences in citation frequency between fields. As noted earlier, the most critical factor in CA is the average number of references cited per paper. Moreover, it has been found that scientific literature grows at different rates from topic to topic and during different periods. Therefore, caution is required in making comparisons between work done in different fields or at different times. Another problem with CA is that although each citation entails recognition of another's work, there is little known about the actual motivations of authors when they cite papers.

Summary of the role of SCI in the evaluation of individual papers

Although some of the problems encountered in CA can and do weaken its strength, they are merely the noise in the measurement procedure. A major advantage of CA is that it is quantitative and, with further research, may be improved and refined. Questions (such as the impact of self-citations) can be isolated and answered. Garfield and Cawkell[42] have stated that statistical routines have been developed to account for derogatory references, self citations, multiple authorship, the stature of the journal in which the article appeared, and unusual technique papers.

CA has its pitfalls when applied to individual papers—particularly recently published ones, where the amount of information available in the SCI is small. Nevertheless, it reflects the real world of science, not a fantasyland where all scientists' work is equally valuable.[42] In the real world of personal economics, the number of citations more strongly correlates with increases in salary than does either professional experience or number of publications.[43]

When evaluating particular papers, readers should combine CA with other techniques described in this book. Its main value for our purposes is that it enables readers to find out other scientists' opinions of cited papers. Second, it serves to make readers suspicious of the significance of noncited papers—a suspicion that will be justified most of the time.

Influencing Judgment: Lower Forms of Rhetorical Life

You will recall that sound conclusions are the result of combining valid logic with reliable data. However, for the conclusions to be accepted, an investigator must persuade his listeners (if giving a seminar) or readers (if writing a paper). Because the social interaction of scientists is said to be that of organized skepticism, the job of listeners and readers, particularly referees, is to criticize the presentation. It is possible for a sound piece of work to remain unrecognized because of poor presentation or inadequate response to criticisms. Conversely, poor science can sometimes be masked by superb showmanship or rhetorical legerdemain. In a satirical paper, Kline[44] has termed some of the techniques used in these lower forms of rhetorical life *factifuging* (ie, putting facts to flight), which he describes as the most successful technique for defending the intuitively correct position against contradictory data. Much of what follows is drawn from Kline's paper, which deals largely with the concerns of psychiatric research. I have condensed his list to three categories that I think are generally applicable to all fields: distraction, denigration, and terminal inexactitude.

Distraction

The point of *distraction* is to so amuse, bore, or confuse the audience that they forget the original question, which may have had a damaging effect on the investigator's arguments. Techniques include:

1. *Joking.* A speaker was once asked whether *contact guidance* (a phenomenon of cell biology) had any effect on his results. Not knowing any cell biology, the speaker replied, "Your point reminds me of the story of an elderly preacher who, having been a bachelor all his life, married a widow. On their honeymoon night, his new bride was anxiously waiting in bed and was surprised when her husband dropped to his knees beside the bed.

   'What are you doing?' she asked.

   'My dear,' replied the preacher, 'I'm praying for guidance.'

   'Don't worry. I'll provide the guidance,' his experienced bride said. 'You pray for strength.'"

The audience remembered the joke but forgot the point of the question.

2. *Individualizing.* Use of the vividness phenomenon. The case is described in excruciating detail in the hope that the concrete effect of the case will overwhelm any abstract statistical information that may contradict the investigator's theories.

3. *Visual-aiding:* Cartoons, photographs of the speaker's university or home, and spectacular color graphics, for example, which are done so well that the audience concludes that the science was done equally well.

4. *Word games.* They come in many forms.

a. *Renaming.* Logicians have long been aware that to avoid contradictions, you must make distinctions. If you are caught in a contradiction, it can be advantageous to assign new meanings to old words or to invent new terms entirely. These can be justified by a dictionary of word origins, the use of which, according to Kline,[44] enables you to show that "everything is either itself or its opposite."

b. *Foreign phrasing.* This is the technique in which phrases in Greek, Latin, French, German, laboratory jargon, or other languages are used to impress and confuse an audience, many of whom will be hesitant to ask what a phrase means.

c. *Apodicting.* This is the art of issuing sententious statements or principles that the speaker feels are self-evident and hence not in need of justification by experimental data.[44] When confronted with a contradictory example, a speaker might reply, "Well, that's the exception that proves the rule." This is obviously a silly statement; the reason for testing a hypothesis and finding an exception is to disprove the rule, yet some people believe the adage. Moreover, there is also the chance that a show-off will point out that the word *prove* in the adage is used in the old Scottish sense of *test.* At this point, the audience will feel erudite, but the thrust of the original attack will have been lost.

5. *Strategic diversions.* When faced with questions for which they have no answers, many speakers prefer to answer some other question, rather than admitting "I don't know." This technique is particularly effective when the question is vaguely worded so that the speaker can answer it any way he or she chooses. The technique can also be used by speakers who are not speaking in their native tongues, since they have a legitimate excuse for misunderstanding questions. Another popular technique is to

say, "I'll deal with that point later in the seminar," and never return to it. Both methods save a speaker from embarrassment.

Denigration

The object of *denigration* is to drag your opponent down to or below your own level. It is used when the attacker cannot disprove the conclusions but feels compelled to question their importance.

1. *Damning with faint praise.* This practice might be called the *English disease.* A North American referee might call a given piece of work *excellent,* whereas an English referee would refer to the same work as *good*—reserving the word *excellent* for contributions that would lead directly to the Nobel Prize. Faint praise can be used in combination with other techniques. An especially devastating combination is lukewarm praise followed by a *but* or an *and* together with a suggestion for future improvement—as in, "thanks for telling us about your interesting work, and I look forward to seeing it being more rigorously pursued in the future." The first part of the sentence lowers the speaker's guard, while the second part delivers the knockout punch.

2. *Holier-than-thou approach.* As a general rule, critics do not have to concern themselves with feasibility or practicality; they can insist on unrealistic standards. For such a critic, there is never enough of anything—the sample size should be larger and there should be more controls, more time points, more sophisticated analysis, and more modern techniques. Until these alterations are made, critics can imply that the work does not meet appropriate standards. The cost of maintaining such standards is cheap if you do not have to bear the expense. In the real world, there are always limitations of time, money, or type of patient, and any sensible evaluation of a paper has to include what is feasible.

3. *Contrarian approach.* Contrarian critics make use of the fact that any study involves making decisions, and each decision means that some other option must be foregone. The instinctive contrarian points out the merits of the other choice. For example, a clinical study can be done with volunteers or nonvolunteers. If a study used volunteers, the contrarian would argue that everyone knows volunteers are a highly unusual group who are not representative of the general population. If the same study had

used nonvolunteers who had somehow been forced or selected to participate, the contrarian would argue that this selection procedure obviously biased the results. Kline[44] notes that subjects have to be something, and whatever it is that they are or are not can be used as the basis for claiming probable bias. The contrarian focuses on the weaknesses of the choice. Like the holier-than-thou critic, the contrarian ignores the information provided by a study on the grounds that it was not the best possible study.

4. *Old-hatting.* The technique of old-hatting denigrates the originality of a study by claiming that, in its essentials, the research has been done before. The technique is most effective if the information being cited was published in an obscure journal or in a hard-to-find thesis at some point in the past, and cannot easily be found. Sometimes an old-hatter will assert that it was he or she who did the work and therefore is glad to see the work confirmed. It has been said that scientists are divided between *splitters,* who like to make distinctions, and *lumpers,* who group everything together. The old-hatters are often great lumpers who show remarkable ability to find parallels in disparate pieces of work.

5. *Nothing-butting/just an example of. . . .* In this form of one-upsmanship, research findings are dismissed as nothing but an example of some more fundamental theory. Nothing-butting has the effect of denigrating the importance of a problem or finding by viewing it as just a subset of other more general problems or findings. Thus, periodontal disease may be regarded as nothing but a minor infection of the mouth. The nothing-butter ignores all of the specifics of a situation and concentrates on the big picture. For periodontal disease, the nothing-butter with training in immunology might ignore the vast economic importance of the problem, as well as the technical difficulties in treating individual teeth, and say that periodontal disease is just an example of an inappropriate immune response.

6. *Devil's advocate.* In the Catholic Church's canonization process, the devil's advocate is responsible for finding weaknesses in the case for the potential saint. As applied to science, the devil's advocate probes the research for weaknesses, including effects or considerations that were outside the original objectives of the study. If a given treatment were applied and produced an effect, the devil's advocate

might want to know why the effect was not larger—or at least as large as some other treatment; whether the treatment had any side effects; or whether, if the treatment was a drug, it works at other dosages, etc. In short, like the holier-than-thou critic, the devil's advocate shows that the research is not ideal. However, unlike the holier-than-thou critic, the devil's advocate makes no pretense that he or she attains such heights. In fact, he or she might even admit, "I'm just being the devil's advocate here but. . . . " The devil's advocate approach can be used constructively by individuals who wish to critique their own work and develop alternate ways of presenting their data. Moreover, it can be used as a tool prior to presentation to develop statements or responses to possible criticisms. Nevertheless, I think the net effect is that the audience becomes less impressed with a speaker after his or her research has been subjected to this type of criticism.

Terminal inexactitude

Remember that the speaker/writer controls the flow of information to an audience, and that this person can be dishonest by not giving all of the available relevant information (as discussed under inductive logic in chapter 6), or can even provide erroneous information. The extent of this problem is actually unknown, but one of the major growth areas in science appears to be writing about scientific fraud. Occasionally, graduate students find themselves in a position where they fear doing one experiment too many—ie, the experiment that disproves their thesis. After years of hard work, it would be tempting for the student who does an experiment disproving his or her thesis to place the results in a file drawer. For the grant-hungry or pre-tenure professor who wants to fatten his or her curriculum vitae, a more effective strategy might be to publish two papers—the first based on the preliminary results and the second a reexamination of the first. *Terminal inexactitudes* carry risks, but some investigators might agree with the comedian who—on considering Lincoln's adage: "You can't fool all of the people all of the time, but you can fool all of the people some of the time, and some of the people all of the time"—concluded "and that's good enough odds for me."

References

1. Dawes RM. You can't systematize human judgment: Dyslexia. In: Shweder RA (ed). Fallible Judgment in Behavioral Research. San Francisco: Jossey-Bass, 1980: 67–98.
2. Gopen GD, Swan JA. The science of scientific writing. Am Sci 1990;78:550–558.
3. Hamilton DW, Brunette DM. The effect of substratum topography on osteoblast adhesion mediated signal transduction and phosphorylation. Biomaterials 2007;28:1806–1819.
4. Horn RE. Teaching philosophy with argumentation maps. Newsletter of the American Philosophical Association, November 2000.
5. Novak JD, Gowin DB. Learning How to Learn. Cambridge: Cambridge Univ Press, 1996.
6. Gehlbach SH. Interpreting the Medical Literature. Lexington, MA: Collamore, 1982:75.
7. Ninio J. The ideology of scientific evaluation. Trends Biochem Sci 1981;6:VII.
8. Watson JD, Crick FHC. A structure for deoxyribose nucleic acid. Nature 1953;171:737–738.
9. Tversky A, Kahneman D. Judgment under uncertainty: Heuristics and biases. Science 1974;185:1124.
10. Nisbett RE, Borgida E, Crandall R, Rago H. Popular induction: Information is not necessarily informative. In: Kahneman D, Slovic P, Tversky A (eds). Judgment Under Uncertainty: Heuristics and Biases. Cambridge: Cambridge Univ Press, 1982:102.
11. Russel BR. Philosophy. New York: WW Norton, 1927.
12. Tversky A, Kahneman D. Causal schemas in judgments under uncertainty. In: Kahneman D, Slovic P, Tversky A (eds). Judgment Under Uncertainty: Heuristics and Biases. Cambridge: Cambridge Univ Press, 1982:117.
13. Ross L, Anderson CA. Shortcomings in the attribution process: On the origins and maintenance of erroneous social assessment. In: Kahneman D, Slovic P, Tversky A (eds). Judgment Under Uncertainty: Heuristics and Biases. Cambridge: Cambridge Univ Press, 1982:129.
14. Spilker B. Guide to the Clinical Interpretation of Data. New York: Raven, 1986:12–18.
15 Ziman J. An Introduction to Science Studies: The Philosophical and Social Aspects of Science and Technology. Cambridge: Cambridge Univ Press, 1984:10.
16. Arkes HR. Impediments to accurate clinical judgment and possible ways to minimize their impact. J Consult Clin Psychol 1981;49:323.
17. Dowie J, Elstein A. Professional Judgment: A Reader in Clinical Decision Making. Cambridge: Cambridge Univ Press, 1988:18–20.
18. Stanovich KE. How to Think Straight About Psychology. New York: HarperCollins, 1992:59–63.
19. Bolender CL. Summation. J Dent Educ 1992;56:873–874.
20. Fung K, Ellen RP, McCulloch CA. Development of a computer program for teaching periodontal diagnosis based on clinical epidemiological principles. J Dent Educ 1995;59:433.
21. Doubilet P, McNeil BJ. Clinical decisionmaking. Med Care 1985;23:648.
22. Llewellyn-Thomas H, Sutherland HJ, Tibshirani R, Ciampi A, Till JE, Boyd NG. The measurement of patients' values in medicine. Med Decis Making 1982;2:449.
23. Holtzman S, Kornman KS. Decision analysis for periodontal therapy. J Dent Educ 1992;56:844–861.
24. Anusavice KJ. Decision analysis in restorative dentistry. J Dent Educ 1992;56:812–27.
25. Hollender L. Decision making in radiographic imaging. J Dent Educ 1992;56:834–842.
26. Mohl ND, Ohrbach R. Clinical decision making for temporomandibular disorders. J Dent Educ 1992;56:823–832.
27. Rohlin M, Mileman PA. Decision analysis in dentistry— The last 30 years. J Dent 2000;20:453–468.
28. Light RJ, Pillemer DB. Summing Up the Science of Reviewing Research. Cambridge, MA: Harvard Univ Press, 1984.
29. DePaola PF. The interpretation of findings in clinical caries trials. ASDC J Dent Child 1974;41:11.
30. Tukey JW. Analyzing data: Sanctification or detective work? American Psychologist 1969;24:83–91.
31. Fisher RA, The Design of Experiments, ed 8. New York: Hafner Publishing, 1966:14.
32. Creugers NH, Van 't Hof MA. An analysis of clinical studies on resin-bonded bridges. J Dent Res 1991;70:146.
33. Löe H. This week's citation classic: Experimental gingivitis in man. Curr Contents September 1982:22.
34. Garfield E. The significant journals of science. Curr Contents June 1977:130–131.
35. Price DJ. Networks of Scientific Papers. Science 1965;149:510.
36. Price DJ. Citation measures of hard science, soft science, technology, and nonscience. In: Nelson CE, Pollock DK (eds). Communication Among Scientists and Engineers. Lexington, MA: Heath, 1970:1–22.
37. Brunette DM, Simon MJ, Reimers MA. Citation records of papers published in the Journal of Periodontology and the Journal of Periodontal Research. J Periodontal Res 1978;13:487.
38. Symington JW, Kramer TR. Does peer review work? Am Sci 1977;65:17.
39. Narin F. Evaluative Bibliometrics: The Use of Publication and Citation Analysis in the Evaluation of Scientific Activity. Cherry Hill, NJ: Computer Horizons, 1976.
40. Sher IH, Garfield E. New tools for improving and evaluating the effectiveness of research. In: Yovits MC, Gilford DM, Wilcox RH, Staveley E, Lemer HD (eds). Research Program Effectiveness: Proceedings of the Conference Sponsored by the Office of Naval Research, Washington, DC, July 27–29, 1965. New York: Gordon and Breach, 1966:135–142.
41. Cronin B. The Citation Process. London: Taylor Graham, 1984.
42. Garfield E, Cawkell AE. Citation analysis studies. Science 1975;189:397.
43. Garfield E. Can researchers bank on citation analysis? Curr Contents October 1988;31:3.
44. Kline NS. Factifuging. Lancet 1962;1:1396.

22 | Exercises in Critical Thinking

It is difficult to overstate the value of practice. For a new skill to become automatic or for new knowledge to become long-lasting, sustained practice, beyond the point of mastery, *is necessary.*

—Daniel T. Willingham
from *Practice makes perfect perfect—
But only if you practice beyond the point of
perfection. Am Educator 2004; Spring:31.*

Problems

The following excerpts from the dental literature are intended to illustrate some of the concepts introduced in the preceding chapters. To keep the section reasonably brief, the examples have been extracted from papers, and much detail has been omitted. In some instances, the authors discuss the weaknesses or strengths of the particular approach they employed in their article, which is not included here. The intent in presenting these examples is not to criticize or commend the articles in question, but rather to show how the arguments, strategies, and ideas discussed in this book appear in the dental (or popular) literature. To provide a wide range of examples in a reasonable amount of space, only select material was extracted from the papers. Often the problems contain a conclusion drawn from the abstract or summary of the paper and select material from other sections of the paper, such as Materials and Methods and Results, relevant to the conclusion. In approaching these problems, you should assume that the aspects of the conclusions that are not concerned with the information presented in the Materials and Methods and Results extracts are not problematic. For example, in Problem 1 assume that bone gain was actually achieved, even though it is not clear from the material that is presented how bone gain was measured, the time fluoride was applied, and so forth.

Problem 1

Biller T, Yosepovitch Z, Gedalia I. Effects of topical fluoride in the healing rate of experimental calvarial defects in rats. J Dent Res 1977;56:53–56.

Summary:

"Bone gain was achieved after topical application of fluoride. Fluoride has a strong promoting effect on osteogenesis and accelerates the repair process of defects in membranous bone. No major histological differences are evident in the newly formed bone."

Materials and Methods:

"In one half of the rats that underwent the procedure, a cotton wool swab soaked in 2% acidulated (0.1 M H_3PO_4) NaF solution was placed in the defect for 20 minutes. The area was then irrigated again with physiological saline solution. The scalp was then sutured. The remaining rats underwent the same local treatment with saline solution and served as controls."

Is this a positive or negative results paper? Is there any explanation, other than the effect of fluoride ions, that could explain the results?

Problem 2

Little JW, Wilson JC, Bickley HC, Bickley C. Effects of parathyroid extract on the rupture strength of intact skin of the rat. J Dent Res 1977;56:46–47.

Summary:

"Rats were injected with parathyroid extract (PTE) to search for possible effects on connective tissue of the skin. Rupture-strength analysis of skin samples showed a significant increase in strength of skin from PTE-treated rats. The explanation for this effect is not understood at present."

From the Results:

"PTE-treated rats lost weight during the 3-day experimental period. The mean starting weight in grams for the PTE-treated groups was 149.75; for the vehicle-treated group, the mean was 148.20; and for the saline solution–treated group, the mean was 153.80. There were no significant differences among groups. At the time of death, the mean weight in grams for the PTE-treated group was 127.63; for the vehicle-treated group it was 162.50; and for the saline solution–treated group, the mean was 163.20. The mean weight at death of the PTE-treated group was significantly different from that of the two control groups . . . (ie, the vehicle-treated group and saline solution–treated group)."

Are there any problems with the interpretation of the increase in rupture strength as a specific effect of PTE?

Problem 3

Nacht M. A devitalizing technique for pulpotomy in primary molars. J Dent Children 1956;22:45–47.

"A review of literature revealed some interesting work done by several men with mummifying pastes. In 1929 Dr Hess, of the University of Zurich, reported negative results in a bacterial analysis of 62 pulps mummified with formaldehyde paste. Dr H. R. Foster of Oakland in 1936 describes a successful treatment using formocresol and paste. Again in 1939 Dr K. A. Easlick used the same treatment substituting paraformaldehyde. In the Handbook of Dental Practice—1948, Dr Charles Sweet describes a treatment using zinc oxide, cresolated formaldehyde and eugenol. Since the principle of mummification had been used by so many of these eminent men at various times, it was decided that this might be the answer to our problem."

Identify the main form of argument used in this paragraph.

Problem 4

Brekke JH, Bresner M, Reitman MJ. Effect of surgical trauma and polylactate cubes and granules on the incidence of alveolar osteitis in mandibular third molar extraction wounds. J Can Dent Assoc 1986;4:315–319.

"The polylactic acid surgical dressing material, in either cube or granular form, substantially reduces the incidence of alveolar osteitis in healthy patients if all other principles of careful surgical technique are observed."

Identify the technique used in this sentence that could deflect possible criticism of the major findings on the dressing material.

Problem 5

Cipes MH, Miraglia M, Gaulin-Kremer E. Habits, monitoring and reinforcement to eliminate thumbsucking. ASDC J Dent Child 1986;53:48–52.

"Although contingency contracting is a widely used strategy for involving parents in modifying their children's behavior, this approach has apparently not been applied to the elimination of thumbsucking. . . . This paper explores monitoring and contingency contracting as alternative treatments for the persistent thumbsucker."

Identify the logical technique used in constructing this approach and the investigational strategy involved in adopting this approach to the problem.

Problem 6

Hoad-Reddick G. Gagging: A chairside approach to control. Br Dent J 1986;161:174–176.

"An attempt was made to help people who were unable to wear dentures owing to an exaggerated gagging reflex. Nineteen patients (7 women and 12 men) were taught a controlled method of breathing based on that recommended by the National Childbirth Trust for use by women in labor. The technique is described and this approach to control is related to work done elsewhere. Fourteen of the patients now wear dentures full time.

"In this study, patients who . . . were unable to wear dentures at all owing to retching problems were encouraged to make one further attempt at denture-wearing, using a breathing technique based on that recommended by the National Childbirth Trust for use by women in labor.

"Landa suggests that the majority of patients show a history of a precipitating cause. In an examination of personalities of dental patients who retched while attempting to wear dentures, Wright used Eysenck Personality Questionnaires. There was no evidence to suggest that retching patients were more neurotic than the control group. Most workers agree that retching is multifactorial in origin.

"All patients were instructed in controlled rhythmic breathing and told to practice it for one or two weeks before prosthetic treatment commenced. . . .

Identify the logical technique used in constructing this approach and the investigational strategy involved in adopting this approach to the problem. Are there any negative results reported here?

Problem 7

Robinson PJ, Shapiro IM. Effect of diphosphonates on root resorption. J Dent Res 1966;55:166.

"These results indicate that under the conditions of this in vivo model system, diphosphonate does not retard the rate of root resorption. In addition, 1.0% pyrophosphate or 2%

sodium fluoride are no more effective than physiological saline in inhibiting root resorption."

Are these positive or negative results? What questions would you want answered when you read the paper?

Problem 8

Grenby TH, Desai T. A trial of lactitol in sweets and its effects on human dental plaque. Br Dent J 1988;164:383–387.

Summary:

"Thirty subjects aged 18–20 years ate boiled sweets made with either sucrose or lactitol in addition to their normal diet over a 3-day experimental period and ceased all oral hygiene. Plaque accumulating on the teeth over the 3 days was assessed by three different methods, all of which showed lower values on the lactitol than on the sucrose sweets ($P < 0.005$ by the photographic method; $P = 0.025$ by the gravimetric method). Plaque collected from the lactitol-sweets group contained less soluble carbohydrate, glucose and sucrose, but was relatively higher in protein, calcium and phosphorous, than that from the sucrose-sweets group. There were unfavorable reactions to the texture and gastric effects of the lactitol sweets. . . ."

Materials and Methods:

"Sweets: These were the popular mint-humbug type, black-and-white striped boiled sweets, weighing approximately 3 g. The conventional sweets were made from a blend of sucrose and glucose syrup, which after boiling, contained 90% sucrose and 10% glucose. The experimental sweets contained 100% lactitol by weight, with additional sweetening by acesulfam-K. They were supplied in 4 oz (113 g) packs, which were identified by the experimental subjects according to color-coding only, not by composition or sweetening agent."

Are there any alternative hypotheses to explain these data?

Problem 9

Kawazoe Y, Kotani H, Hamada T, Yamada S. Effect of occlusal splints on the electromyographic activities of masseter muscles during maximum clenching in patients with myofacial-pain-dysfunction syndrome. J Prosthet Dent 1980;43:578–580.

"If the elimination of occlusal interferences causes a decrease in the degree of tactile afferent impulses from periodontal receptors, the masseter muscle activity during maximum clenching with the splint should be reduced more than without a splint (intracuspal clenching) in patients with MPD syndrome having occlusal interferences."

Identify the form of the deductive argument used and, if relevant, any additional premises that might be added to make the argument valid.

Problem 10

Eggleston DW. The interrelationship of stress and degenerative diseases. J Prosthet Dent 1980;44:541–544.

"If dental plaque were the only etiologic factor for caries and periodontal disease then all people with dental plaque would have these diseases. Such is not the case. Primitive humans on their natural diet have the lowest incidence of dental caries and periodontal disease even though they have no devices for removal of plaque."

Identify the form of deductive argument used here and any additional rhetorical technique that contributes to the force of the argument.

Problem 11

Following up on the argument on chalones presented in chapter 5: *Iversen OH. Comments on chalones and cancer. Mech Ageing Dev 1980;12:211–212.*

"The correct syllogism is:

Chalones cause proliferation decay and thus tumor regression.
Tumor regression is most often not followed by cure in human cancer cases.
Ergo: Chalones will most often not cure cancer."

Is this syllogism valid?

Problem 12

Sussman MI. Tooth reimplantation when it follows unintentional evulsion utilizing synthetic bone. Oral Health 1986;76:29.

"Since all 32 teeth were present, it was decided to attempt to save this tooth via periodontal surgery."

Comment on the logic used in this sentence.

Problem 13

Kontturi-Närhi V, Markkanen S, Markkanen H. Effects of airpolishing on dental plaque removal and hard tissues as evaluated by scanning electron microscopy. J Periodontol 1990;61:334–338.

In this paper, the following scale was described.

"The condition of enamel surface was classified into three groups on the basis of photographs.

1. No abrasion: Smooth normal enamel surface.
2. Mild abrasion: Few micropits or prism ends (ameloblastic pits) visible between perikymata lines.

3. Severe abrasion: Distinct perikymata lines with many prism ends and/or micropits visible on the whole surface occasional fracturing of perikymata edge."

Discuss this measurement and indicate the type of statistical test that would be used to compare surfaces before and after airpolishing.

Problem 14

Henderson CW, Schwartz RS, Herbold ET, Mayhew RB. Evaluation of the barrier system, an infection control system for the dental laboratory. J Prosthet Dent 1987;58:517–521.

"On that particular day a different technician was used and the results did not agree with the rest of the data. . . . If the results on that day were eliminated from the data, after the first cleansing there would be no positive cultures for sodium hypochlorite, and after the second cleansing only one positive culture. This would improve the results of 3.25% sodium hypochlorite."

Identify the type of error alluded to by the author in this excerpt.

Problem 15

Meinig DA. Removable partial dentures without rests. J Prosthet Dent 1994;71:350–358.

"Very poor—could lose their remaining teeth in two to three years

Poor—could lose their remaining teeth in 3 to 5 years

Fair—could lose several teeth but not all of them

Good—probably will keep all of their teeth for their lifetime."

Comment on the classification system for periodontal condition used in this study. Is this an operational definition?

Problem 16

Stach DJ, Cross-Poline GN, Newman SM, Tilliss TS. Effect of repeated sterilization and ultrasonic cleaning on curet blades. J Dent Hyg 1995;69:31–39.

"The blades pretreated with the anticorrosive and then autoclaved were the most difficult to evaluate via SEM photographs because the product itself appears to leave a visible residue on the blade surface."

Identify the type of measurement problem experienced in this study.

Problem 17

Novak MJ, Polson AM, Adair SM. Tetracycline therapy in patients with early juvenile periodontitis. J Periodontol 1988;59:366–372.

"1. The distance from the cementoenamel junction (CEJ) to the alveolar bone crest. The CEJ was designated as that point where the outer edge of the crown intersected the outer edge of the dentin of the root. The alveolar bone crest for a specific tooth surface was defined as the most coronal point of bone adjacent to the tooth surface where the periodontal ligament space had a uniform width. If an oblique flaring of the periodontal ligament space occurred coronally, the alveolar crest was taken as the point immediately subjacent to the flare, where the ligament space still exhibited uniform width."

Comment on this measurement. Does it meet Wilson's criteria (see page 122)?

Problem 18

Murray ID, McCabe JF, Storer R. Abrasivity of denture cleaning pastes in vitro and in situ. Br Dent J 1986;16:137–141.

Summary:

"The six-month abrasion scores . . . show a similar result to that recorded at one month except that differences between materials have diminished. This is due to the fact that the maximum possible abrasion score is 4 and a number of G and K dentures reached this value well before six months."

Identify the experimental tactical problem that occurred in this study.

Problem 19

Triol CW, Mandanas BY, Juliano GF, Yraolo B, Cano-Arevalo M, Volpe AR. A clinical study of children comparing anticaries effect of two fluoride dentifrices. A 31-month study. Clin Prev Dent 1987; 9:22–24.

Summary:

"A negative control dentrifice (nonfluoridated) was not used in this program, since the water supply was below [optimal] levels of fluoridation, and total abstention from fluoride was considered not to be good dental practice. "

Comment on the use of controls in this study.

Problem 20

Cao CF, Aeppli DM, Bloomquist WF, Bandt CL, Wolff LF. Comparison of plaque microflora between Chinese and Caucasian population groups. J Clin Periodontol 1990;17:115–118.

From the Abstract:

"This investigation was designed to compare the predominant plaque micro-organisms from a Chinese group of patients exhibiting periodontitis with an age-, sex- and periodontal disease–matched Caucasian group of patients. In addition to race, the 2 population groups differed with respect to diet and oral hygiene habits, or effectiveness at removing plaque. Clinical measurements were determined along with an evaluation for micro-organisms in supragingival and subgingival

Table P-1 Mean severity scores of ulcers*

Parameter	Chlorhexidine gel	Placebo gel
A/P sequence	.84	1.31
P/A sequence (9)	1.03	1.11
All patients (20)	.93	1.22
Adjusted means	0.94	1.21
Difference in means = 0.27	—	—
SE of the difference = 0.115	—	—

*Used with permission from Addy M, Carpenter R, Roberts WR. Br Dent J 1976;141:118.

plaque. Although the Chinese and Caucasian population groups were similar with respect to composition of microorganisms in subgingival plaque, notable differences were observed in supragingival plaque. The microbial differences observed in supragingival plaque may be explained at least in part, if not totally, by the higher plaque index scores of the Chinese versus Caucasian population groups. "

From Materials and Methods:

"10 visiting male Chinese students or scholars at the University of Minnesota, aged 25 to 40 years (mean age + SD = 31.3 + 4.4 years), with symptoms of gingival bleeding, were evaluated for periodontal disease. The criteria for selection of Chinese patients included less than 2.5 years residence in the USA. . . . Caucasians were selected from previous studies for comparison. . . . There was no statistically significant difference between Chinese and Caucasians in this study with respect to the gingival index."

From the Results:

"The proportions of spirochetes, motile rods and cocci in plaques are shown . . . . The 2 groups differ significantly with respect to all three microbial forms in supragingival plaque. . . ."

From the Discussion:

"The greater amount of plaque in the Chinese subjects can probably best be explained by differences in oral hygiene habits. Differences in the microbial composition of supragingival plaque between Chinese and Caucasians is likely attributable to the age and quantity of plaque, since old plaque is inhabited by a more complicated microflora. . . . However, the general similarity of subgingival cultivatable flora in the two population groups suggests that subgingival plaque is more dependent on its microenvironment than on the composition of the adjacent supragingival plaque, race or diet."

How would you classify this study design? What are some of the difficulties in coming to definitive conclusions with this approach?

Problem 21

Addy M, Carpenter R, Roberts WR. Management of recurrent aphthous ulceration: A trial of chlorhexidine gluconate gel. Br Dent J 1976;141:118–120.

Some relevant information extracted from the paper includes:

"Thirty patients agreed to participate in the trial. They were chosen from a larger group of aphthous-ulcer sufferers who regularly attended dental school and who experienced regular and frequent ulceration. The trial was conducted in a double-blind crossover manner employing an active gel containing 1 percent chlorhexidine gluconate in an aqueous base. Each gel was used for a period of 35 days with 14 days between the two preparations to avoid carry-over effects. At the commencement of the trial each patient was examined and then verbally instructed on the use of gels. Thus, each gel was to be used 3 times a day after meals. The patients were requested to place approximately 2.5 cm of the gel on the index finger, carry it to the mouth and allow the gel to distribute itself throughout the mouth, any residue being swallowed. The patients were also instructed to record the number and duration of the ulcers and to describe the discomfort experienced according to an arbitrary scale of: 1 = uncomfortable; 2 = fairly painful; 3 = very painful."

See the results in Table P-1. The difference in means of 0.27 between the chlorhexidine treatment and the placebo treatment was significant ($P \leq .05$).

From the Discussion:

"Chlorhexidine gluconate as a 1 percent gel produced a significant reduction in the duration and discomfort of ulcers in a group of 20 patients when compared with a placebo gel."

Identify the experimental design and discuss any problems that there might be in the analysis of the data.

Problem 22

Addy M, Moran J, Davies RM, Beak A, Lewis A. The effect of single morning and evening rinses of chlorhexidine on the development of tooth staining and plaque accumulation. J Periodontol 1982;9:134–140.

From the Materials and Methods:

"Verbal and written instructions were given at the commencement of each period. Thus, during the rinsing period subjects refrained from all forms of oral hygiene and excluded from their diet coffee, red wine and port. Each was provided with a supply of a branded tea in bags and re-

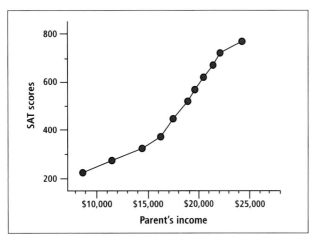

Fig P-1 Relationship of income to aptitude test scores. (From the *Ubyssey*, October 7, 1980.)

quested to consume eight cups per day. An attempt to standardize the teas was made by suggesting that one bag should be placed in a cup of boiling water for 2 min. The resulting infusion was then sweetened to taste and all volunteers agreed to add milk."

Identify the experiment tactic used in this study on tooth staining.

Problem 23

On October 7, 1980, the *Ubyssey* (a student newspaper at the University of British Columbia) reported that aptitude tests (such as SAT, CSAT, MSAT) show an economic slant. The most striking test bias, they claimed, was the tendency to rank people by income. The following data were presented (Fig P-1).

Give various interpretations of the data in Fig P-1.

Problem 24

Lindeberg RW. Combined management of mucogingival defects with citric acid root conditioning, lateral pedicle grafts, and free gingival grafts. Compend Contin Educ Dent 1985;6:265–266, 268, 270–272.

From the Abstract:

"This article describes a new technique for managing mucogingival defects. The procedure uses a lateral pedicle graft along with citric-acid root conditioning to gain better connective-tissue attachment to denuded root surfaces; it also uses a free gingiva at the donor tissue site. The technique has been used successfully in five patients, demonstrating good esthetics and root coverage with sound clinical attachment, stable for an extended period of time."

From Materials and Methods:

"Five patients, two men and three women, ranging in age from 26–45 with a mean of 36, were included in this study. Nine teeth with mucogingival defects demonstrating localized gingival recession were treated. The case described below involved a mandibular central incisor. . . . " (Twenty-two clinical photos were presented.)

Summary:

"This clinical study demonstrates an effective technique to eliminate mucogingival defects by a combination approach of lateral pedicle graft, free gingival graft, and citric-acid root conditioning. It has been shown that lateral pedicle grafts should not be performed without first conditioning the root with citric acid to guarantee good clinical attachment to the exposed root."

Comment on the relationship between the conclusions as presented in the summary and the evidence presented in this paper.

Problem 25

Havenaar R. The anti-cariogenic potential of xylitol in comparison with sodium fluoride in rat caries experiments. J Dent Res 1984;62:120–123.

"On the anti-cariogenic potential of xylitol in rat caries experiments: From day zero, the experimental diet and drinking water were supplied ad libitum. On day two the animals were inoculated once with a suspension of *Streptococcus mutans* strain 50 B4, serotype d, containing at least 108 CFU/mL."

Comment on the experiment tactics.

Problem 26

Douglas WH, Fields RP, Fundingsland J. A comparison between the microleakage of direct and indirect composite restorative systems. J Dent 1989;17:184–188.

In a study on microleakage, the authors varied the type of resin and whether the resin was applied directly or indirectly (ie, the composite is cured outside the mouth and cemented into the prepared cavity using a dual-cure resin-based cement). Their data provides microleakage in micrometers ($\pm$ SD) (Table P-2).

"Statistical analysis was done by a one-way analysis of variance and comparison between the means using the Bonferroni test (see Table [P-3])."

Identify the experiment design and suggest another approach to the statistical analysis of these data.

Problem 27

Jensen ME, Kohout F. The effect of a fluoridated dentifrice on root and coronal caries in an older adult population. J Am Dent Assoc 1988;117:829–832.

Table P-2 Microleakage of various resins

	Group			
	1	2	3	4
	Resin 1 Direct	Resin 2 Direct	Resin 1 Indirect	Resin 2 Indirect
	772 (257)	338 (105)	171 (117)	27 (22)

*Used with permission from Douglas WH, Fields RP, Fundingsland J. J Dent 1989;17:184.

Table P-3 Obtained differences between means and significance levels*

Groups	1	2	3	4
1	—	P < 0.001	P < 0.001	P < 0.001
2	434.5	—	P < 0.01	P < 0.001
3	595.6	161.1	—	P < 0.01
4	744.6	310.1	149.0	—

*Used with permission from Douglas WH, Fields RP, Fundingsland J. J Dent 1989;17:184.

Table P-4 Postoperative pain incidence for emergency treatment of symptomatic pulpitis*†

	Pulpotomy	Partial pulpotomy	Complete pulpectomy
Pain	30	44	14
No pain	364	302	202
Total	394	346	216

*Total no. of patients is 956.
†Data from Oguntebi BR, DeSchepper EJ, Taylor TS, White CL, Pink FE. Oral Surg Oral Med Oral Pathol 1992;73:479–483.

From Methods and Materials:

"A total of 810 volunteers were selected who were 54 years of age and older, had at least ten natural teeth, and were living in nonfluoridated communities. Individuals currently receiving fluoride therapy, antibiotics, or those with severe periodontal disease were excluded from the study. . . .

"After baseline examinations, the subjects were separated by gender, intervals of age (≤ 64, > 64), and arrayed by intervals of clinical root caries (0, ≥ 1). Within strata, subjects were assigned to treatment groups by random permutations of 2."

Comment on the procedure used to allocate the subjects into groups. What are the advantages and costs of using this approach?

Problem 28

Sheiham A, Smales FC, Cushing AM, Cowell CR. Changes in periodontal health in a cohort of British workers over a 14-year period. Br Dent J 1986;60:125–127.

"Of the 659 people examined in 1966, 120 were contacted and 89 accepted the invitation to be examined."

Identify the possible sources of invalidity in this study.

Problem 29

Former Vancouver Canucks' head coach Rick Ley once coached the Hartford Whalers. It was reported on February 3, 1990, in the *Globe and Mail* that he commented as follows on motivating the Whalers:

"Every time I throw them bouquets, it comes back to haunt me. But when I praise them, they don't play well the next game. Evidently this team would rather be kicked than stroked."

What statistical phenomenon would appear to be at work that would explain Coach Ley's observations?

Problem 30

Oguntebi BR, DeSchepper EJ, Taylor TS, White CL, Pink FE. Postoperative pain incidence related to the type of emergency treatment of symptomatic pulpitis. Oral Surg Oral Med Oral Pathol 1992;73: 479–483.

From the data in Table P-4, how could you determine if pain was associated with type of treatment? Assuming that you obtained a statistically significant result what would be a difficulty in interpreting it?

Table P-5 Effects of a mouthrinse on dental caries in children

Treatment	DMFT	SD	n
Mouthrinse + placebo	4.78	4.66	87
Mouthrinse + fluoride	5.06	5.41	87

DMFT = decayed, missing, or filled teeth.

Table P-6 Results of calcium hydroxide pulp capping done on Group 1 and Group 2 patients*

	Anesthetic used	Teeth treated (no.)	Unsuccessful procedures (no.)	Rate of unsuccessful procedures (%)
Group 1	Local anesthetic	9	2	27.2
Group 2	General anesthetic (no local anesthetic)	8	1	12.5

*Data from Gallieu GS Jr, Schuman NJ. J Am Dent Assoc 1985;111:599–601.

Problem 31

Review data taken from a study on the effects of a mouthrinse on dental caries in children (Table P-5).

Why do you think the investigators used 87 per group?

Problem 32

A study examined the fluoride-releasing pattern of five glass ionomers (identified here as A, B, C, D, and E), each type being cured for 20, 40, and 60 seconds and then measured for the fluoride released after 24, 48, 72 hours as well as 7 days. The authors state, "The statistical analyses were performed only for the materials light-cured for 40 seconds, in view of the reports that the best polymerization and physical characteristics are achieved after light curing for 40 seconds." The authors calculated t scores for the 10 possible comparisons (ie, A-B, A-C, A-D, A-E, B-C, B-D,B-E, C-D, C-E, D-E) at two times: 24 hours and 1 week. The t scores were then used to determine whether there were statistically significant differences between the amounts of fluoride released by the different ionomers.

Comment on the statistical analysis.

Problem 33

Evans DJ, Rugg-Gunn AJ, Tabari ED, Butler T. The effect of 25 years of water fluoridation in Newcastle assessed in four surveys of 5-year-old children over an 18-year period. Br Dent J 1995;178:60–64.

a) From the Materials and Methods:

"The criteria for the clinical examination for caries used in the previous studies was modified to reflect the criteria used in surveys co-ordinated by the British Association for the Study of Community Dentistry."

From the Results:

"Comparison with data from previous studies is tentative due to the change in criteria adopted."

What kind of threat to validity does this statement "comparison with" exemplify?

b) From the Results:

"However data collected from the 110 duplicate examinations by the two examiners allowed a comparison to be made between the results using two different criteria. . . . This difference was not statistically significant."

Identify the type of result reported in this segment. Does it alleviate the concern over the change of criteria?

c) Judging from the title of the paper, what other possible threats to validity would you suspect?

Problem 34

Gallien GS Jr, Schuman NJ. Local versus general anesthesia: A study of pulpal response in the treatment of cariously exposed teeth. J Am Dent Assoc 1985;111:599–601.

Review Table P-6 from the Results section. What rule of presentation of data is violated here?

Problem 35

Martin JA, Bader JD. Five-year treatment outcomes for teeth with large amalgams and crowns. Oper Dent 1997;22:72–78.

"In 1988 a total of 7,687 target restorations were placed in 5,901 enrolled adult patients. Of these, 4,735 restorations were placed in 3,655 members whose eligibility was continuous from

1988 to 1993. Thus we were able to follow 62% of both the patients and eligible target restorations placed in 1988 to 1993."

The restorations of those who dropped out of the program were not followed for the entire 5-year period. What is the main threat to the internal validity of this study? How can the authors attempt to determine if the threat seriously compromises their conclusions?

Problem 36

Sherman PR, Hutchens LH Jr, Jewson LG, Moriarty JM, Greco GW, Mc-Fall WT Jr. The effectiveness of subgingival scaling and root planing. I. Clinical detection of residual calculus. J Periodontol 1990; 61:3–8.

a) From Methods of Measurement:

"An unsatisfactory surface was defined as, 'that surface which in the individual evaluator's judgment could be made smoother with further instrumentation.' . . . For use in comparison of the clinical and microscopic detection of calculus, a surface was considered clinically positive for calculus when at least two of the three evaluators determined the surface to be satisfactory."

Using the criteria on page 122, in what stage in the development of a measurement scale does this fall? What do you think the next step in the development of this measurement should be?

b) "A second appointment, approximately 1 week later, was scheduled to allow the operator an opportunity to evaluate the instrumented surfaces and accomplish any additional scaling and root planing. Although no time constraints were imposed, the total amount of time spent in the use of ultrasonics and the time spent in hand instrumentation per tooth were recorded."

What principle in experiment design is illustrated here?

Problem 37

Yankell SL, Emling RC. A study of gingival irritation and plaque removal following a three-minute toothbrushing. J Clin Dent 1994; 5:1–4.

"If there are 'no significant differences' among new designs in efficacy, perhaps safety of use factors should be given increased attention and reporting."

Comment on the logic of this sentence and how it may be criticized.

Problem 38

The following rhetorical strategies can be found in the following problem (some more than once): authority, data manipulation, scarcity, proposing of alternatives, credibility, agenda control, law of cognitive response, contrast, concreteness, liking, and social validation. Identify the locations where they occur.

Persuading the Professor

This cautionary tale demonstrates the various rhetorical strategies routinely employed by salespeople to persuade consumers to part with their hard-earned funds. While the bill of goods in this story is a mutual fund, the same strategies are applied every day in the selling of dental equipment, cars, and other necessities and luxuries of life. More importantly, they are also used in science: Persuasion is a key element of scientific papers, and scientists regularly interact in decision-making situations, such as when serving on grant committees and tenure boards. In each of these arenas, they use their persuasive abilities to convince their colleagues of the rightness of their beliefs.

Paragraph 1

Professor Brunette felt a strong tug of jealousy as he stood in the doorway of his office chatting about financial matters with his colleagues Waterfield and Tonzetich. Both of these men had discovered a path to wealth and had long since left Brunette behind, choking on their dust. Waterfield had reached financial nirvana by the clever stratagem of having his wife work in a company with stock options that had multiplied in value. Tonzetich had arrived at his comfortable position by a lifetime of rigorous financial discipline. As a young married man, for example, he had abstained from purchasing a car so that he could save for a house. Brunette had neither the foresight of a Waterfield to marry a woman employed by a thriving corporation nor the self-discipline of a Tonzetich. Yet he felt that he deserved more; he believed he worked as hard as his friends and was equally intelligent. What could he do?

Paragraph 2

At that moment a courier approached and asked Brunette to sign for a package. Inside the package he found a letter and an audio cassette. The letter explained that the cassette contained information about the financial services provided by Mr Edgar Endwater, who specialized in selling investments to faculty of the University of British Columbia (UBC). His credentials included a BA (commerce), CA (Chartered Accountant), and CFP (Certified Financial Planner). The investments that Mr Endwater sold would then be integrated into the UBC pension plan—a plan that he described in his letter as "conservative with historically low rates of return." Now, Brunette had recently served as an expert witness at a trial and was looking for a place to invest the $25,000 he had been paid. He called Endwater.

Paragraph 3

One day later, Mr Endwater appeared at his door. Tall, lean, and clad in an impeccable English-tailored suit, he made Brunette feel stumpy and distinctly unfashionable in his casual attire characteristic of academics. But it turned out they had much in common. Both lived in the fashionable Point Grey area and coached in the soccer club. Mr Endwater enthused about how much he liked working with the children and their parents. Brunette could only admire such a selfless soul; he had found many of the children to be spoiled brats and their parents pretentious yuppies. He felt that Endwater must be quite a good fellow not to mind some of the annoyances associated with coaching Point Grey children.

Paragraph 4

Mr Endwater outlined his qualifications and explained why he had decided to specialize in working with UBC professors. "The amount you can save from your salary is, as you know, quite small. What I'm really interested in is being your agent when you retire and you're ready to invest your UBC pension fund. I don't really make any money from these small investments," he sniffed. (Brunette had mentioned that he wanted to invest $20,000, and, in response to an earlier request, had provided Endwater with a copy of his UBC pension statement.) "But I want to do a good job on the small investments so that you'll have the confidence to make me your financial planner when you retire."

Paragraph 5

When Brunette questioned why UBC professors, who would be expected to be intelligent people, didn't handle their own investments, Mr Endwater replied "That's a very astute question. UBC professors are indeed very intelligent people—no doubt much smarter than me—but they generally don't have the time, the interest, or the background to do all the work necessary to evaluate investments." He paused and looked around Brunette's office. "Judging by all the awards you've received, you've worked very hard; you couldn't have accomplished what you have without working hard. Particularly," he added with a smile, "when you're busy participating in sports with your children. But I don't want to take too much of your time, so let's get down to business." He sat in the seat opposite Brunette.

Paragraph 6

"You mentioned that you're interested in equity investments in US dollars—a very wise move in my opinion; it's common knowledge that the US dollar is more stable than the Canadian. Moreover, as you know, RRSP (Registered Retirement Savings Plan) are limited by Canadian law in the number of US stocks they can hold so they don't appreciate as quickly because the Canadian stocks don't increase as rapidly as the US ones. Many financial planners believe Canadians should invest in US stocks. I recommend the McTavish St Bernard Action Research Plan." He underlined the S–t–A–R. "This plan will make you an investment 'StAR.'"

Paragraph 7

The StAR plan was a collection of funds from the McTavish company. With a flourish, Mr Endwater handed Brunette a stack of brochures for each of the funds. The brochures featured colorful graphs and detailed the names of all the stocks purchased by the funds. Mr Endwater continued, "The sophisticated StAR plan involves reallocating assets among the plans on a strategic basis. In this way the volatility of the funds is reduced, hence lowering your risk of losing your investment. The StAR plan is designed by a professor of finance from McGill. His research has appeared in a high-impact financial journal." He rose from his chair and walked a few steps to examine a painting on the wall. "Of course, having the advantage of this StAR system costs a bit more because more administration is required, but the additional 0.5% added to the standard management expense ratio of 3% is well worthwhile, in my opinion, particularly when you can expect such high rates of return. Twenty percent is possible."

Paragraph 8

"I've heard that the Templeton funds are very good," Brunette said. "How does the StAR plan compare to those?" "Oh, it's better," said Mr. Endwater. "Last year StAR made more money than Templeton Growth. Moreover, I suggest that you move immediately. The market is poised to move up. Better for you to get that October growth spurt than to buy in later and pay a premium. Just let me know what you decide, and I can send a courier to pick up your check."

That night, during his nightly walk with his dog Brutus, Brunette visited Mr Endwater's house and delivered the check. Mr Endwater's house looked rather more expensive than his own, Brunette noticed.

Conclusion

What happened to St Bernard Action Research Plan? It did not do well. Brunette took to calling it "Dog-of-My-Heart Mutual Fund." Only later did Brunette learn that investing guru Warren Buffet had predicted that, over time, the most likely return on equities would be around 6%. That, combined with high management expense ratios (MERs) of 3.5%, meant that the fund managers were benefitting more from the investors' wealth than the investors themselves. By receiving "trailer commissions," agents received a chunk of the MER for themselves for as long as the investor held the fund. Mr Endwater thus did well on Brunette's investment. Brunette himself did not do so well; although he didn't actually lose money on StAR, neither did he make as much money as he could have through other strategies. Moreover, he got out in time. When the stock market declined sharply in 2000, many funds, including StAR, were folded. Today, when McTavish distributes the performance of its funds, StAR isn't listed because it no longer exists. Like a bad doctor, McTavish has buried its mistake.

Comments on Problems

These comments should be viewed as neither the definitive nor indeed the only answer to the questions posed in the problem set. Other views are possible, and I suspect that in some instances the authors would be prepared to argue with these comments.

Comment on problem 1

This question illustrates the often complex nature of treatments as applied. Considered as a treatment, the results of this positive-effects paper indicate that fluoride treatment promotes bone formation. However, it is difficult to ascribe the effect solely to the fluoride ion because the treatment is complex, for an acidated (0.1 M H_3PO_4) solution is used. An alternative hypothesis is that the acid, rather than the fluoride treatment, promotes bone formation. This concern could be alleviated by introducing another control in which only acid is applied.

Comment on problem 2

The usual reason for using specific biologic response modifiers such as PTE is to look for specific effects. In this example there was an effect on rupture strength of intact skin but also weight loss in the PTE-treated group. It thus appears that there were some more general effects on the animals' metabolism and the authors rightly conclude that the explanation for the increase in strength of skin produced by PTE is not understood.

Comment on problem 3

This is a clear example of argument to authority. An aspect of this excerpt that I find charming is that it includes a compliment to the cited authorities, quite different from the common style today where such compliments are absent and grudging citations common.

Comment on problem 4

The phrase "if all other principles of careful surgical technique are observed" exemplifies the technique of using an auxiliary hypothesis. If anyone failed to repeat the findings on polylactate, the authors could question their surgical technique.

Comment on problem 5

This study exemplifies analogy as a method of designing studies. Every parent—or at least every parent that I know—at some point descends to the level of striking deals with their children as opposed to maintaining the high moral ground of insisting their children do the right thing on principle alone. This paper argues that a similar deal-making (or contingency-contracting) approach could be used by oral health professionals. The outcome is not guaranteed because, as in all analogies, similarity is not identity. Healthcare professionals share with parents a need to modify children's behavior sometimes, but the relationship between the child and the parent is different from that between the child and the healthcare worker. The analogy, however, provides perfectly reasonable grounds for doing the study.

Comment on problem 6

This example involves analogy but also shows the use of the transfer method in research design. In brief, it builds on clinical traditions that gagging can sometimes be controlled by breathing techniques and transfers the techniques developed for women in labor to gaggers. The advantages of such an approach are many. For example, the authors do not have to undergo all of the problems that were involved in developing the method. Moreover, because they are dealing with an established method, readers will probably be less skeptical than if the authors introduced a new method for this study. The negative result was a finding of no difference in the neurotic dimension between the retching and control patients. This finding enables the authors to interpret their results more specifically. They do not have to consider the neuroses of the subjects as influencing the results.

Comment on problem 7

This is a negative-results paper. The question of interest would be: What size effect could the authors have seen using their methods?

Comment on problem 8

Two types of questions emerge. First, the lactitol "treatment" consists of two treatments (ie, lactitols and an artificial sweetener acesulfam-K), so that in theory at least, either could be responsible for effects. Experts in this topic could judge whether the acesulfam-K was a *plausible* as opposed to a *possible* explanation. Similarly, another possible problem is whether the unfavorable gastric effects of the lactitol caused the subjects to alter other aspects of their diet in ways that might affect plaque.

287

Comment on problem 9

I construct the argument in formal terms as a valid pure hypothetical syllogism as follows:

> If splint, then occlusal interferences (OIs) decrease (a suppressed premise that would appear to be true in many instances).
> If OIs decrease, then afferent impulses (AIs) decrease.
> If AIs decrease, then masseter muscle activity decreases.

Comment on problem 10

I construct the argument in formal terms as follows:

> If dental plaque were the only etiologic factor . . . then all people . . . with plaque have these diseases (ie, if P then Q).
> It is not the case that all people with plaque have the disease (ie, not Q).

This step involves a suppressed premise assuming through the sentence "Primitive humans . . ." that plaque is correlated negatively with the presence of devices for removing plaque. (This may not be the case; a number of investigators have demonstrated devices used by so-called primitive peoples. Devices include such things as twigs that contain antimicrobial agents that might inhibit plaque.)
Therefore:

> Plaque is not the only etiologic factor (ie, not P).

The conclusion, which is not stated explicitly in the excerpt, is valid (modus tollens). Because of the uncertainty of the suppressed premise, however, it may not be sound.

Comment on problem 11

Although I believe the first part of Iversen's analysis given in chapter 5 to be correct, I do not agree with the second part. Translating his syllogism into standard form, I get:

> All chalones are tumor regressors (A proposition).
> Some tumor regressors are not cancer cures (O proposition).
> Chalones are not cancer cures.

This syllogism is invalid because the middle term (tumor regressors) is not distributed in either premise. Readers should recall that an invalid conclusion does not necessarily mean a wrong conclusion; invalidity merely means that the truth of the conclusion is not guaranteed by the truth of the premises.

Comment on problem 12

This is an example of a suppressed premise. To justify saving the tooth via periodontal surgery, some additional assumptions must be added about the 32 teeth being present. One assumption that would satisfy this need would be "it is necessary to maintain the complete dental arch." Another might be "and since the patient has demonstrated sufficient oral care to keep the other 31 teeth in good shape, chances are he or she will be able to look after this tooth properly after surgery." But some may disagree with either of these premises, so it is clear that additional explanation would be helpful.

Comment on problem 13

This is an example of ordinal scale data. Statistical purists would not like the authors to average such data and would prefer that the statistical testing use nonparametric methods such as the Mann-Whitney test.

Comment on problem 14

This is an example of error due to an assignable cause (the different technician). It is a comparatively rare event to see such an error acknowledged so explicitly. But it is certainly better for the authors to state, as they did, how the data are affected by eliminating the suspect points than it is simply not to report the suspect data at all—probably the more common approach.

Comment on problem 15

This classification fulfills the first step in Wilson's criteria for a full-fledged operational definition (that of an intuitive feeling for the quantity). However, given the uncertainties in estimating the survival time of individual teeth, it seems it would be difficult to get agreement between observers. Moreover, verifying the classifications would be difficult because, in all probability, ethics would dictate that treatment be done now, and validation of the classifications would require observing the teeth with no treatment for a considerable time.

Comment on problem 16

This is an instance of observational reactivity. The anticorrosive treatment interfered with the SEM observations.

Comment on problem 17

I think this is a good operational definition that specifies precisely how the measurement was done. Length (in this example mm) is part of an international system of standards.

Comment on problem 18

The problem that occurred here was the "ceiling effect." After groups G and K got to the ceiling value of 4, they had nowhere higher to go, and other groups started to catch up to them, diminishing the difference between groups.

Comment on problem 19

This is an instance where ethical considerations eliminate a preferred experiment design; this example illustrates that real-world experimentation often necessarily involves compromises.

Comment on problem 20

In this case-control study, the outcome variable is the plaque microflora. A possible concern is that a number of other factors, such as diet, are not controlled and would be expected to vary systematically between the groups. As in all case-control designs, such differences are potential alternative explanations. Note that the authors argue that such differences are not important because the subgingival flora is similar, but there is still the possibility of a specific interaction between type of plaque and one of the uncontrolled factors.

Comment on problem 21

The power of the crossover design is illustrated in this study in which a small effect could be demonstrated in a relatively small sample of 20. It appears that the authors were taking means of ordinal scale data and analyzing the data using parametric statistics, a procedure that would not necessarily garner the approval of most statisticians.

Comment on problem 22

This is an example of a cardinal rule of experimentation, namely, to make sure that things are set up so that you will see something. In this instance, the authors ensured that tooth staining would occur by the simple expedient of having the subjects drink eight cups of tea a day. If tea drinking had been left to chance, there would have been much more variability, and effects would have been more difficult to demonstrate.

Comment on problem 23

This is an example of the problems of interpreting causation from correlational data. If simply being rich leads to higher SAT scores and thus entrance into desired programs, then there is a problem, since most people would agree that entrance into programs should be based on merit. There may be a hidden variable in that the wealthier homes may be wealthier because the parents are, in fact, smarter, and these smarter parents produce smarter children. Seligman seems to advocate the latter view in his book, *A Question of Intelligence*. Others would argue the validity of the SAT tests or the accuracy of the reports of parents' income. In any case, it is clear that such data cannot be interpreted simplistically.

Comment on problem 24

This case series demonstrates two features often associated with clinical presentations:

1. A complex treatment in which a clinician conscientiously tries to combine the best of several approaches in an attempt to produce the best outcome. The difficulty, from the point of view of determining causes of any successes that occur, is that there are multiple variables of treatment, and one does not know which parts of the treatment are necessary. In this example, the author would have to have a control group in which the roots were not treated with citric acid to demonstrate the necessity of citric acid conditioning.
2. This problem reveals an emphasis on concrete information (clinical photographs) and a lack of statistical analysis. The vividness of the clinical photos tends to convince readers of the efficacy of the treatment even though the case series itself is fairly small (five patients).

Comment on problem 25

This is another example of an investigator taking no chances and setting up conditions so that something will happen. Who knows how long the investigator would have to wait for those rats to develop caries if he hadn't given them 10^8 CFU/mL *Streptococcus mutans*?

Comment on problem 26

Although not treated as such, this experiment appears to employ factorial design with two factors (ie, resin and mode of application) each at two levels (ie, resins 1 and 2, direct and indirect methods of application). If the experiment were analyzed as a factorial design, the authors could have tested for an interaction between resin and mode of application, and indeed inspection of the data indicates that such an interaction was present. A positive aspect of their analysis was the use of Bonferroni, a correction for multiple comparisons.

Comment on problem 27

The blocking procedure used here should enable the investigators to determine the effects of treatment on specific groups in terms of age, sex, and root caries score. Note that the cost of this inferential power is that they had to obtain 810 volunteers to get sufficient sample size in the subgroups.

Comment on problem 28

This is a clear instance of sample mortality—the sample shrank to 89 from 659. The problem is that one cannot be sure that the 89 remaining subjects are randomly selected and thus representative of the original 659. Another possible source of invalidity is history, because the cohort marched along 14 years together in a particular period of time; in a different 14-year period, it is possible that different results would be obtained. Sometimes there is nothing investigators can do to deal with such problems. They cannot, for example, force subjects to be examined. In such instances, the most common approach is to discuss the problem and make allowance for it in the interpretation of results.

Comment on problem 29

It looks like Coach Ley is a victim of statistical regression. He thinks his praise results in decreased performance, but in all likelihood after an exceptionally good game his team merely regresses to their mean performance level. In the instance of the Hartford Whalers, that level was not very high, and Coach Ley had to seek employment elsewhere.

Comment on problem 30

One way of interpreting the data would be to use a contingency table (Table CP-1). Using the formula on page 112, we can calculate the expected values for each of the cells and the χ^2 value.

$\chi^2 = 8.22$
$df = 2$
$P = .016$

Thus pain is significantly associated with type of treatment.

A difficulty associated with the interpretation might be what is called *confounding by indication*. In other words, the choice of treatment might be influenced by the signs and symptoms of the patient, so it may be the pre-existing condition of the patient that is causing the association of pain and treatment.

Table CP-1 Expected values

	Pulpotomy	Partial pulpotomy	Complete pulpectomy
Pain	36.3	31.8	19.9
No pain	358	314	196

Comment on problem 31

This is an example of a treatment that produces only a small effect, so to have any hope of seeing a statistically significant difference, the investigator has to study a large number of subjects. Using the formula for effect size on page 252:

$$d_S = \frac{\bar{X}_a - \bar{X}_b}{S_p} \qquad S_p = \sqrt{\frac{(n_a - 1)s_a^2 + (n_b - 1)s_b^2}{n_a + n_b - 2}}$$

$$S_p = \sqrt{\frac{86(4.66)^2 + 86(5.41)^2}{172}} = 5.04$$

$$d = \frac{5.06 - 4.78}{5.04} = 0.055$$

It is indeed a very small effect size, and it needs a large sample size to be demonstrated.

Comment on problem 32

The use of multiple t tests is inappropriate since it increases the risk of type I error. ANOVA and a multiple comparison test, such as Tukey's HSD (honestly significantly different) test would be the preferred approach. An unusual feature of the paper was that only $\approx$ 17% of the data collected in the paper was subjected to statistical analysis. The reader must wonder whether other analyses were done and the comparisons showed no significant differences.

Comment on problem 33

a) Changing the criteria would be an example of what Campbell and Stanley called "instrumentation," ie, your measuring instrument is changing.

b) This is a negative result, ie, one in which the null hypothesis is accepted. Indeed, it is a negative result that the authors would have been happy to obtain, because it makes interpretation of their study more straightforward. As for all negative results, one worries about how small a difference could have been detected. The authors, however, alleviate that concern by conducting a comparison involving quite a large number of children (110). Thus, it seems that the authors looked very hard for a possible difference and did not find it.

c) Eighteen years is a relatively long time, and one would suspect that history in various forms could be operative. For example, was there a change during that time in the socio-economic status of the residents being examined.

Comment on problem 34

The presentation of data has violated Huth's rule of 50; that is, percentages are allowed to be reported when the fraction used in calculating them has a denominator (in this case the number of teeth treated) greater than 50. The basis for the rule is that one wants to avoid pseudo-precision such as that implied by the 1/8 = 12.5% reported in Table P-6 for Group 2. When the denominator of the fraction is less than 50, the confidence interval (CI) for the reported percentage will be very large. Using the table given in appendix 2, we can calculate that the 95% CI for the rate of unsuccessful procedures (reported as 27.2% in Group 1) ranges from 2.8 % to 60%. Similarly for Group 2 (reported as 12.5%), the CI ranges from 0.32% to 53%.

Comment on problem 35

The main threat to the validity of this study is mortality. In brief, we wonder whether the 62% who were studied differed in significant ways from those who dropped out. For example, if loss of employment is a prime reason for dropping out of the plan, it seems plausible that patients who dropped out of the plan may differ in socioeconomic status from those who remain; that factor could be linked to treatment outcomes through some intervening variable, such as diet or oral hygiene practices. Thus, there is the possibility that treatment outcomes observed in those who stayed in the plan cannot be reliably extrapolated to the target population (ie, all patients enrolled in a plan).

The authors attempted to deal with this problem by 1) comparing the demographic and dental characteristics of those who stayed with those who dropped out of the plan, and 2) comparing the outcomes of the dropouts with the outcomes of stay-ins to the extent that it was possible with the limited data available for the dropouts.

Comment on problem 36

a) The evaluation of root surface smoothness is a necessary component of practice as well as instruction in clinical periodontics. Thousands of evaluations of this type must be done every day. However, because the methods used in this study are less than ideal, a vote must be taken among the evaluators to measure the property. Thus, it appears that the method used is not much better than the lowest rank of an "intuitive feeling for the quantity."

From the latter part of the sentence, it appears that the authors are working on a method involving microscopy that would take them to the next level, that is "a method of comparison so that it can be said that A has more of the property than B." Given the importance of this measurement, one imagines that it might become a fertile research area where modification of the types of instruments used in surface science (such as profilometry) might be employed to get standardized readings.

b) The principle adopted here seems to be sound—controlling those factors that you can and measuring the rest. The principal aim in this study was to determine the ability of clinicians to detect residual calculus, and because the investigators wanted to include surfaces that had been evaluated as satisfactory, they could not necessarily limit the time spent on preparing the surface. But by measuring the time spent using ultrasonics and hand scaling, they gave themselves the opportunity to gain other insights into the problem—for example, the frequency of satisfactory surfaces as a function of time of hand scaling.

Comment on problem 37

Considered as a deductive argument, this statement makes a number of assumptions.

1. The studies that reported "no significant differences" were powerful enough to detect clinically meaningful effects.
2. The designs that were investigated were the only ones possible or at least likely to improve plaque removal.
3. The only important considerations are plaque removal and safety.

A formal analysis of the logic might be cast along the lines of a disjunctive syllogism as follows:

Either new designs or efficacy should be studied (suppressed disjunctive premise).
New designs should NOT be studied (as they do not differ in efficacy).
Therefore, safety and efficacy should be studied.

The logic could be criticized as an example of the UFO fallacy; surely there are other reasons besides the ones stated for studying new designs including appearance, price, and composition, among others. To be fair, the authors hedge their conclusion by including the word "perhaps," so maybe they were not attempting a definitive conclusion.

Comment on Problem 38

A list of the strategies used in each paragraph follows.

Paragraph 1
Cognitive dissonance. Brunette experiences discomfort on realizing that his friends, who overtly are no smarter or harder-working than he, are nonetheless wealthier. This makes him

vulnerable to persuasion from a credible person who offers a simple solution (in this case, a mutual fund). Note that it is Brunette who creates this discomforting state for himself; not uncommonly, the most effective salesman is the customer.

Cognitive dissonance also occurs when scientists become dissatisfied with contradictions or gaps in our knowledge and perform experiments to try to resolve them. But sometimes scientists become so enamored of their theories that they fail to undertake critical experiments, or even adjust their data, to avoid contradiction with their favored hypothesis and the cognitive dissonance that it entails. Cognitive dissonance, then, can be used for good or evil.

Paragraph 2
Endwater's degrees serve as obvious appeals to *authority*.

Paragraph 3
The fact that Endwater wears a suit, silly as it may seem, does add *authority* to his pronouncements. (I once knew a senior academic administrator, who, I strongly suspected, must have worn his suit to bed. He was a terrible administrator, the numbers in his budget reports never added up, bureaucratic staff multiplied without reason, and, although he was allegedly an academic, no one could really figure out his record in teaching or research—except that he never seemed to have done much of either. But he did look good in a suit and that seemed to form the basis of his authority.)

Clothing as a basis for authority is not restricted to academe. The *Fortune* columnist Stanley Bing has commented that some star CEO's seem to wear shirts that are whiter and crisper than the rest of us. According to Bing, CEO's also have better hair. The moral of this paragraph is to beware of men of fine suits but limited substance.

A second rhetorical device is demonstrated in this paragraph; Endwater seems to be a friendly guy to whom Brunette takes a *liking*. Cialdini tells us that liking is one of the tools of effective persuasion.

Paragraph 4
Endwater's methods of establishing *credibility* and *opinion movement* are subtle. Endwater (as a salesman) clearly has an agenda: Sales form the basis of his salary. This self-interest reduces the credibility of his advice somewhat. Under conditions of limited credibility, the best strategy for a persuader is to attempt only moderate movement—in this case, get the $20,000 sale and move to the large sale later.

Paragraph 5
This is unabashed *flattery*, pure and simple. People like flattery; they even like flattery that they know to be inaccurate. Flattery leads to *liking* and, Cialdini tells us, liking leads to persuasion.

Paragraph 6
Social validation. Brunette receives some social validation of his thoughts. Phrases such as "common knowledge" and "many planners believe" serve as social validation of

Brunette's plans and make it easier for Endwater to sell products that conform to those plans.

The use of "StAR," an easily memorable acronym, is an example of the value of *vivid concrete examples*.

More important, Endwater *controls the agenda* by introducing the MacTavish product and thus directing Brunette's thoughts along a specific line (*law of cognitive response*). Out of a universe of mutual funds, Brunette's thoughts are focused on one.

Paragraph 7
Authority is used again in the allusion to the McGill professor. Argument from authority is strictly valid only if all reasonable, well-qualified experts agree. It is highly unlikely that all professors of commerce would agree with their McGill colleague.

Contrast (another of Cialdini's tools of persuasion) can be found in the difference between the possible 20% return and the mere 0.5% additional cost of opting for StAR. The problem, of course, is that the 0.5% cost is a certainty whereas the 20% is only a possibility, and an unlikely one at that. But by placing 0.5% in context with 20%, the 0.5% appears small.

Paragraph 8
Brunette makes an abortive attempt to consider *alternative proposals*. If one considers the hypothesis that StAR is the best investment, and given that the supporting evidence comprises brochures from just one firm, it is certainly a good logical approach to criticize the proposal by considering alternatives. However, Brunette's knowledge is limited and his approach tentative. It is an easy matter for Endwater, with his superior financial credentials, to brush it aside. In fact, history shows that Templeton Growth was a superior fund and that the comparison selected by Endwater (looking to last year) was anomalous. This exchange shows that an expert has a significant advantage when discussing alternatives.

Survivorship bias. The average return of the MacTavish funds that survive are better than the average of all their funds, because the number calculated for the survivors does not include the numbers generated by the dogs, like StAR, that have been sacrificed to the gods of public relations. Survivorship bias is always an important factor in evaluating experiments or clinical trails where the drop-out rate of participants is high.

In addition, *scarcity* (another Cialdini tool of persuasion) can be a strong motivator. Here, the scarce element is time. In science, scarcity appears as a tool of persuasion when an author who is attempting to persuade reviewers of the high quality of his work emphasizes publications in general interest journals (such as *Science* or *Nature*). These journals have limited space, and any article that appears in them is thus generally associated with high quality.

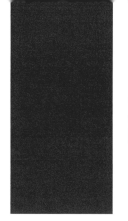

Appendices

Appendix 1

Library of Congress Classification System

Main Classifications

A.	General Works
B.	Philosophy; Religion
C.	History
D.	World History
G.	Geography; Anthropology
H.	Social Sciences
I.	(Vacant)
J.	Political Science
K.	Law
P.	Language

Expanded Classifications
(subject areas of interest in oral health research)

Q. Science

QH	Biology
QR	Microbiology
QS	Human Anatomy
QT	Physiology
QU	Biochemistry
QV	Pharmacology
QW	Bacteriology and Immunology
QX	Parasitology
QY	Clinical Pathology
QZ	Pathology

R. Medicine

RA	Public Aspects of Medicine
RB	Pathology
RC	Internal Medicine
RD	Surgery
RE	Ophthalmology
RF	Otorhinolaryngology
RG	Gynecology and Obstetrics
RJ	Pediatrics
RK	DENTISTRY
RL	Dermatology
RM	Therapeutics; Pharmacology
RS	Pharmacy and Materia Medica
RT	Nursing

W. General and Miscellaneous Material Relating to the Medical Profession

WA	Public Health
WB	Practice of Medicine
WC	Infectious Diseases
WD	Deficiency Diseases
WE	Musculoskeletal System
WF	Respiratory System
WG	Cardiovascular System
WH	Hemic and Lymphatic System
WI	Gastrointestinal System
WJ	Urogenital System
WK	Endocrine System
WL	Nervous System
WM	Psychiatry
WN	Radiology
WO	Surgery
WP	Gynecology
WQ	Obstetrics
WR	Dermatology
WS	Pediatrics
WT	Geriatrics
WU	DENTISTRY, ORAL SURGERY
WV	Otorhinolaryngology
WW	Ophthalmology
WX	Hospitals
WY	Nursing
WZ	History of Medicine

Appendix 2

Limits of Binomial Population Percentages of Xs Estimated from Random Samples—No. of Xs in Sample: 0–50; Sample Sizes: 1–100*

This table of binomial population limits can be used to indicate the confidence interval, that is, the zone that we would accept any population as being a possible parent of the sample. Thus if a treatment yielded three failures in the six patients treated, we would look up the values grouped to the right of X = 3 (the number of failures), and find the number 6 (the number in the sample). This entry reads "12; 88," that is, the failure rate could lie anywhere between 12% and 88%. To save space, the table does not show values above 50%; these must be calculated by taking the opposite class and then subtracting from 100%. For example, suppose there were four failures out of six patients. We would first calculate the confidence interval using the opposite class, ie, successes, which equal two out of six. Referring to the table at X = 2 and moving across to 6, we find "4.3; 78." Then, subtracting from 100, we find that for failures, the lower limit for percentage of failures is 100 – 78 (upper limit for percentage of success) = 22%. The upper limit for percentage of failures is 100 – 4.3 = 95.7%.

Maximum risks of overestimating lower limit and of underestimating upper limit = 2.5%. X = No. of Xs in sample. Bold-faced figures are sample sizes. Lower and upper limits are separated by semicolons. For explanation and method of use, see chapters 11 and 12.

X = 0	**1** 0; 97.5	**2** 0; 84	**3** 0; 71	**4** 0; 60	**5** 0; 52
	6 0; 46	**7** 0; 41	**8** 0; 37	**9** 0; 34	**10** 0; 31
	12 0; 26	**14** 0; 23	**16** 0; 21	**18** 0; 19	**20** 0; 17
	25 0; 14	**30** 0; 12	**35** 0; 10	**40** 0; 8.8	**50** 0; 7.1
	60 0; 6.0	**70** 0; 5.1	**80** 0; 4.5	**90** 0; 4.0	**100** 0; 3.62

X = 1	**2** 1.3; 98.74	**3** 0.84; 91	**4** 0.63; 81	**5** 0.51; 72	**6** 0.42; 64
	7 0.36; 58	**8** 0.32; 53	**9** 0.28; 48	**10** 0.25; 44.5	**12** 0.21; 38.5
	14 0.18; 34	**16** 0.16; 30	**18** 0.14; 27	**20** 0.13; 25	**22** 0.12; 23
	25 0.10; 20	**30** 0.08; 17	**35** 0.07; 15	**40** 0.06; 13	**50** 0.05; 11
	60 0.04; 9.0	**70** 0.04; 7.7	**80** 0.03; 6.8	**90** 0.03; 6.0	**100** 0.025; 5.45

X = 2	**4** 6.8; 93	**5** 5.3; 85	**6** 4.3; 78	**7** 3.7; 71	**8** 3.2; 65
	9 2.8; 60	**10** 2.5; 56	**11** 2.3; 52	**12** 2.1; 48	**14** 1.8; 43
	16 1.6; 38	**18** 1.4; 35	**20** 1.2; 32	**22** 1.1; 29	**24** 1.0; 27
	26 0.95; 25	**28** 0.88; 24	**30** 0.82; 22	**35** 0.70; 19	**40** 0.61; 17
	50 0.49; 14	**60** 0.41; 12	**70** 0.35; 10	**80** 0.30; 9	**90** 0.27; 8
	100 0.24; 7.04				

X = 3	**6** 12; 88	**7** 9.9; 82	**8** 8.5; 75.5	**9** 7.5; 70	**10** 6.7; 65
	12 5.5; 57	**14** 4.7; 51	**16** 4.0; 46	**18** 3.6; 41	**20** 3.2; 38
	22 2.9; 35	**24** 2.7; 32	**26** 2.4; 30	**28** 2.3; 28	**30** 2.1; 27
	35 1.8; 23	**40** 1.6; 20	**45** 1.4; 18	**50** 1.3; 17	**60** 1.0; 14
	70 0.89; 12	**80** 0.78; 11	**90** 0.69; 9	**100** 0.62; 8.53	

X = 4	**8** 16; 84	**9** 14; 79	**10** 12; 74	**11** 11; 69	**12** 9.9; 65
	14 8.4; 58	**16** 7.3; 52	**18** 6.4; 48	**20** 5.8; 44	**22** 5.2; 40
	24 4.8; 37	**26** 4.4; 35	**28** 4.0; 33	**30** 3.8; 31	**32** 3.5; 29
	35 3.2; 27	**40** 2.8; 24	**45** 2.5; 21	**50** 2.2; 19	**60** 1.9; 16
	70 1.6; 14	**80** 1. 4; 12	**90** 1.2; 11	**100** 1.10; 9.93	

X = 5	**10** 19; 81	**11** 17;77	**12** 15;72	**14** 13;65	**16** 11; 59
	18 9.7; 53	**20** 8.7; 49	**22** 7.8; 45	**24** 7.1; 42	**26** 6.6; 39
	28 6.1; 37	**30** 5.6; 35	**32** 5.3; 33	**35** 4.8; 30	**40** 4.2; 27
	45 3.7; 24	**50** 3.3; 22	**60** 2.8; 18	**70** 2.4; 16	**80** 2.1; 14
	90 1.8; 12.5	**100** 1.64; 11.29			

*Used with permission from Mainland D. Elementary Medical Statistics. Philadelphia: WB Saunders; 1952:359—360.

Appendix 2 (continued)

X = 6	12 21; 79	13 19; 75	14 18; 71	15 16; 68	16 15; 65
	18 13; 59	20 12; 54	22 11; 50	24 9.8; 47	26 9.0; 44
	28 8.3; 41	30 7.7; 39	32 7.2; 36	35 6.6; 34	37 6.2; 32
	40 5.7; 30	45 5.1; 27	50 4.5; 24	60 3.8; 20.5	70 3.2; 18
	80 2.8; 16	90 2.5; 14	100 2.24; 12.60		

X = 7	14 23; 77	15 21; 73	16 20; 70	18 17; 64	20 15; 59
	22 14; 55	24 13; 51	26 12; 48	28 11; 45	30 9.9; 42
	32 9.3; 40	34 8.7; 38	37 8.0; 35	40 7.3; 33	42 7.0; 31
	45 6.5; 29	50 5.8; 27	55 5.3; 24	60 4.8; 23	65 4.4; 21
	70 4.1; 20	80 3.6; 17	90 3.2; 15	100 2.86; 13.90	

X = 8	16 25; 75	17 23; 72	18 22; 69	19 20; 66.5	20 19; 64
	22 17; 59	24 16; 55	26 14; 52	28 13; 49	30 12; 46
	32 11; 43	35 10; 40	37 9.8; 38	40 9.0; 36	42 8.6; 34
	45 8.0; 32	50 7.2; 29	55 6.5; 27	60 5.9; 25	65 5.5; 23
	70 5.1; 21	80 4.4; 19	90 3.9; 17	100 3.51; 15.16	

X = 9	18 26; 74	19 24; 71	20 23; 68	22 21; 64	24 19; 59
	26 17; 56	28 16; 52	30 15; 49	32 14; 47	34 13; 44
	37 12; 41	40 11; 38	42 10; 37	45 9.6; 35	47 9.2; 33
	50 8.6; 31	55 7.8; 29	60 7.1; 27	65 6.5; 25	70 6.1; 23
	80 5.3; 20	90 4.7; 18	100 4.20; 16.40		

X = 10	20 27; 73	21 26; 70	22 24; 68	24 22; 63	26 20; 59
	28 19; 56	30 17; 53	32 16; 50	34 15; 47	37 14; 44
	40 13; 41	42 12; 39	45 11; 37	47 11; 36	50 10; 34
	55 9.1; 31	60 8.3; 29	65 7.6; 26	70 7.1; 25	80 6.2; 22
	90 5.5; 19	100 4.90; 17.62			

X = 11	22 28; 72	24 26; 67	26 23; 63	28 21; 59	30 20; 56
	32 19; 53	34 17; 51	36 16; 48	38 15; 46	40 15; 44
	42 14; 42	45 13; 40	47 12; 38	50 12; 36	55 10; 33
	60 9.5; 30	65 8.8; 28	70 8.1; 26	80 7.1; 23	90 6.3; 21
	100 5.62; 18.83				

X = 12	24 29; 71	25 28; 69	26 27; 67	28 24; 63	30 23; 59
	32 21; 56	34 20; 53.5	36 19; 51	38 18; 49	40 17; 47
	42 16; 45	45 15; 42	47 14; 40	50 13; 38	55 12; 35
	60 11; 32	65 9.9; 30	70 9.2; 28	80 8.0; 25	90 7.1; 22
	100 6.36; 20.02				

X = 13	26 30; 70	27 29; 68	28 28; 66	29 26; 64	30 25; 63
	32 24; 59	34 22; 56	36 21; 54	38 20; 51	40 19; 49
	42 18; 47	45 16; 44	47 16; 43	50 15; 40	55 13; 37
	60 12; 34	65 11; 32	70 10; 30	75 9.6; 28	80 9.0; 26
	90 7.9; 23	100 7.11; 21.20			

X = 14 | **28** 31; 69 | **30** 28; 66 | **32** 26; 62 | **34** 25; 59 | **36** 23; 57
38 22; 54 | **40** 21; 52 | **42** 20; 50 | **45** 18; 47 | **47** 17; 45
50 16; 42 | **55** 15; 39 | **60** 13, 36 | **65** 12; 33 | **70** 11; 31
75 11; 29 | **80** 9.9; 28 | **90** 8.8; 25 | **100** 7.87; 22.37

X = 15 | **30** 31; 69 | **32** 29; 65 | **34** 27; 62 | **36** 26; 59 | **38** 24; 57
40 23; 54 | **42** 22; 52 | **44** 21; 50 | **46** 20; 48 | **48** 19; 46
50 18; 45 | **55** 16; 41 | **60** 15; 38 | **65** 14; 35 | **70** 13; 33
75 12; 31 | **80** 11; 29 | **85** 10; 27 | **90** 10; 26 | **100** 8.645; 23.53

X = 16 | **32** 32; 68 | **34** 30; 65 | **36** 28; 62 | **38** 26; 59 | **40** 25; 57
42 23; 54 | **44** 22; 52 | **46** 21; 50 | **48** 20; 48 | **50** 20; 47
55 18; 43 | **60** 16; 40 | **65** 15; 37 | **70** 14; 34 | **75** 13; 32
80 12; 30 | **90** 11; 27 | **100** 9.45; 24.66

X = 17 | **34** 32; 68 | **36** 30; 65 | **38** 29; 61 | **40** 27; 59 | **42** 26; 57
44 24; 55 | **46** 23; 52 | **48** 22; 51 | **50** 21; 49 | **55** 19;45
60 17; 41 | **65** 16; 39 | **70** 15; 36 | **75** 14; 34 | **80** 13; 32
85 12; 30 | **90** 11; 28 | **100** 10.25; 25.79

X = 18 | **36** 33; 67 | **38** 31; 64 | **40** 29; 62 | **42** 28; 59 | **44** 26; 57
46 25; 55 | **48** 24; 53 | **50** 23; 51 | **55** 21; 47 | **60** 19; 43
65 17; 40 | **70** 16; 38 | **75** 15; 35 | **80** 14; 33 | **85** 13; 31
90 12; 30 | **100** 11.06; 26.92

X = 19 | **38** 33; 67 | **40** 32; 64 | **42** 30; 61 | **44** 28; 59 | **46** 27; 57
48 26; 55 | **50** 25; 53 | **55** 22; 49 | **60** 20; 45 | **65** 19; 42
70 17; 39 | **75** 16;37 | **80** 15; 35 | **85** 14; 33 | **90** 13; 31
100 11.86; 28.06

X = 20 | **40** 34; 66 | **42** 32; 64 | **44** 30; 61 | **46** 29; 59 | **48** 28; 57
50 26; 55 | **55** 24; 50 | **60** 22, 47 | **65** 20; 43 | **70** 18; 41
75 17; 38 | **80** 16; 36 | **85** 15; 34 | **90** 14; 32 | **100** 12.66; 29.19

X = 21 | **42** 34; 66 | **44** 32; 63 | **46** 31; 61 | **48** 29; 59 | **50** 28; 57
55 25; 52 | **60** 23; 48 | **65** 21; 45 | **70** 20; 42 | **75** 18; 40
80 17;37 | **85** 16; 35 | **90** 15; 33 | **100** 13.51; 30.28

X = 22 | **44** 35; 65 | **46** 33; 63 | **48** 31; 61 | **50** 30; 59 | **55** 27; 54
60 25; 50 | **65** 23; 47 | **70** 21; 44 | **75** 19; 41 | **80** 18; 39
85 17; 36 | **90** 16; 35 | **95** 15; 33 | **100** 14.35; 31.37

X = 23 | **46** 35; 65 | **48** 33; 63 | **50** 32; 61 | **55** 29; 56 | **60** 26; 52
65 24; 48 | **70** 22; 45 | **75** 20; 42 | **80** 19; 40 | **85** 18; 38
90 17; 36 | **95** 16; 34 | **100** 15.19; 32.47

X = 24 | **48** 35; 65 | **50** 34; 63 | **55** 30; 58 | **60** 28; 53 | **65** 25; 50
70 23; 47 | **75** 22; 44 | **80** 20; 41 | **85** 19; 39 | **90** 18; 37
95 17; 35 | **100** 16.03; 33.56

X = 25 | **50** 36; 64 | **55** 32; 59 | **60** 29; 55 | **65** 27; 51 | **70** 25; 48
75 23; 45 | **80** 21; 43 | **85** 20; 40 | **90** 19; 38 | **95** 18; 36
100 16.88; 34.66

Appendix 2 (continued)

X = 26	52 36; 64	55 34; 61	60 31; 57	65 28; 53	70 26; 50
	75 24; 47	80 22; 44	85 21; 42	90 20; 39	95 19; 37
	100 17.75; 35.72				

X = 27	54 36; 64	55 35; 63	60 32; 58	65 29; 54	70 27; 51
	75 25; 48	80 24; 45	85 22; 43	90 21.41	95 20; 39
	100 18.62; 36.79				

X = 28	56 36; 64	60 34; 60	65 31; 56	70 28; 52	75 26; 49
	80 25; 46	85 23; 44	90 22; 42	95 21; 40	100 19.50; 37.85

X = 29	58 37; 63	60 35; 62	65 32; 57	70 30; 54	75 28; 51
	80 26; 48	85 24; 45	90 23; 43	95 21; 41	100 20.37; 38.92

X = 30	60 37; 63	65 34; 59	70 31; 55	75 29; 52	80 27; 49
	85 25; 46	90 24; 44	95 22; 42	100 21.24; 39.98	

X = 31	62 37; 63	65 35; 60	70 32; 57	75 30; 53	80 28; 50
	85 26; 48	90 25; 45	95 23; 43	100 22.14; 41.02	

X = 32	64 37; 63	65 37; 62	70 34; 58	75 31; 55	80 29; 52
	85 27; 49	90 26; 46	95 24; 44	100 23.04; 42.06	

X = 33	66 37; 63	70 35; 59	75 33; 56	80 30; 53	85 28; 50
	90 27; 47	95 25; 45	100 23.93; 43.10		

X = 34	68 38; 62	70 36; 61	75 34; 57	80 32; 54	85 30; 51
	90 28; 49	95 26; 46	100 24.83; 44.15		

X = 35	70 38; 62	75 35; 59	80 33; 55	85 31; 52	90 29; 50
	95 27; 47	100 25.73; 45.19			

X = 36	72 38; 62	75 36; 60	80 34; 57	85 32; 54	90 30; 51
	95 28; 48	100 26.65; 46.20			

X = 37	74 38; 62	75 38; 61	80 35; 58	85 33; 55	90 31; 52
	95 29; 49	100 27.57; 47.22			

X = 38	76 38; 62	80 36; 59	85 34; 56	90 32; 53	95 30; 51
	100 28.49; 48.24				

X = 39	78 38; 62	80 37; 60	85 35; 57	90 33; 54	95 31; 52
	100 29.41; 49.26				

X = 40	80 39; 61	85 36; 58	90 34; 55	95 32; 53	100 30.33; 50.28

X = 41	82 39; 61	85 37; 59	90 35; 56	95 33; 54	100 31.27; 51.28

X = 42	84 39; 61	85 38; 60	90 36; 57	95 34; 55	100 32.21; 52.28

X = 43 | **86** 39; 61   **90** 37; 59   **95** 35; 56   **100** 33.15; 53.27

X = 44 | **88** 39; 61   **90** 38; 60   **95** 36; 57   **100** 34.09; 54.27

X = 45 | **90** 39; 61   **95** 37; 58   **100** 35.03; 55.27

X = 46 | **92** 39; 61   **95** 38; 59   **100** 35.99; 56.25

X = 47 | **94** 40; 60   **95** 39; 60   **100** 36.95; 57.23

X = 48 | **96** 40; 60   **100** 37.91; 58.21

X = 49 | **98** 40; 60   **100** 38.87; 59.19

X = 50 | **100** 39.83; 60.17

Appendix 3

Critical Values of the t Distribution*

α (2):	0.50	0.20	0.10	0.05	0.02	0.01	0.005	0.002	0.001
ν α (1):	0.25	0.10	0.05	0.025	0.01	0.005	0.0025	0.001	0.0005
1	1.000	3.078	6.314	12.706	31.821	63.657	127.321	318.309	636.619
2	0.816	1.886	2.920	4.303	6.965	9.925	14.089	22.327	31.599
3	0.765	1.638	2.353	3.182	4.541	5.841	7.453	10.215	12.924
4	0.741	1.533	2.132	2.776	3.747	4.604	5.598	7.173	8.610
5	0.727	1.476	2.015	2.571	3.365	4.032	4.773	5.893	6.869
6	0.718	1.440	1.943	2.447	3.143	3.707	4.317	5.208	5.959
7	0.711	1.415	1.895	2.365	2.998	3.499	4.029	4.785	5.408
8	0.706	1.397	1.860	2.306	2.896	3.355	3.833	4.501	5.041
9	0.703	1.383	1.833	2.262	2.821	3.250	3.690	4.297	4.781
10	0.700	1.372	1.812	2.228	2.764	3.169	3.581	4.144	4.587
11	0.697	1.363	1.796	2.201	2.718	3.106	3.497	4.025	4.437
12	0.695	1.356	1.782	2.179	2.681	3.055	3.428	3.930	4.318
13	0.694	1.350	1.771	2.160	2.650	3.012	3.372	3.852	4.221
14	0.692	1.345	1.761	2.145	2.624	2.977	3.326	3.787	4.140
15	0.691	1.341	1.753	2.131	2.602	2.947	3.286	3.733	4.073
16	0.690	1.337	1.746	2.120	2.583	2.921	3.252	3.686	4.015
17	0.689	1.333	1.740	2.110	2.567	2.898	3.222	3.646	3.965
18	0.688	1.330	1.734	2.101	2.552	2.878	3.197	3.610	3.922
19	0.688	1.328	1.729	2.093	2.539	2.861	3.174	3.579	3.883
20	0.687	1.325	1.725	2.086	2.528	2.845	3.153	3.552	3.850
21	0.686	1.323	1.721	2.080	2.518	2.831	3.135	3.527	3.819
22	0.686	1.321	1.717	2.074	2.508	2.819	3.119	3.505	3.792
23	0.685	1.319	1.714	2.069	2.500	2.807	3.104	3.485	3.768
24	0.685	1.318	1.711	2.064	2.492	2.797	3.091	3.467	3.745
25	0.684	1.316	1.708	2.060	2.485	2.787	3.078	3.450	3.725
26	0.684	1.315	1.706	2.056	2.479	2.779	3.067	3.435	3.707
27	0.684	1.314	1.703	2.052	2.473	2.771	3.057	3.421	3.690
28	0.683	1.313	1.701	2.048	2.467	2.763	3.047	3.048	3.674
29	0.683	1.311	1.699	2.045	2.462	2.756	3.038	3.396	3.659
30	0.683	1.310	1.697	2.042	2.457	2.750	3.030	3.385	3.646
31	0.682	1.309	1.696	2.040	2.453	2.744	3.022	3.375	3.633
32	0.682	1.309	1.694	2.037	2.449	2.738	3.015	3.365	3.622
33	0.682	1.308	1.692	2.035	2.445	2.733	3.008	3.356	3.611
34	0.682	1.307	1.691	2.032	2.441	2.728	3.002	3.348	3.601
35	0.682	1.306	1.690	2.030	2.438	2.724	2.996	3.340	3.591
36	0.681	1.306	1.688	2.028	2.434	2.719	2.990	3.333	3.582
37	0.681	1.305	1.687	2.026	2.431	2.715	2.985	3.326	3.574
38	0.681	1.304	1.686	2.024	2.429	2.712	2.980	3.319	3.566
39	0.681	1.304	1.685	2.023	2.426	2.708	2.976	3.313	3.558
40	0.681	1.303	1.684	2.021	2.423	2.704	2.971	3.307	3.551
41	0.681	1.303	1.683	2.020	2.421	2.701	2.967	3.301	3.544
42	0.680	1.302	1.682	2.018	2.418	2.698	2.963	3.296	3.538
43	0.680	1.302	1.681	2.017	2.416	2.695	2.959	3.291	3.532
44	0.680	1.301	1.680	2.015	2.414	2.692	2.956	3.286	3.526
45	0.680	1.301	1.679	2.014	2.412	2.690	2.952	3.281	3.520
46	0.680	1.300	1.679	2.013	2.410	2.687	2.949	3.277	3.515
47	0.680	1.300	1.678	2.012	2.408	2.865	2.946	3.273	3.510
48	0.680	1.299	1.677	2.011	2.407	2.682	2.943	3.269	3.505
49	0.680	1.299	1.677	2.010	2.405	2.680	2.940	3.265	3.500
50	0.679	1.299	1.676	2.009	2.403	2.678	2.937	3.621	3.496

ν = degrees of freedom.
$\alpha(2)$ = α for two-tailed test.
$\alpha(1)$ = α for one-tailed test.

*Used with permission from Zar JH. Biostatistical analysis, ed 3. Englewood Cliffs, NJ: Prentice-Hall; 1996:App18.

Critical Values of the t Distribution

ν	α (2): α (1):	0.50 0.25	0.20 0.10	0.10 0.05	0.05 0.025	0.02 0.01	0.01 0.005	0.005 0.0025	0.002 0.001	0.001 0.0005
52		0.679	1.298	1.675	2.007	2.400	2.674	2.932	3.255	3.488
54		0.679	1.297	1.674	2.005	2.397	2.670	2.927	3.248	3.480
56		0.679	1.297	1.673	2.003	2.395	2.667	2.923	3.242	3.473
58		0.679	1.296	1.672	2.002	2.392	2.663	2.918	3.237	3.466
60		0.679	1.296	1.671	2.000	2.390	2.660	2.915	3.232	3.460
62		0.678	1.295	1.670	1.999	2.388	2.657	2.911	3.227	3.454
64		0.678	1.295	1.669	1.998	2.386	2.655	2.908	3.223	3.449
66		0.678	1.295	1.668	1.997	2.384	2.652	2.904	3.218	3.444
68		0.678	1.294	1.668	1.995	2.382	2.650	2.902	3.214	3.439
70		0.678	1.294	1.667	1.994	2.381	2.648	2.899	3.211	3.435
72		0.678	1.293	1.666	1.993	2.379	2.646	2.896	3.207	3.431
74		0.678	1.293	1.666	1.993	2.378	2.644	2.894	3.204	3.427
76		0.678	1.293	1.665	1.992	2.376	2.642	2.891	3.201	3.423
78		0.678	1.292	1.665	1.991	2.375	2.640	2.889	3.198	3.420
80		0.678	1.292	1.664	1.990	2.374	2.639	2.887	3.195	3.416
82		0.677	1.292	1.664	1.989	2.373	2.637	2.885	3.193	3.413
84		0.677	1.292	1.663	1.989	2.372	2.636	2.883	3.190	3.410
86		0.677	1.291	1.663	1.988	2.370	2.634	2.881	3.188	3.407
88		0.677	1.291	1.662	1.987	2.369	2.633	2.880	3.185	3.405
90		0.677	1.291	1.662	1.987	2.368	2.632	2.878	3.183	3.402
92		0.677	1.291	1.662	1.986	2.368	2.630	2.876	3.181	3.399
94		0.677	1.291	1.661	1.986	2.367	2.629	2.875	3.179	3.397
96		0.677	1.290	1.661	1.985	2.366	2.628	2.873	3.177	3.395
98		0.677	1.290	1.661	1.984	2.365	2.627	2.872	3.175	3.393
100		0.677	1.290	1.660	1.984	2.364	2.626	2.871	3.174	3.390
105		0.677	1.290	1.659	1.983	2.362	2.623	2.868	3.170	3.386
110		0.677	1.289	1.659	1.982	2.361	2.621	2.865	3.166	3.381
115		0.677	1.289	1.658	1.981	2.359	2.619	2.862	3.163	3.377
120		0.677	1.289	1.658	1.980	2.358	2.617	2.860	3.160	3.373
125		0.676	1.288	1.657	1.979	2.357	2.616	2.858	3.157	3.370
130		0.676	1.288	1.657	1.978	2.355	2.614	2.856	3.154	3.367
135		0.676	1.288	1.656	1.978	2.354	2.613	2.854	3.152	3.364
140		0.676	1.288	1.656	1.977	2.353	2.611	2.852	3.149	3.361
145		0.676	1.287	1.655	1.976	2.352	2.610	2.851	3.147	3.359
150		0.676	1.287	1.655	1.976	2.531	2.609	2.849	3.145	3.357
160		0.676	1.287	1.654	1.975	2.350	2.607	2.846	3.142	3.352
170		0.676	1.287	1.654	1.974	2.348	2.605	2.844	3.139	3.349
180		0.676	1.286	1.653	1.973	2.347	2.603	2.842	3.136	3.345
190		0.676	1.286	1.653	1.973	2.346	2.602	2.840	3.134	3.342
200		0.676	1.286	1.653	1.972	2.345	2.601	2.839	3.131	3.340
250		0.675	1.285	1.651	1.969	2.341	2.596	2.832	3.123	3.330
300		0.675	1.284	1.650	1.968	2.339	2.592	2.828	3.118	3.323
350		0.675	1.284	1.649	1.967	2.337	2.590	2.825	3.114	3.319
400		0.675	1.284	1.649	1.966	2.336	2.588	2.823	3.111	3.315
450		0.675	1.283	1.648	1.965	2.335	2.587	2.821	3.108	3.312
500		0.675	1.283	1.648	1.965	2.334	2.586	2.820	3.107	3.310
600		0.675	1.283	1.647	1.964	2.333	2.584	2.817	3.104	3.307
700		0.675	1.283	1.647	1.963	2.332	2.583	2.816	3.102	3.304
800		0.675	1.283	1.647	1.963	2.331	2.582	2.815	3.100	3.303
900		0.675	1.282	1.647	1.963	2.330	2.581	2.814	3.099	3.301
1000		0.675	1.282	1.646	1.962	2.330	2.581	2.813	3.098	3.300
∞		0.6745	1.2816	1.6449	1.9600	2.3263	2.5758	2.8070	3.0902	3.2905

Appendix 4

Critical Values of the χ^2 Distribution*

ν	0.001	0.005	0.01	0.025	0.05	0.10	0.25	0.50	0.75	0.90	0.95	0.975	0.99	0.995	0.999
1	10.828	7.879	6.635	5.024	3.841	2.706	1.323	0.455	0.102	0.016	0.004	0.001	0.000	0.000	0.000
2	13.816	10.597	9.210	7.378	5.991	4.605	2.773	1.386	0.575	0.211	0.103	0.051	0.020	0.010	0.002
3	16.266	12.838	11.345	9.348	7.815	6.251	4.108	2.366	1.213	0.584	0.352	0.216	0.115	0.072	0.024
4	18.467	14.860	13.277	11.143	9.488	7.779	5.385	3.357	1.923	1.064	0.711	0.484	0.297	0.207	0.091
5	20.515	16.750	15.086	12.833	11.070	9.236	6.626	4.351	2.675	1.610	1.145	0.831	0.554	0.412	0.210
6	22.458	18.548	16.812	14.449	12.592	10.645	7.841	5.348	3.455	2.204	1.635	1.237	0.872	0.676	0.381
7	24.322	20.278	18.475	16.013	14.067	12.017	9.037	6.346	4.255	2.833	2.167	1.690	1.239	0.989	0.599
8	26.124	21.955	20.090	17.535	15.507	13.362	10.219	7.344	5.071	3.490	2.733	2.180	1.646	1.344	0.857
9	27.877	23.589	21.666	19.023	16.919	14.684	11.389	8.343	5.899	4.168	3.325	2.700	2.088	1.735	1.152
10	29.588	25.188	23.209	20.483	18.307	15.987	12.549	9.342	6.737	4.865	3.940	3.247	2.558	2.156	1.479
11	31.264	26.757	24.725	21.920	19.675	17.275	13.701	10.341	7.584	5.578	4.575	3.816	3.053	2.603	1.834
12	32.909	28.300	26.217	23.337	21.026	18.549	14.845	11.340	8.438	6.304	5.226	4.404	3.571	3.074	2.214
13	34.528	29.819	27.688	24.736	22.362	19.812	15.984	12.340	9.299	7.042	5.892	5.009	4.107	3.565	2.617
14	36.123	31.319	29.141	26.119	23.685	21.064	17.117	13.339	10.165	7.790	6.571	5.629	4.660	4.075	3.041
15	37.697	32.801	30.578	27.488	24.996	22.307	18.245	14.339	11.037	8.547	7.261	6.262	5.229	4.601	3.483
16	39.252	34.267	32.000	28.845	26.296	23.542	19.369	15.338	11.912	9.312	7.962	6.908	5.812	5.142	3.942
17	40.790	35.718	33.409	30.191	27.587	24.769	20.489	16.338	12.792	10.085	8.672	7.564	6.408	5.697	4.416
18	42.312	37.156	34.805	31.526	28.869	25.989	21.605	17.338	13.675	10.865	9.390	8.231	7.015	6.265	4.905
19	43.820	38.582	36.191	32.852	30.144	27.204	22.718	18.338	14.562	11.651	10.117	8.907	7.633	6.844	5.407
20	45.315	39.997	37.566	34.170	31.410	28.412	23.828	19.337	15.452	12.443	10.851	9.591	8.260	7.434	5.921
21	46.797	41.401	38.932	35.479	32.671	29.615	24.935	20.337	16.344	13.240	11.591	10.283	8.897	8.034	6.447
22	48.268	42.796	40.289	36.781	33.924	30.813	26.039	21.337	17.240	14.041	12.338	10.982	9.542	8.643	6.983
23	49.728	44.181	41.638	38.076	35.172	32.007	27.141	22.337	18.137	14.848	13.091	11.689	10.196	9.260	7.529
24	51.179	45.559	42.980	39.364	36.415	33.196	28.241	23.337	19.037	15.659	13.848	12.401	10.856	9.886	8.085
25	52.620	46.928	44.314	40.646	37.652	34.382	29.339	24.337	19.939	16.473	14.611	13.120	11.524	10.520	8.649
26	54.052	48.290	45.642	41.923	38.885	35.563	30.435	25.336	20.843	17.292	15.379	13.844	12.198	11.160	9.222
27	55.476	49.645	46.963	43.195	40.113	36.741	31.528	26.336	21.749	18.114	16.151	14.573	12.879	11.808	9.803
28	56.892	50.993	48.278	44.461	41.337	37.916	32.620	27.336	22.657	18.939	16.928	15.308	13.565	12.461	10.391
29	58.301	52.336	49.588	45.722	42.557	39.087	33.711	28.336	23.567	19.768	17.708	16.047	14.256	13.121	10.986
30	59.703	53.672	50.892	46.979	43.773	40.256	34.800	29.336	24.478	20.599	18.493	16.791	14.953	13.787	11.588
31	61.098	55.003	52.191	48.232	44.985	41.422	35.887	30.336	25.390	21.434	19.281	17.539	15.655	14.458	12.196
32	62.487	56.328	53.486	49.480	46.194	42.585	36.973	31.336	26.304	22.271	20.072	18.291	16.362	15.134	12.811
33	63.870	57.648	54.776	50.725	47.400	43.745	38.058	32.336	27.219	23.110	20.867	19.047	17.074	15.815	13.431
34	65.247	58.964	56.061	51.966	48.602	44.903	39.141	33.336	28.136	23.952	21.664	19.806	17.789	16.501	14.057
35	66.619	60.275	57.342	53.203	49.802	46.059	40.223	34.336	29.054	24.797	22.465	20.569	18.509	17.192	14.688
36	67.985	61.581	58.619	54.437	50.998	47.212	41.304	35.336	29.973	25.643	23.269	21.336	19.233	17.887	15.324
37	69.346	62.883	59.893	55.668	52.192	48.363	42.383	36.336	30.893	26.492	24.075	22.106	19.960	18.586	15.965
38	70.703	64.181	61.162	56.896	53.384	49.513	43.462	37.335	31.815	27.343	24.884	22.878	20.691	19.289	16.611
39	72.055	65.476	62.428	58.120	54.572	50.660	44.539	38.335	32.737	28.196	25.695	23.654	21.426	19.996	17.262
40	73.402	66.766	63.691	59.342	55.758	51.805	45.616	39.335	33.660	29.051	26.509	24.433	22.164	20.707	17.916
41	74.745	68.053	64.950	60.561	56.942	52.949	46.692	40.335	34.585	29.907	27.326	25.215	22.906	21.421	18.576
42	76.084	69.336	66.206	61.777	58.124	54.090	47.766	41.335	35.510	30.765	28.144	25.999	23.650	22.138	19.239
43	77.419	70.616	67.459	62.990	59.304	55.230	48.840	42.335	36.436	31.625	28.965	26.785	24.398	22.859	19.906
44	78.750	71.893	68.710	64.201	60.481	56.369	49.913	43.335	37.363	32.487	29.787	27.575	25.148	23.584	20.576
45	80.077	73.166	69.957	65.410	61.656	57.505	50.985	44.335	38.291	33.350	30.612	28.366	25.901	24.311	21.251
46	81.400	74.437	71.201	66.617	62.830	58.641	52.056	45.335	39.220	34.215	31.439	29.160	26.657	25.041	21.929
47	82.720	75.704	72.443	67.821	64.001	59.774	53.127	46.335	40.149	35.081	32.268	29.956	27.416	25.775	22.610
48	84.037	76.969	73.683	69.023	65.171	60.907	54.196	47.335	41.079	35.949	33.098	30.755	28.177	26.511	23.295
49	85.351	78.231	74.919	70.222	66.339	62.038	55.265	48.335	42.010	36.818	33.930	31.555	28.941	27.249	23.983
50	86.661	79.490	76.154	71.420	67.505	63.167	56.334	49.335	42.942	37.689	34.764	32.357	29.707	27.991	24.674

n = degrees of freedom.

*Used with permission from Zar JH. Biostatistical analysis, ed 3. Englewood Cliffs, NJ: Prentice Hall; 1996:App13.

Appendix 5

Sources of invalidity*

	H	MAT	T	INST	R	S	MORT	INTER
Pre-experimental designs:								
1. One-shot case study X O	—	—				—	—	
2. One-group pretest posttest design O X O	—	—	—	—	?	+	+	—
3. Static-group comparison X O O	+	+	+	+	+	+	+	+
True experimental designs:								
4. Pretest-posttest control group design R O X O R O O	+	+	+	+	+	—	—	—
5. Solomon four-group design R O X O R O O R X O R O	+	+	+	+	+	+	+	+
6. Posttest-only control group design R X O R O	+	+	+	+	+	+	+	+
Quasi-experimental designs:								
7. Time series O O O OXO O O O	—	+	+	?	+	+	+	+
8. Equivalent time samples design X_1O X_2O X_1O X_0O, etc.	+	+	+	+	+	+	+	+
9. Nonequivalent control design O X O O O	+	+	+	+	?	+	+	—

Note: In the tables, (—) indicates a definite weakness, (+) indicates that the factor is controlled, (?) indicates a possible source of concern, and a blank indicates that the factor is not relevant.

Sources of Invalidity
H = History
MAT = Maturation
T = Testing
INST = Instrumentation
R = Regression
S = Selection
MORT = Mortality
INTER = Interaction of Selection and Maturation, etc.

Design
R = Randomization of subjects into separate groups
X = Treatment
O = Observation or measurement

*Used with permission from Campbell DT, Stanley JC. Experimental and Quasi-Experimental Designs for Research. Chicago: Rand-McNally College Publishing; 1963.

Appendix 5 (continued)

Sources of invalidity

	H	MAT	T	INST	R	S	MORT	INTER
10. Counterbalanced designs X_1O X_2O X_3O X_4O X_2O X_4O X_1O X_3O X_3O X_1O X_4O X_1O X_4O X_3O X_2O X_1O	+	+	+	+	+	+	+	?
11. Separate-sample pretest-posttest design R O (X) R X O	−	−	+	?	+	+	−	−
12. Separate-sample pretest-posttest control group design R O (X) R X O ———————— R O R O	+	+	+	+	+	+	+	−
13. Multiple time-series O O OXO O O ———————— O O OXO O O	+	+	+	+	+	+	+	+

Appendix 6

Approximate total number of subjects required for significance for different values of d. Note that the values given are for the total number of subjects in the two groups, so that if an investigator suspected an effect size of d = 0.4 and decided on a significance level of 5%, 100 subjects would be required with 50 in each group.*

	Total no. of subjects	
d	5% level	1% level
0.4	100	200
0.5	77	132
0.6	56	97
0.7	38	72
0.8	29	52
0.9	24	38
1.0	20	30
1.2	15	24
1.4	13	20
1.6	11	17
1.8	10	15
2.0	8	12
2.2	8	11
2.4	7	10
2.6	7	9
2.8	7	8
3.0	7	8

*Used with permission from Plutchik R. Foundations of Experimental Research, ed 2. New York; Harper and Row; 1974.

Appendix 7

The degree of overlap of experimental and control group distribution for different values of d with corresponding percent of variance accounted for (σ^2).*

d	Degree of overlap (%)	σ^2
0.0	100.00	.00
0.1	92.3	.00
0.2	85.3	.01
0.3	78.7	.02
0.4	72.6	.04
0.5	67.0	.06
0.6	61.8	.08
0.7	57.0	.11
0.8	52.6	.14
0.9	48.4	.17
1.0	44.6	.20
1.1	41.4	.23
1.2	37.8	.26
1.3	34.7	.30
1.4	31.9	.33
1.5	29.3	.36
1.6	26.9	.39
1.7	24.6	.42
1.8	22.6	.45
1.9	20.6	.47
2.0	18.9	.50
2.2	15.7	.55
2.4	13.0	.59
2.6	10.7	.63
2.8	8.8	.66
3.0	7.2	.69
3.2	5.8	.72
3.4	4.7	.74
3.6	3.7	.76
3.8	3.0	.78
4.0	2.3	.80

*Used with permission from Plutchik R. Foundations of Experimental Research, ed. 2. New York: Harper and Row; 1974.

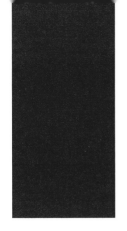

Index